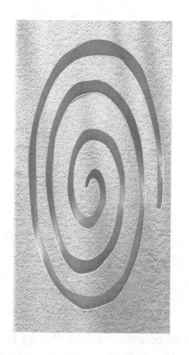

perspectives

Health

Academic Editor

Judy Baker

Texas Woman's University

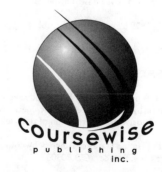

coursewise
publishing
inc.

Boulder • Bellevue • Dubuque • Madison

Our mission at **coursewise** is to help students make connections—linking theory to practice and the classroom to the outside world. Learners are motivated to synthesize ideas when course materials are placed in a context they recognize. By providing gateways to contemporary and enduring issues, **coursewise** publications will expand students' awareness of and context for the course subject.

For more information on **coursewise** visit us at our web site: www.coursewise.com

coursewise publishing editorial staff

Thomas Doran, ceo/publisher: Journalism/Marketing/Speech
Edgar Laube, publisher: Geography/Political Science/Psychology/Sociology
Linda Meehan Avenarius, publisher: CourseLinks
Sue Pulvermacher-Alt, publisher: Education/Health/Gender Studies
Victoria Putman, publisher: Anthropology/Philosophy/Religion
Tom Romaniak, publisher: Business/Criminal Justice/Economics

Cover photo Copyright © 1997 T. Teshigawara/Panoramic Images, Chicago, All Rights Reserved.

Interior design and cover design by Jeff Storm

Copyright © 1998 by **coursewise publishing**, Inc. All rights reserved

Library of Congress Catalog Card Number: 97-075315

ISBN 0-395-902479

Printed in the United States of America by **coursewise publishing**, Inc.
1379 Lodge Lane, Boulder, CO 80303

10 9 8 7 6 5 4 3 2

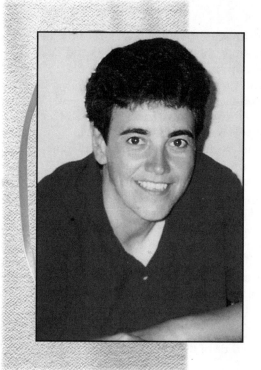

from the
Publisher

coursewise publishing

Sue Pulvermacher-Alt

I'm baaaack!

Over ten years ago I started my career in publishing as an editor in health education. Through the years I moved on to editorial work in other discipline areas. When I joined the creative team at **coursewise publishing** I had the chance to get back into a discipline I enjoy. I'm glad to be back in health education.

Being an editor in health education means I'm knee-deep (sometimes neck-deep) in gaining a better understanding of issues important to health educators. On a personal level, working in the discipline of health education reminds me to take better care of myself. I think I lead a more balanced life when I'm constantly seeing messages about how important it is to lead a balanced life!

Another reason I'm glad to be back in this discipline is that I get to work with the *people* in health education. I immensely enjoy the positive nature and determined attitude I see in health educators as a group. This group of individuals is out to make the world a healthier place—one student and one class and one issue at a time.

I've enjoyed working with one health educator in particular—Judy Baker, the Academic Editor for this volume. I've found Judy speedy, professional, opinionated, efficient, technologically savvy, and gutsy. She is passionate about her profession and not willing to shy away from controversy. You'll see articles here that touch upon many issues in health education that are sometimes glossed over—minority health, equity in medical research, sexual harassment, homophobia, and ageism to name a few.

Dr. Baker brings an impressive background to this project. She's taught graduate and undergraduate courses at Texas Woman's University since 1987 (coincidentally the year I entered the world of publishing). She earned her Ph.D. in Community Health Education from the University of Texas at Austin, her M.S.W. in Health Planning from the School of Social Work, Virginia Commonwealth University and her B.A. in Sociology from the College of William and Mary. She is currently the chair of the university's Task Force on Emerging Instructional Technologies. Her knowledge of the content and the technology, magnified by her professional passion, is capped by her diligence to meet deadlines and get the job done right.

I also had the chance to work with other health educators on this project—members of our Editorial Board. At **coursewise** we're working hard to publish **R**elevant, **E**xciting, **A**pproved, and **L**inked (what we call R.E.A.L.) learning tools. Articles and web sites have been selected with these criteria in mind. We worked with a top-notch editorial board. They offered some hard feedback and posed some interesting challenges. They know their content and are a web-savvy bunch. The result is a R.E.A.L. learning tool. My thanks to Judy and the entire Editorial Board.

As I've returned to the field of health education I've been struck by the ton of information available to the consumer about health products and health services. In magazines and newspapers, on radio and TV, we're bombarded by advertisements for health products and services—HMOs, allergy products, massage therapists, headache medications, dentists—all trying to grab our dollars to improve our health. We've tried to put together articles in this volume that help you to sort out the important issues and become a critical health consumer. In each section, articles are presented in order from general health concepts and problem identification to specific applications and solutions—our goal being to inform you and help you become a wiser health consumer.

Not only are we given unsolicited advice through advertising, we can solicit information on any health topic we choose using the Internet. The R.E.A.L. Sites you'll find throughout this *Perspectives* volume and at the **courselinks**™ Site have been chosen because they are particularly useful sites. You, however, still need to be the critical consumer. Read our annotations and decide if the site is worth visiting. Do the activities so you can get to know the site better. Search our **courselinks** Site by key topic and find the information you need to be a better health consumer.

In closing I want to leave you with the words of the philosopher Publius Syrus, 42 B.C.:

"Good health and good sense are two of life's greatest blessings."

With *Perspectives: Health* and the **courselinks**™ Site for Health we want to help you improve your good sense so that you might in turn be blessed by good health. Have we helped you? It's good to be back; let me know how we're doing.

suepa@coursewise.com

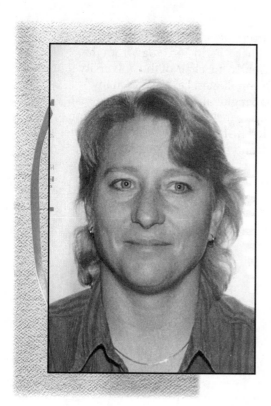

from the
Academic Editor

coursewise publishing
Judy Baker

Most of us value good health. We have yet to agree, however, as to whether health is an individual or a societal responsibility and if health care is a right or a privilege. This is a reader for all of us who are curious about and challenged by contemporary health issues. *Perspectives: Health* provides health articles that span the continuum from the personal to the political. The selection is intended to address the complexities of many health issues, including health behaviors, health risk factors, sexual health, consumer health, the health care system, minority health, access to health care, and managed care.

Each of the six sections contains commentaries and reports that can be used to encourage critical thinking and to stimulate dialogue about controversial health issues. The first four sections in this reader include articles that address personal health concerns, while the last two sections contain articles about the health care system. Within each section, articles are presented in order from general health concepts and problem identification to specific applications and solutions.

Articles in the first section describe ways that we can incorporate positive health habits into our daily routines so as to make them an integral part of our lives. In the second section, we can find out how to recognize and reduce our risk of developing illness and disease. The section on sexual and reproductive health addresses birth control, pregnancy, safer sex, sexual hygiene, and homosexuality. Another section deals with ways we can make the most of health care opportunities when we encounter conditions such as heart disease and cancer. Articles in the remaining two sections remind us that inequities and other problems exist in the current health care system, and they offer some solutions.

With the increasing popularity of the Internet, we have a unique opportunity to change our approach to learning. Universal and immediate access to health information, made possible with the Internet, allows health consumers to get relevant and timely health information when we are ready and when we need it. *Perspectives: Health* is part of a larger effort by **coursewise** to meet this challenge by integrating classroom and textbook instruction with distance learning via the Internet. The information age demands that educators shift from teacher-centered instruction to student-directed learning in colleges and universities. My participation as Academic Editor allowed me to take an active part in this exciting process.

Judy is a Professor of Health Studies and Affiliate Faculty in the Women's Studies Program at Texas Woman's University. She's taught graduate and undergraduate courses at TWU since 1987. She earned her Ph.D. in Community Health Education from the University of Texas at

Austin, her M.S.W. in Health Planning from the School of Social Work, Virginia Commonwealth University and her B.A. in Sociology from the College of William and Mary. She is currently the chair of the university's Task Force on Emerging Instructional Technologies. Dr. Baker's many presentations and workshops at national, regional, and state professional conferences have covered a variety of topics including distance education, women's health, aging, computer-assisted instruction for health educators, diversity awareness, teaching strategies, and program evaluation.

Editorial Board

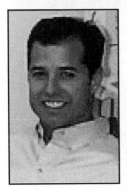
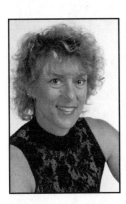
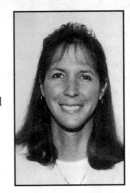
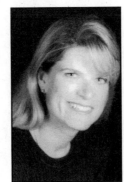

LeaVonne Pulley

University of Alabama

Dr. Pulley is an Assistant Professor in the Department of Health Behavior and Director of the Survey Research Unit within the UAB Center for Health Promotion. She has been active in designing, implementing and evaluating theory-based interventions for minority populations over the past 12 years. Prior to relocating to Alabama she was an investigator or project director with several NCI-funded cancer control studies in Texas. Her educational background includes a B.A. in Anthropology, an M.Ed. in Health Education and an interdisciplinary Ph. D. focusing on Health Behavior.

Jill Black

Cleveland State University

Dr. Jill Black joined the faculty of Health, Physical Education, Recreation and Dance as an Assistant Professor in 1994. She holds a B.A. in Mass Communications, a B.S. in Health, Physical Education and Recreation, a master's degree in Health Promotion from the University of Oklahoma and received her Ph.D. in Community Health from Southern Illinois University at Carbondale in 1992. She came to Cleveland State University from Springfield College where she was director of the Health Promotion Wellness Management Graduate Program. Specific areas of specialization include program planning and evaluation, health promotion and wellness, foundations and methods of community health, aging and gerontology issues, stress management and related issues.

Critical Thinking and Bumper Stickers

The bumper sticker said: Question Authority. This is a simple directive that goes straight to the heart of critical thinking. The issue is not whether the authority is right or wrong; it's the questioning process that's important. Questioning helps you develop awareness and a clearer sense of what you think. That's critical thinking.

Critical thinking is a new label for an old approach to learning—that of challenging all ideas, hypotheses, and assumptions. In the physical and life sciences, systematic questioning and testing methods (known as the scientific method) help verify information, and objectivity is the benchmark on which all knowledge is pursued. In the social sciences, however, where the goal is to study people and their behavior, things get fuzzy. It's one thing for the chemistry experiment to work out as predicted, or for the petri dish to yield a certain result. It's quite another matter, however, in the social sciences, where the subject is ourselves. Objectivity is harder to achieve.

Although you'll hear critical thinking defined in many different ways, it really boils down to analyzing the ideas and messages that you receive. What are you being asked to think or believe? Does it make sense, objectively? Using the same facts and considerations, could you reasonably come up with a different conclusion? And, why does this matter in the first place? As the bumper sticker urged, question authority. Authority can be a textbook, a politician, a boss, a big sister, or an ad on television. Whatever the message, learning to question it appropriately is a habit that will serve you well for a lifetime. And in the meantime, thinking critically will certainly help you be course wise.

`Question Authority`

Getting Connected

This reader is a tool for connected learning. This means that the readings and other learning aids explained here will help you to link classroom theory to real-world issues. They will help you to think critically and to make long-lasting learning connections. Feedback from both instructors and students has helped us to develop some suggestions on how you can wisely use this connected learning tool.

WiseGuide Pedagogy

A wise reader is better able to be a critical reader. Therefore, we want to help you get wise about the articles in this reader. Each section of *Perspectives* has three tools to help you: the WiseGuide Intro, the WiseGuide Wrap-Up, and the Putting It in *Perspectives* review form.

WiseGuide Intro

In the WiseGuide Intro, the Academic Editor introduces the section, gives you an overview of the topics covered, and explains why particular articles were selected and what's important about them.

Also in the WiseGuide Intro, you'll find several key points or learning objectives that highlight the most important things to remember from this section. These will help you to focus your study of section topics.

WiseGuide Intro

At the end of the Wiseguide Intro, you'll find questions designed to stimulate critical thinking. Wise students will keep these questions in mind as they read an article (we repeat the questions at the start of the articles as a reminder). When you finish each article, check your understanding. Can you answer the questions? If not, go back and reread the article. The Academic Editor has written sample responses for many of the questions, and you'll find these online at the **courselinks**™ site for this course. More about **courselinks**™ in a minute. . . .

WiseGuide Wrap-Up

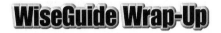

Be course wise and develop a thorough understanding of the topics covered in this course. The WiseGuide Wrap-Up at the end of each section will help you do just that with concluding comments or summary points that repeat what's most important to understand from the section you just read.

In addition, we try to get you wired up by providing a list of select Internet resources—what we call R.E.A.L. web sites because they're Relevant, Exciting, Approved, and Linked. The information at these web sites will enhance your understanding of a topic. (Remember to use your Passport and start at http://www.courselinks.com so that if any of these sites have changed, you'll have the latest link.)

Putting It in *Perspectives* Review Form

At the end of the book is the Putting It in *Perspectives* review form. Your instructor may ask you to complete this form as an assignment or for extra credit. If nothing else, consider doing it on your own to help you critically think about the reading.

Prompts at the end of each article encourage you to complete this review form. Feel free to copy the form and use it as needed.

The courselinks™ Site

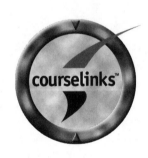

The **courselinks**™ Passport is your ticket to a wonderful world of integrated web resources designed to help you with your course work. These resources are found at the **courselinks**™ site for your course area. This is where the readings in this book and the key topics of your course are linked to an exciting array of online learning tools. Here you will find carefully selected readings, web links, quizzes, worksheets, and more, tailored to your course and approved as connected learning tools. The ever-changing, always interesting **courselinks**™ site features a number of carefully integrated resources designed to help you be course wise. These include:

- **R.E.A.L. Sites** At the core of a **courselinks**™ site is the list of R.E.A.L. sites. This is a select group of web sites for studying, not surfing. Like the readings in this book, these sites have been selected, reviewed, and approved by the Academic Editor and the Editorial Board. The R.E.A.L. sites are arranged by topic and are annotated with short descriptions and key words to make them easier for you to use for reference or research. With R.E.A.L. sites, you're studying approved resources within seconds—and not wasting precious time surfing unproven sites.

- **Editor's Choice** Here you'll find updates on news related to your course, with links to the actual online sources. This is also where we'll tell you about changes to the site and about online events.

- **Course Overview** This is a general description of the typical course in this area of study. While your instructor will provide specific course objectives, this overview helps you place the course in a generic context and offers you an additional reference point.

- **www.orksheet** Focus your trip to a R.E.A.L. site with the www.orksheet. Each of the 10 to 15 questions will prompt you to take in the best that site has to offer. Use this tool for self-study, or if required, email it to your instructor.

- **Course Quiz** The questions on this self-scoring quiz are related to articles in the reader, information at R.E.A.L. sites, and other course topics, and will help you pinpoint areas you need to study. Only you will know your score—it's an easy, risk-free way to keep pace!

- **Topic Key** The Topic Key is a listing of the main topics in your course, and it correlates with the Topic Key that appears in this reader. This handy reference tool also links directly to those R.E.A.L. sites that are especially appropriate to each topic, bringing you integrated online resources within seconds!

- **Web Savvy Student Site** If you're new to the Internet or want to brush up, stop by the Web Savvy Student site. This unique supplement is a complete **courselinks**™ site unto itself. Here, you'll find basic information on using the Internet, creating a web page, communicating on the web, and more. Quizzes and Web Savvy Worksheets test your web knowledge, and the R.E.A.L. sites listed here will further enhance your understanding of the web.

- **Student Lounge** Drop by the Student Lounge to chat with other students taking the same course or to learn more about careers in your major. You'll find links to resources for scholarships, financial aid, internships, professional associations, and jobs. Take a look around the Student Lounge and give us your feedback. We're open to remodeling the Lounge per your suggestions.

Building Better Perspectives!

Please tell us what you think of this *Perspectives* volume so we can improve the next one. Here's how you can help:

1. Visit our **coursewise** site at: http://www.coursewise.com

2. Click on *Perspectives*. Then select the Building Better *Perspectives* Form for your book.

3. Forms and instructions for submission are available online.

Tell us what you think—did the readings and online materials help you make some learning connections? Were some materials more helpful than others? Thanks in advance for helping us build better *Perspectives*.

Student Internships

If you enjoy evaluating these articles or would like to help us evaluate the **courselinks**™ site for this course, check out the **coursewise** Student Internship Program. For more information, visit:

http://www.coursewise.com/intern.html

Brief Contents

Contents

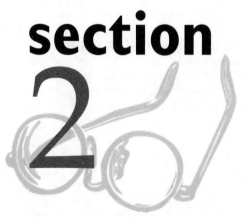

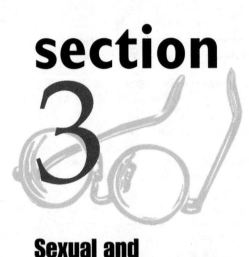

section
3

Sexual and Reproductive Health

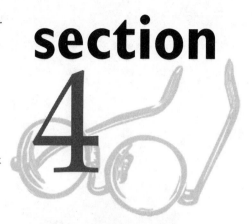

section 4

Living Well with Illness, Disease, and Challenge

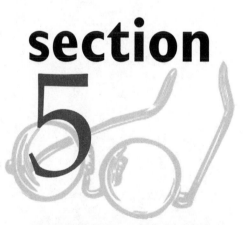

section 5

Health for All: Access to Healthcare

section

6

Making Your World a Healthier Place

Topic Key

This Topic Key is an important tool for learning. The Topic Key will help you integrate this reader into your course studies. Listed below, in alphabetical order, are important topics covered in this volume. Below the topic you'll find the article or articles and one or more R.E.A.L. sites relating to that topic. Note that the Topic Key might not include every topic your instructor chooses to emphasize. If you don't find the topic you're looking for in the Topic Key, check the index or the OnLine Topic Key at The **courselinks**™ Site for your course.

Activism & Advocacy
4   Food Police
26 A Burst of Light
35 Give Your HMO Checkup
39 Partnerships: The Prescription for Healthier Communities

National Organization for Women
http://www.now.org/
HMO Home Page
http://www.hmopage.org

Aging
26 A Burst of Light

American Association for Retired Persons
http://www.aarp.org:80/

Alcohol & Drugs
7   OTC Medication Errors
8   Medication Decision-Making and Management
9   Self-Presentation Can Be Hazardous to Your Health

Prevline: Prevention Hotline and National Clearinghouse for Alcohol and Drug Information
http://www.health.gov/
Federal Drug Administration
http://www.fda.gov/

Alternative Medicine
38 Whatever Works

Office of Alternative Medicine-NIH
http://altmed.od.nih.gov

Cancer
25 Winning the War on Cancer
26 A Burst of Light

American Cancer Society
http://www.cancer.org/
OncoLink at The University of Pennsylvania Cancer Center
http://oncolink.upenn.edu

Community Agency
4   Food Police
37 Checking Up on Your Doctor

American Lung Association
http://www.lungusa.org/

Consumer Health
6   Which Indoor Exercise Is Best?
7   OTC Medication Errors
8   Medication Decision-Making and Management
13 Rethinking Birth Control

Healthfinder
http://www.healthfinder.gov
NOAH
http://www.noah.cuny.edu/qksearch.html

Disease
15 Misunderstanding of Safer Sex by Heterosexually Active Adults
19 Redefining Health for People with Chronic Disabilities
23 Mysterious Maladies
24 Women and Their PCPs Lack Understanding of Heart Disease Symptoms and Risks
25 Winning the War on Cancer
26 A Burst of Light
32 Concern About AIDS in Minority Communities

Medical Matrix
http://www.medmatrix.org

Empowerment
5   Strong Is Beautiful
8   Medication Decision-Making and Management
22 To Get Top Health Care, Be Sure to Consult a Trusted Advisor—Yourself
33 Power to the Patient
39 Partnerships: The Prescription for Healthier Communities

Community Toolbox
http://ctb.lsi.ukans.edu/

Environmental Health
Environmental Protection Agency
http://www.epa.gov/epahome/students.htm

Evaluation
13 Rethinking Birth Control
20 An FDA Guide to Choosing Medical Treatments
35 Give Your HMO a Checkup

The Web as a Research Tool: Evaluation Techniques
http://www.science.widener.edu/~withers/evalout.htm

Fitness & Physical Activity
1   Weight Management
2   Race and the Role of Weight
5   Strong Is Beautiful
6   Which Indoor Exercise Is Best?
9   Self-Presentation Can Be Hazardous to Your Health
19 Redefining Health for People with Chronic Disabilities

FitLife
http://www.fitlife.com/

General Health & Wellness
9   Self-Presentation Can Be Hazardous to Your Health
19 Redefining Health for People with Chronic Disabilities
38 Whatever Works

Health A to Z
http://www.HealthAtoZ.com/

ACHOO
http://www.achoo.com/index.htm

Governmental Agency
Healthy People 2000
http://ofphp.osophs.dhhs.gov/pubs/hp2000

Centers for Disease Control and Prevention
http://www.cdc.gov/diseases/diseases.html

Health Insurance & Managed Care
30 How Women Pay More Than Men for Less Health Coverage

section

1

Key Points

- Preoccupation with diet and exercise defeats the purpose of healthy living.

- Weight management and body image have a cultural context.

- Nutrition has significant impact on health status and healthcare costs.

- Building physical strength can be empowering for women.

- In order to be successful, exercise regimens need to be tailored to individual preferences.

Good Health as a Way of Life

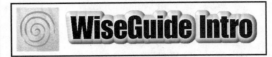 WiseGuide Intro

Good health comes with a balanced and realistic approach to healthy living. A nutritious diet, regular physical activity, and appropriate weight management are ways to live longer and better. Sometimes, however, in our eternal quest to improve the quality of our lives, we allow the pursuit to assume greater importance than the goal.

We have begun to attach meanings to eating and activity choices that extend well beyond their actual health benefits. Those who believe that diets or exercise can magically transform their lives may experience inevitable disappointment and frustration when the expected outcomes fail to materialize. Instead of recognizing that their preoccupation with diet and exercise defeats the purpose of healthy living, they blame themselves. As a result, healthy living has become regarded as synonymous with denial, sacrifice, guilt, and failure.

However, when faced with the choice between pleasure and sacrifice, pleasure will win every time. Until eating and exercise choices become devoid of moral judgment, health will remain an elusive goal. True healthy living involves celebration, self-acceptance, and balance.

The readings selected for Section 1 provide alternative views of weight management, nutrition, and physical activity in contrast to unrealistic and self-defeating approaches.

Jon Robison ("Weight Management: Shifting the Paradigm") poses a new view of weight management that shifts focus from self-sacrifice to a more balanced and pleasure-based approach. The cultural context of weight management and body image issues is addressed in a study by Abood and Chandler ("Race and the Role of Weight, Weight Change, and Body Dissatisfaction in Eating Disorders").

While Frazao ("The American Diet: A Costly Health Problem") clearly delineates the importance of nutrition on health status, Morse ("Food Police") personalizes the eating dilemmas posed by knowing the health risks and benefits of specific foods. Gloria Steinem ("Strong Is Beautiful") urges women to transcend the limitations on physical activity imposed by adherence to traditional sex roles by building physical strength. And, finally, Hoffman ("Which Indoor Exercise Is Best?") emphasizes the need to tailor exercise regimens to individual preferences.

Questions

R1. How do the concepts of the current weight management paradigm compare with the alternative paradigm? What will be necessary to achieve the goals of the alternative weight management paradigm?

R2. What is the relationship of race, weight, and desired weight change to body dissatisfaction? Who has greater body dissatisfaction according to the study conducted by Abood and Chandler: African-American or white women?

R3. How are poor diets associated with leading causes of death? In what ways can even small dietary changes yield large benefits?

R4. What role has the Center for Science in the Public Interest taken in changing the nutritional health of Americans? What are some of the tactics used by the Center for Science in the Public Interest to achieve its goals?

R5. In what way is physical strength among women a political issue? How does strength training provide an alternative to the fat-versus-thin dichotomy for women?

R6. What factors make certain modes of exercise more appropriate than others for some individuals?

How do the concepts of the current weight management paradigm compare with the alternative paradigm?
What will be necessary to achieve the goals of the alternative weight management paradigm?

Weight Management
Shifting the paradigm

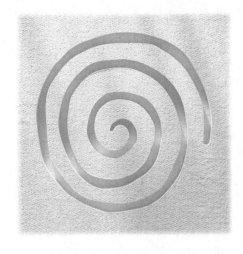

Jon Robison

Jon Robison is with the Michigan Center for Preventive Medicine, Lansing, MI 48910.

General agreement that weight loss regimens are ineffective in producing lasting results for the vast majority of participants led the recent National Institutes of Health Consensus Conference to conclude that treatment for obesity should focus on "strategies that can produce health benefits independently of weight loss" (National Institutes of Health, 1992). Nevertheless, research on and treatment for obesity continue to focus on the promotion of short term weight loss, particularly through dietary restriction.

An alternative paradigm for weight management has been developing as a result of the work of professionals from a variety of disciplines. Unfortunately, much of this information has not been widely disseminated to health educators, resulting in a continuation of approaches that are not beneficial and are potentially harmful (Garner & Wooley, 1991; Burgard & Lyons, 1994). The pur-

pose of this article is to summarize for health educators: (1) the need for and conceptual basis of this alternative paradigm and (2) the potential ramifications of this paradigm for research and programming.

A paradigm is a model for looking at the world. Paradigms provide a framework for scientific investigation, focusing attention and guiding inquiry in certain areas to the exclusion of others (Sloan, 1987). It has been suggested that scientific revolutions are driven by paradigmatic shifts resulting from repeated experiences with limitations and failures of existing paradigms (Kuhn, 1962). Such shifts result in creation of a new framework that serves to redirect inquiry, guiding both the selection of topics for research, and the manner in which that research is conducted.

The ancient Greeks were confronted with scientific phenomena that could not be explained using the existing flat-earth paradigm. Why were different stars visible from different points on the earth? Why did ships disappear hull first with the sails still visible and irrespective

of the direction in which they travelled? The failure of the existing paradigm to explain these and other phenomenon prompted the Greeks to hypothesize that the earth was not flat, but spherical. This shift provided a new framework for further scientific inquiry that eventually led to discoveries involving the true nature of the solar system (Asimov, 1980). It was not until many centuries later, when the first ships sailed around the world and did not fall off, that the concept of the spherical earth was validated.

Weight Management: The Current Paradigm

The failure of the existing paradigm underlying weight management research and intervention is at least as striking as the failure of the flat earth paradigm previously described. It is estimated that 65 million Americans are dieting at any one time (Lustig, 1991), spending nearly 50 billion dollars a year on weight loss products and services (Begley, 1991). Many of these produce short-term weight loss for participants. Yet, despite the best efforts of re-

This article is reprinted with permission from *Journal of Health Education*, January/February 1997, pages 28-34. The *Journal of Health Education* is a publication of the American Alliance for Health, Physical Education, Recreation and Dance, 1900 Association Drive, Reston, Virginia 22091.

searchers in medicine, nutrition, exercise, and psychology, "one-third to two-thirds of the weight is regained within one year, and almost all is regained within five years" (National Institutes of Health, 1992). Recent evidence suggests that weight fluctuation is strongly associated with negative psychological effects in normal weight and obese individuals (Foreyt, 1995). In addition, the latest national survey data demonstrate a striking increase in obesity in all segments of the population during the last 20 years (Kuczmarski, Flegal, Campbell, & Johnson, 1994). Further, approximately 50 percent of adolescent and young women are dieting at any one time, even though at least half of these individuals are at or below normal weight (Centers for Disease Control, 1991). Dieting in normal weight individuals is associated with adverse psychological and physiological consequences in men and women (Rosen & Gross, 1987; Keys, Brozek, Herschel, Michelsen, & Taylor, 1950). Finally, the present epidemic of dieting may be promoting the spread of eating disorders as well as an increase in the prevalence of obesity (Council on Scientific Affairs, 1988; Wilson, 1992; Foreyt, 1995; Polivy, 1996.).

Perhaps the explanation for these failures lies in the faulty paradigm underlying weight management research and intervention efforts. The conceptual basis of the existing paradigm for weight management is summarized in Table 1. The basic assumptions are that everyone should be thin because thinness is necessary for good health and happiness, and that individuals who are not thin, must lack will power and either eat too much

and/or not exercise enough (Ritenbaugh, 1991). According to this paradigm, anyone can correct these problems and be thin by dieting and exercising more (Allan, 1994). Within this framework, research continues to focus on the development of interventions designed to produce weight loss.

In recent years, there have been some attempts to modify traditional approaches to weight management to address the mythological nature of some of these underlying assumptions. Almost everyone agrees, in principle, that diets don't work. Additionally, the important contributions of genetics and physiological mechanisms to body size and shape are more commonly accepted, resulting in a somewhat decreased morality around weight-related issues (Sobal, 1995). Further, there has been increased discussion concerning the contribution of our cultural pressure for thinness to the current epidemic of dangerous eating disorders. As a result, some programs now describe themselves as "lifestyle change" interventions rather than diets, while others focus on so-called "new" paradigms like counting fat grams instead of calories (Hawks & Richins, 1994).

There is scant evidence, however, that the basic underlying assumptions of the paradigm have been altered significantly. That is, our society continues to be obsessed with an intense fear of fat that far outweighs anything that can be justified in terms of potential health consequences. The pressure (particularly on women) to conform to unrealistic notions of "ideal" body shape and size shows few signs of diminishing. There are numerous journal articles (Powers, 1988; Czajka-Narins & Parham, 1990; Garner & Wooley, 1991; Nichter & Nichter, 1991; Cassell, 1995) and a number of excellent books (Erdman, 1995; Johnson, 1995; Goodman, 1995) that explore these issues in great detail. Recent treatment of the much heralded Nurse's Study (Manson, 1995) provides a clear example from the scientific literature. While the data show no significant health risk to women until they achieved a body mass index (BMI) of greater than 27, the message that emerged was that the "ideal" was a BMI of 19 or less, a body size that would be unhealthy for many, potentially

Table 1 Current and Alternative Weight Management Paradigms Comparison of Conceptual Bases

Current Paradigm	Alternative Paradigm
Everyone needs to be thin for good health and happiness.	Thin is not intrinsically healthy and beautiful, nor is fat intrinsically unhealthy and unappealing.
People have different body shapes and sizes because they lack will power, eat too much, and move too little.	People naturally have different body shapes and sizes. These differences may be exacerbated by a culture that promotes unhealthy living.
Everyone can be thin, happy, and healthy by dieting.	Dieting invariably leads to weight gain, decreased self-esteem, and increased risk for disordered eating. Health and happiness include mental, social, and spiritual as well as physical considerations.

dangerous for some, and clearly unattainable for the vast majority of women (Byers, 1995; Berg, 1996).

Though more than 30 percent of women in America wear a size 16 or larger, the majority of Miss America contestants and Playboy centerfolds are now at least 15 percent below the recommended body weight for height, one commonly accepted indicator of anorexia nervosa (Wiseman et al., 1992). One only has to peruse the shelves of local book stores, flip through the pages of women's magazines, or observe the size of women in flattering roles on television to comprehend the pervasiveness of the current paradigm. Even in women's magazines that include articles concerning the dangers of slimness addiction and anorexia, these articles often are sandwiched between "lavish fashion spreads or advertisements depicting ultra-slim models living the fantasy of the perfect life" (Nichter & Nichter). In the advertisements for weight loss programs that claim to no longer promote dieting, the *before* pictures often still depict women of average or below average size. Regardless of what the program is called, the message is still that women can and should reduce their body weight by restricting the intake of food—a reasonable definition of dieting (Heatherton, 1991). Prescribing diets disguised as food plans or fitness programs may exacerbate physical and psychological problems (Elam, 1995). Finally, there is considerable evidence that health professionals' attitudes toward larger individuals reflect, or are even harsher than, general societal beliefs (Powers, 1988; Garner & Wooley, 1992; Oberrieder et al., 1995).

In summary, though there has been some movement in recent years in our understanding and treatment of the complex issues surrounding weight management, the current paradigm is still firmly entrenched in the fabric of our society. While it cannot be stated with certainty that new treatments arising from this paradigm will continue to fail, it is possible that an alternative paradigm is needed to redirect research and treatment and increase the likelihood of long-term success.

An Alternative Paradigm

It was more than a decade and a half ago that two major reviews first questioned the effectiveness and social appropriateness of traditional treatment for obesity (Stunkard & Pennick, 1979; Wooley, Wooley, & Dyrenforth, 1979). Since that time, numerous papers and books have continued to challenge the basic assumptions underlying the current paradigm (Bennett & Gurin, 1982; Ernsberger & Haskew, 1987; Polivy & Herman, 1987; Seid, 1988; Garner & Wooley, 1991; Schroeder, 1992; Robison, 1995; Erdman, 1995; Goodman, 1995; Johnson, 1994; Hirschmann & Munter, 1989, 1995).

An alternative paradigm for weight management has been developing from the work of these and other professionals from a variety of disciplines (Berg, 1992). This paradigm is beginning to make some inroads into traditional practice. In 1988, Health and Welfare Canada initiated a policy advocating acceptance of a wide range of healthy weights and challenging health professionals to deal more effectively with weight prejudice (Berg, 1992). At least one respected insurance company in the United States, Kaiser Permanente, has implemented a major revision of their approach to weight management, acknowledging the failure of dieting and the myth that healthy must mean thin (Lyons, 1995). In addition, numerous anti-dieting and self-acceptance organizations, for both lay people and professionals alike, have been formed and are active in promoting this new paradigm (Erdman, 1995). Nevertheless, the arguments put forth by this alternative paradigm have not been embraced, and in many cases not even addressed by most health care professionals who work with people concerned with weight management (Garner & Wooley, 1992).

The underlying concepts of this alternative paradigm for weight management are contrasted with those of the current paradigm in Table 1. The paradigm proposes that thinness is not intrinsically healthy or beautiful, and that fat is not intrinsically unhealthy or ugly. Standards of body size and beauty are strongly influenced by cultural norms. Throughout history, most cultures have regarded fatness as a sign of success, health, and beauty (Furnham & Alibhai, 1983; Brown & Konner, 1987). Even in the United States, standards of beauty and body size have changed dramatically in a short period of time. Full-figured women like Jane Russell, Jayne Mansfield, and Marilyn Monroe were considered the ideals of feminine beauty. It is informative that Marilyn Monroe maintained a size 12 figure for her movies only through constant dieting and often was larger (Nadelson, 1995). Yet she was worshipped by most men and emulated by most women in America at the time. Fifty years later, these women applying for jobs in the same industry would likely not be hired, but instead be told to "go on a diet [and] get a trainer" (Schneider, 1996).

Unlike the current paradigm, this alternative paradigm emphasizes that people have different body shapes and sizes by nature. When these naturally existing differences are exacerbated to the point that health is endangered, usually it is not as a result of a lack of individual initiative or will power. Rather, the underlying causes can be traced to a culture that promotes sedentary living and fast-food, high-fat eating, while at the same time applying tremendous pressure to achieve unrealistic body shapes and sizes (Robison et al., 1995).

The final contrast between the two paradigms is likely the most important. Recall that the basic assumption of the current paradigm is that everyone can be thin, happy, and healthy by dieting. First, it is clear that dieting for the vast majority of people *does not* result in sustained weight loss. Secondly, while for some individuals weight is associated with increased medical risks and health problems, for many people it is not. Although much has been made about the health benefits of being thin, there remains considerable controversy concerning the actual health risks that can be attributed to fatness (Ernsberger & Haskew 1987; Garner & Wooley, 1991; Gaesser, 1996). Finally, health is concerned with the integration and balance of the mental, emotional, and spiritual as well as physical aspects of life. Weight is only one component of physical health, and physical health is only one component of total health. Focusing excessively on one component of health, particularly when there are no effective methods to alter that component, may lead to imbalances and create a "medical terrorism" that may carry with it its own negative health implications (Ornstein & Sobel, 1989).

Practical Implications

This alternative paradigm proposes three major foci for people with weight concerns and the health professionals with whom they are working (Table 2). All focus on a holistic view of wellness that promotes "feeling good about oneself, eating well in a natural, relaxed way, and being comfortably active" (Berg, 1992). Burgard & Lyons, 1994). The underlying assumption of the paradigm is that people can improve the quality of their lives with these approaches, regardless of their size.

The first and most important focus is self acceptance. This term is often misunderstood when used in the context of weight-related issues. Self acceptance is not a denial of the potential health risks of excess weight for some individuals. Self acceptance is an affirmation that, just as human worth is not based on race, color, or creed, it also is not dependent on body weight, shape, or size. It is an affirmation that self-esteem is an essential part of the foundation for building a healthy lifestyle. Motivation for successful behavior change is enhanced when individuals accept and value themselves just as they are (Kornfield, 1993; Johnson, 1994). For larger individuals, this is acknowledged as a difficult but necessary goal in a culture obsessed with thinness and dieting (Polivy & Herman, 1987). Health professionals can encourage self-acceptance by honoring the natural diversity in body shape and size, and exposing societal prejudice and discrimination against larger individuals.

Although the current paradigm generally has minimized the link between weight and underlying psychological problems, methodologic and interpretive shortcomings may have resulted in premature closure on this issue (Brownell, 1993). Recent studies suggest that individuals seeking treatment for weight-related concerns may be more psychologically distressed than the general population (Fitzgibbon, Stollet, & Kirschenbaum, 1993; Telch & Agras, 1994; Sullivan et al., 1993). Further, binge eaters, who constitute 20 to 46 percent of those participating in weight loss programs, appear to have higher levels of psychological dysfunction than nonbinging larger individuals and persons who have never been large (Marcus et al., 1993). Kuehnel & Wadden, 1994; de Zwaan et al., 1993). Unfortunately, it is not possible at this time to determine causality. For some individuals, underlying psychological issues may contribute to weight problems (Felliti, 1993). However, it also has been suggested that the shame, discrimination, and isolation encountered by large individuals living in a thin-obsessed society, combined with the constant preoccupation with dieting, may contribute significantly to development of both physical and psychological problems (Schroeder, 1992). The emphasis on self-acceptance in this alternative paradigm acknowledges the primacy of mental health concerns and the complex, multi-faceted nature of weight-related problems. Psychological is-

Table 2	Alternative Paradigm for Weight Management: Major Foci for Health Educators

Self-Acceptance

Provide affirmation and reinforcement of human worth irrespective of differences in physical size and shape.

Physical Activity

Provide skills and support for increasing social, pleasure-based movement for enjoyment and enhanced quality of life.

Normalized Eating

Provide skills and support for discarding externally imposed rules and regimens for eating and attaining a more peaceful relationship with food by relearning to regulate intake in response to physiological hunger and satiety cues.

The Goal

Health educators should use these approaches to empower clients to live healthier, more fulfilled lives in the bodies they presently have.

sues need to be addressed whether they arise from trauma related to family dysfunction, societal discrimination, or any combination thereof.

The second major focus, physical activity, is widely recognized as an important element in human health and a critical factor in weight management, yet the majority of Americans of all sizes remain sedentary. Part of the explanation may be that traditional approaches to increasing participation have promoted vigorous, continuous exercise as essential for good health. The latest scientific evidence indicates that the primary determinant of health benefits is the total quantity of physical activity performed, rather than the type, duration, and intensity of the activity itself (Pate et al., 1993). Therefore, the paradigm focuses on promoting movement that is social, playful, and pleasurable, including everyday activities such as walking and gardening. Movement is engaged in for enjoyment and improved quality of life, not calorie burning and weight loss (Lyons & Burgard, 1988). Evidence supports

that physical activity can positively affect health and longevity regardless of weight status (Krotkiewski et al., 1979; Tremblay et al., 1991; Barlow et al., 1995). In addition, this alternative paradigm acknowledges the prevalence of sedentary living in our society as largely a cultural phenomenon that can be significantly impacted only by addressing cultural barriers (Robison & Rogers, 1994). This is especially true for larger individuals, many of whom are deterred from engaging in physical activity by fear of the ridicule and humiliation that they have endured as a regular, ongoing part of their lives (Garner & Wooley, 1992; For many such individuals, movement can be a means of beginning to rediscover and reconnect to the bodies they have for so long been taught to hate and ignore (Lyons, 1995).

The third focus of this alternative paradigm involves the concept of normal eating. Although proper eating is an important component of good health, the externally focused methods used by most diet programs rarely succeed in changing people's eating

habits permanently. Dieters learn not to eat when they are hungry and to stop eating before they are satisfied. Such arbitrary rules and regulations often lead to an elaborate "morality" involving "good" and "bad" foods, and feelings of virtuosity and guilt related to eating (Garner & Wooley, 1992). This "diet mentality" (Omichinski & Harrison, 1995) has contributed to increased anxiety and disordered eating in the general population as well as a precipitous rise in clinical eating disorders (Polivy & Herman, 1987). Further, the chronic disuse of hunger and satiety signals leads to an inability to use these normal physiological cues to guide food intake (Satter, 1987). Normalizing eating involves reducing anxiety about food, calories, fat, etc. and relearning to regulate food intake in response to physiological hunger and satiety cues. External controls, such as calorie-and fat-gram counting, are discouraged in this alternative approach, in favor of increased attention to internal needs and mindful eating (Satter, 1987). Hirschman, & Munter, 1988, 1995; Kano, 1989).

The underlying goal of current paradigm approaches to weight management is for people to be smaller, i.e. lose weight. The goal for health educators in the alternative paradigm is to use the approaches introduced in this article to empower people to live healthier, more fulfilled lives *in the bodies they presently have* (Erdman, 1995). This focus on health includes the need to screen for and treat potential underlying metabolic and or psychological problems in individuals when these pathologies are compromising their quality of life.

Future Directions

Research is needed to test the components of this alternative approach. With a paradigm focused on a comprehensive definition of health, the first step will be to redefine success. Weight loss is not a valid indicator of success, because it is not associated with long-term maintenance and because health benefits can be obtained through behavior change independently of changes in weight. Long-term amelioration of health risks and medical problems, with or without weight loss, should be the most important indicator of success (Robison, Hoerr, Strandmark, & Mavis, 1993; Atkinson, 1993). Given that weight loss is rarely maintained, a more holistic view of success that focuses on health, comfort, and self-esteem may be more productive and help to ameliorate the present unhealthy cultural obsession with thinness (Parham, 1991; Allan, 1994).

Programs that focus on discouraging the "diet mentality" and improving quality of life have met with some initial success. Results of these preliminary investigations indicate improvements in self-esteem and body image, and normalization of eating behaviors (Ciliska, 1989; Roughan, Seddon, & Vernon-Roberts, 1990; Carrier, Steinhardt, & Bowman, 1993; Armstrong & King, 1993; Hirschmann & Munter, 1995; Omichinski & Harrison, 1995; Rosen, 1995). There also is some suggestion that positive psychological changes may be maintained following treatment (Roughan, Seddon, & Vernon-Roberts, 1990; Carrier, Steinhardt, & Bowman, 1993, though additional studies are needed to validate and determine generalizability of these findings. Given the potential health risks

associated with both weight fluctuation and obesity, the long-term effects of these interventions on weight stability also need to be established (Carrier, Steinhardt, & Bowman, 1993).

Effective approaches to help people increase physical activity need to be incorporated into alternative paradigm interventions. Though many diets now include exercise components, maintenance remains a significant barrier, and it has been suggested that exercise that is not coupled with dieting may be more easily maintained (Garner & Wooley, 1991).

Finally, it is imperative that interventions respect the tremendous investment participants are likely to have in weight loss. Many individuals still firmly believe they will feel good about themselves only by losing weight, and they must be helped to explore alternatives in a caring and sensitive manner (Garner & Wooley, 1992). Ultimately, changes in cultural norms may be necessary to help people permanently reduce the chronic dieting and low-self-acceptance resulting from the failure to achieve society's unrealistic standards of body shape and size.

Perhaps it is again time to throw off the shackles of an invalid and non-productive paradigm. This alternative paradigm offers a marked departure from tradition, just the kind of change from which scientific revolutions arise. The validity of the approaches suggested will be determined by rigorous scientific evaluation over time. Given the lack of success and potential dangers of the current paradigm, we must hope that it will not take centuries to learn the outcome.

Allan, J.D. (1994). A biomedical and feminist perspective on women's experiences with weight management. *Western Journal of Nursing Research, 16*(5), 524-543.

Armstrong, D., & King, A. (1993). "Demand feeding" as diabetes treatment. *Obesity and Health, 7*, 109-110,115.

Asimov, I. (1980). The universe: From flat earth to black holes—and beyond. New York: Walker and Company.

Atkinson, R.L. (1993). Proposed standards for judging the success of the treatment of obesity. *Annals of Internal Medicine, 119*(7), 677-680.

Barlow, C.E., & Kohl, H.W., Gibbons, L.W., & Blair, S.N. (1995). Physical fitness, mortality, and obesity. *International Journal of Obesity, 19*(sup4):S41-S44.

Begley, C.E. (1991). Government should strengthen regulation in the weight loss industry. *Journal of the American Dietetics Association, 91*, 1255-1257.

Bennett, W.I., & Gurin, J. (1982). *The dieter's dilemma*. Basic Books: New York.

Berg, F.M. (1989). *Obesity and health*, March, 7-24.

Berg, F.M. (1992). Nondiet movement gains strength. *Obesity and Health*, Sept/Oct.

Brown, P.J., & Konner, M. (1987). An anthropological perspective on obesity. *Annals of The New York Academy of Sciences, 499*, 29-46.

Brownell, K.D. (1993). Whether obesity should be treated. *Health Psychology, 12*, 339-341.

Burgard, D., & Lyons, P. (1994). Alternatives in Obesity Treatment: Focusing on health for fat women. In Fallon, P, Katzman, M, & Wooley, S. (eds.), *Feminist perspectives in eating disorders*. The Guilford Press: New York, 212-230.

Carrier, K.M., Steinhardt, M.A., & Bowman, S. (1993). Rethinking traditional weight management programs: A 3-year follow-up evaluation of a new approach. *Journal of Psychology, 128*(5), 517-535.

Cassell, J.O. (1995). Social anthropology and nutrition: A different look at obesity in America. *Journal of the American Dietetics Association, 95*, 424-427.

Centers for Disease Control. (1991). Leads from the morbidity and mortality weekly report. *Journal of The American Medical Association, 266*, 2811-2812.

Ciliska, D.K. (1989). The effects of a group intervention on self-esteem, body dissatisfaction, and restrained eating of obese women. Unpublished doctoral dissertation, University of Toronto.

Council on Scientific Affairs. (1988). Treatment of obesity in adults. *Journal of The American Medical Association, 260,* 2547-2551.

Czajka-Narins, D.M., & Parham, E.S. (1990). Fear of fat: Attitudes toward obesity: The thinning of America. *Nutrition Today, Jan/Feb,* 26-32.

de Zwaan, M., Mitchell, J.E., Seim, H.C., Specker, S.M., Pyle, R.L., Raymond, N.C., & Crosby, R.B. (1994). Eating related and general psychopathology in obese females with binge eating disorder. *International Journal of Eating Disorders, 15,* 43-52.

Elam, P., & Kimbrell, D. (1995). Size, lies, and measuring tape. *Cognitive and Behavioral Practice, 2,* 233-248.

Erdman, C.K. (1995). *Nothing to Lose: A guide to sane living in a larger body.* Harper: San Francisco.

Ernsberger, P., & Haskew, P. (1987). "Rethinking obesity: An alternative view of it's health implications. *Journal of Obesity and Weight Regulation, 6,*(2),1-81.

Felitti, V. (1993). Childhood sexual abuse, depression, and family dysfunction in adult obese patients: A case control study. *Southern Medical Journal, 86,* 732-736.

Fitzgibbon, M.L., Stolley, M.R., & Kirschenbaum, D.S. (1993). Obese people who seek treatment have different characteristics than those who do not seek treatment. *Health Psychology, 12,* 342-345.

Foreyt, J.P., Brunner, R.L., Goodrick, G.K., Cutter, G., Brownell, K.D., & St. Jeor ST. (1995). Psychological correlates of weight fluctuation. *International Journal of Eating Disorders, 17*(3), 263-275.

Furnham, A., & Alibhai, N. (1983). Cross-cultural differences in the perception of female body types. *Psychological Medicine, 13,* 829-837.

Garner, D., & Wooley, S. (1991). Confronting the failure of behavioral and dietary treatments for obesity. *Clinical Psychology Review, 11,* 729-780.

Gaesser, G. (1996). *Big fat lies: The truth about your weight and your health.* Fawcett Columbine: New York.

Goodman, W.C. (1995). *The invisible women: Confronting weight prejudice in America.* Gurze Books: California.

Hawks, S.R., & Richins, P. (1994). Toward a new paradigm for the management of obesity. *Journal of Health Education, 25*(3), 147-153.

Hirschmann, J.R., & Munter, C.H. (1988). *Overcoming overeating.* Fawcett Columbine.

Hirschmann, J.R., & Munter, C.H. (1995). *When women stop hating their bodies: Freeing yourself from food and weight obsession.* Ballantine Books: New York.

Increasing prevalence of overweight among U.S. adults: The national health and nutrition examination surveys, 1960-1991. Kuczmarski, R.J., Flegal, K.M., Campbell, S.M., & Johnson, C.L. (1994). *Journal of The American Medical Association, 272,* 205-211.

Johnson, C. (1995). *Self-esteem comes in all sizes: How to be happy and healthy at your natural weight.* Doubleday: New York.

Kano, S. (1989). *Making peace with food.* Harper & Row.

Keys, A., Brozek, J., Herschel, A., Michelsen, O., & Taylor, H.L. (1950). *The biology of human starvation.* Minneapolis, MN: University of Minnesota Press.

Kornfield, J. (1993). *A path with heart: A guide through the perils and promises of spiritual life.* New York: Bantam Books.

Krotkiewski, et al. (1979). Effects of long-term physical training on body-fat, metabolism, and blood pressure in obesity. *Metabolism, 28,* 650-658.

Kuehnel, R.H., & Wadden, T.A. (1994). Binge eating disorder, weight cycling, and psychopathology. *International Journal of Eating Disorders, 15,* 321-329.

Kuhn, T.S. (1962). *The structure of scientific revolutions.* Chicago: University of Chicago Press.

Lustig, A. (1991). Weight loss programs: Failing to meet ethical standards? *Journal of the American Dietetic Association, 91,* 1252-1254.

Lyons, P., & Burgard, D. (1988). *Great shape: The first fitness guide for large women.* Bull Publishing.

Lyons, P. (1995). Weight and health: A new approach for the new year. Wellness Management: Newsletter of the National Wellness Association, 11(4),1,5-7.

Marcus, M.D., Wing, R.R., Ewing, L., Kern, E., Gooding, W., & McDermott, M. (1990). Psychiatric disorders among obese binge eaters. *International Journal of Eating Disorders, 9,* 69-77.

Nadelson, R. (1995). Marilyn Monroe: Was she really a size 16? *In Style Magazine; Sept.,* 88-91.

Nichter, M., & Nichter, M. (1991). Hype and weight. *Medical Anthropology, 13,* 249-284.

National Institutes of Health Technology Assessment Conference. (1992). Methods for voluntary weight loss and control. *Annals of Internal Medicine, 116,* 942-949.

Omichinski, L., & Harrison, K.R. (1995). Reduction of dieting attitudes and practises after participation in a non-diet lifestyle program. *Journal of The Canadian Dietetic Association, 56*(2), 81-85.

Ornstein, R., & Sobel, D. (1989). *Healthy pleasures.* Addison-Wesley Publishing: Reading, MA.

Parham, E.S. (1991). Alternative goals render successful outcomes likely. *Obesity and Health, 5,* 57-58.

Pate, R.R., Pratt, M., Blair, S.N., Haskell, W.L., et al. (1995). Physical activity and public health: A recommendation from the Centers for Disease Control and Prevention and the American College of Sports Medicine. *Journal of The American Medical Association, 273*(5), 402-407.

Polivy, J., & Herman, C.P. (1987). Diagnosis and treatment of normal eating. *Journal of Consulting and Clinical Psychology, 55*(5), 635-644.

Polivy, J. (1996). Psychological consequences of feed restriction. *Journal of The American Dietetic Association, 96*(6), 589-592.

Powers, P.S. (1988). Social issues in obesity. In Burrows, Beumont, and Casper (eds.), *Handbook of eating disorders, part 2.* Elsivier Science Publishers, 27-41.

Rittenbaugh, C. (1991). Body size and shape: A dialogue of culture and biology. *Medical Anthropology, 13,* 173-180.

Robison, J.I., Hoerr, S.L., Petersmarck, K.A., & Anderson, J.V. (1995). Redefining success in obesity intervention. *Journal of the American Dietetic Association, 95*(4), 422-423.

Robison, J.I., & Rogers, M.A. (1994). Adherence to exercise programmes: Recommendations. *Sports Medicine, 17*(1), 39-52.

Robison, J.I., Hoerr, S.L., Strandmark, J., & Mavis, B. (1993). Obesity, weight loss, and health. *Journal of the American Dietetic Association, 93,* 445-449.

Rosen, J.C., & Gross, J. (1987). Prevalence of weight reducing and weight gaining in adolescent girls and boys. *Health Psychology, 6,* 131-147.

Rosen, J.C., Orosan, P., & Reiter, J. (1995). Cognitive behavior therapy for negative body image in obese women. *Behavior Therapy, 26,* 25-42.

Roughan, P., Seddon, E., & Vernon-Roberts, J. (1990). Long term effects of a psychologically based group programme for women preoccupied with body weight and eating behavior. *International Journal of Obesity, 14,* 137-147.

Satter, E. (1987). *How to get your kid to eat—but not too much.* Bull Publishing Co.

Schneider, K.S. (1996). Too fat? Too thin? How media images of celebrities teach kids to hate their bodies. *People Magazine, June 3,* 65-74.

Schroeder, C.R. (1992). *Fat is not a four-letter word.* Chronimed: Minneapolis.

Seid, R.P. (1989). *Never too thin: Why women are at war with their bodies.* Prentice Hall: New York.

Sloan, R.P. (1987). Workplace health promotion: A commentary on the evolution of a paradigm. *Health Education Quarterly, 14*(2), 181-194.

Sobal, J. (1995). The Medicalization and demedicalization of obesity. In Maurer, Sobal (eds.). *Eating agendas: Food and nutrition as social problems.* Aldine de Gruyter: Hawthorne, NY, 67-89.

Stunkard, A.J., & Penick, S.B. (1979). Behavior modification in the treatment of obesity: The problem of maintaining weight loss. *Archives of General Psychiatry, 36,* 801-806.

Sullivan, M., Karlsson, J., Sjostrom, L., Backman, L., Bengtsson, C., Bouchard, C., Dahlgren, S., Jonsson, E., Larsson, B., Lindstedt, S., Naslund, I., Olbe, L., & Wedel, H. (1993). Swedish obese subjects (SOS)—an intervention study of obesity. Baseline evaluation of health and psychosocial functioning in the first 1743 subjects examined. *International Journal of Obesity, 17,* 503-512.

Telch, C.F., & Agras, W.S. (1994). Obesity, binge eating, and psychopathology: Are they related? *International Journal of Eating Disorders, 15,* 53-61.

Tremblay, A., Despres, J.P., Maheux, J., Pouliot, M.C., Nadeau, A., Moorjani, S., Lupien, P.J., & Bouchard, C. (1991). Normalization of the metabolic profile in obese women by exercise and a low fat diet. *Medicine and Science in Sports and Exercise, 23,* 1326-1331.

Wilson, G.T. (1992). Short-term psychological benefits and adverse effects of weight loss. Methods for voluntary weight loss and control. *National Institutes of Health Technology Assessment Conference,* 134-137.

Wiseman, C.V., Gray, J.J., Mosimann, J.E., & Ahrens, A.H. (1992). Cultural expectations of thinness in women: An update. *International Journal of Eating Disorders, 11*(1), 85-89.

Wooley, O.W., Wooley, S.C., & Dyrenforth, S.R. (1979). Obesity and women II. A neglected feminist topic. *Women's International Quarterly, 2,* 81-92.

 Article Review Form at end of book.

What is the relationship of race, weight, and desired weight change to body dissatisfaction?
Who has greater body dissatisfaction: African-American or white women according to the study conducted by Abood and Chandler?

Race and the Role of Weight, Weight Change, and Body Dissatisfaction in Eating Disorders

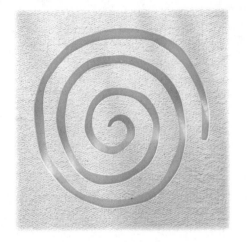

Doris A. Abood, EdD;
Steve B. Chandler, PhD

Doris A. Abood, EdD, Associate Professor, Health Education, Florida State University, Department of Nutrition, Food and Movement Sciences, 214U WJB, Tallahassee, FL; Steve B. Chandler, PhD, Associate Professor, Florida A&M University, Department of Health, Physical Education and Recreation, Tallahassee, FL.

ABSTRACT: This study assessed the relationship of race, weight, and desired weight change to body dissatisfaction and the relationship of desired weight change and body dissatisfaction to Eating Attitude Test (EAT-26) scores. Subjects were 373 white and 80 black college females. Results indicated that for both black and white women, current weight and desire to change weight were related to body dissatisfaction. White women, however, had significantly higher body dissatisfaction scores than did black women. For both black and white women, desired weight change and body dissatisfaction were related to EAT-26 scores. However, white women had significantly higher EAT-26 scores than did black women.

Symptoms of body-image disturbances have been recognized as essential characteristics of anorexia and bulimia nervosa.[1] The diagnostic criteria for anorexia nervosa include body-image distortion (e.g., claiming to "feel fat" even when emaciated), a weight phobia (e.g., intense fear of gaining weight or becoming fat), and preference for thinness (e.g., refusal to maintain normal body weight). The diagnostic criteria for bulimia nervosa include a persistent overconcern with body shape and weight, suggesting that body-image disturbances are symptomatic of bulimia nervosa as well.

It has been suggested that body image should be considered in a cultural context.[2] Cultural ideals can shape an individual's body-image experiences and the extent to which the individual utilizes dieting, exercising, restricting, and other measures to manage these body-image experiences.[3,4] The importance of thinness and the pressures placed on women to be thin in Western societies have been implicated as important predisposing factors in the greater prevalence of both body-image and eating disorders among women than men.[4,5-9]

In the United States, it has been reported that black women in the general population[10-13] and in college[14-16] develop eating disorders to a much lesser extent than do white women. Although black women may binge eat and diet to manage their weight, they are not as likely to engage in the pathogenic weight-loss behaviors that constitute anorexia and bulimia nervosa.[15] Despite a greater prevalence of obesity, black women appear to experience less body dissatisfaction than do white women and do not strive for thinness to the same extent as white women.[17-19] It has been reported that the observed differences may be due to a more positive body image held by black females and a greater acceptance of a larger body size among blacks.[15, 20]

It has been argued that the notion that black females are afforded a certain invulnerability to eating disorders may be due to cultural stereotypes and an internal adoption of cultural norms within therapeutic settings.[20] It has also been suggested that prevalent stereotypes of the white upper-class victim may undermine early identification of eating disorders in people of color.[21] Indeed, a recent study of readers of a popular black magazine may indicate that black women have levels of abnormal eating attitudes and behaviors at least comparable to those of white women, as well as experience some degree of body-size distortion and dissatisfaction.[22] In light of the equivocal findings related to the experience of eating disorders by blacks and whites, the present study was designed to answer the following questions: (a) What is the relationship of race, weight, and desired weight change to body dissatisfaction? (b) What is the relationship of race, desired weight change, and body dissatisfaction to eating difficulties?

Methods

Subjects

Questionnaires were distributed to students in personal health and nutrition courses at a historically black southeastern university and a neighboring predominantly white university. The students completed the questionnaire during class. A general explanation of the research was given, including a description of the questionnaire and aspects of voluntary participation, consent, confidentiality, and anonymity. Subjects for this study included black females (n = 80), and white females (n = 373). The mean ages of black and white females were 19.2 years (SD = 3.4) and 20.1 years (SD = 2.7), respectively. The average height and weight of white females was 1.661 m (SD = .065) and 60.0 kg (SD = 10.058), black females 1.663 m (SD = .077) and 64.1 kg (SD = 12.762).

Procedures

The questionnaire examined demographic and anthropometric characteristics as well as attitudes and behaviors associated with eating disorders as operationalized by the abbreviated Eating Attitudes Test (EAT-26).[22] The EAT-26 consists of 26 items designed to evaluate a broad range of attitudes and behaviors characteristic of anorexia nervosa and bulimia. In addition, the questionnaire examined body dissatisfaction as operationalized by the body dissatisfaction scale (BDS) of the Eating Disorder Inventory.[23] This scale has nine items that reflect the belief that specific body parts associated with shape change or increased "fatness" at puberty are too large. In this study, the BDS was used to assess dissatisfaction with aspects of the body-related size, shape, and weight. Subjects were divided into three groups according to their scores on the BDS as follows: a score of 10 or less was considered "low" 11-20 "moderate," and 21 or greater "high" dissatisfaction.

Self-reported height and weight information was utilized to group subjects into weight categories of below, at, or above optimum weight based on guidelines described by Zeman.[24] The weight categories of "above" and "below" deviate from optimum weight by 10%. The categories are commonly used in nutritional assessment when measuring body composition is not practical. The categories are not sensitive to racial differences in body composition.

Statistical Analysis

Analysis of variance was used to test the relationship of race, weight, and desired weight change to body dissatisfaction as well as the relationship of race, weight change, and body dissatisfaction to pathogenic eating attitudes and behaviors as operationalized by the EAT-26. Post hoc analyses were performed using Scheffe's test. Student's t-test was used to test for differences in weight between blacks and whites.

Table 1 Body Dissatisfaction (BDS) Means and Standard Deviations for Black and White Females

	White Females (N=373)	Black Females (N=80)
BDS		
Mean	12.4	10.2
SD	7.4	7.5

Note: F = 4.8584, p <.05

		White				**Black**		
		N	**M**	**SD**		**N**	**M**	**SD**
Weight	10% below ideal	67	9.01	6.61		10	6.36	7.10
Category	Ideal	215	11.66	7.07		17	5.48	13.17
	10% above ideal	91	16.58	7.24		53	13.92	6.94
Desired Weight	Lose	294	14.07	6.93		50	14.14	6.71
Change	Gain	24	6.52	6.63		13	4.54	4.56
	Neither	55	5.07	4.85		17	3.00	4.06

Table 2 BDS Means and Standard Deviations by Weight Category and Desired Weight Change

Results

BDS means and standard deviations can be seen in Table 1. White women were significantly more dissatisfied with their bodies than were black women (12.4 vs. 10.2; $F = 4.858$, $p < .05$). This was especially interesting in light of the fact that black women weighed more than white women (64.1 kg and 60.0 kg, respectively; $F = 1.49$, $p < .01$). BDS means and standard deviations by weight category and desired weight change can be seen in Table 2. ANOVA results revealed that weight ($F = 16.684$, $p < .05$), weight change ($F = 43.397$, $p < .05$), and race ($F = 14.121$, $p < .05$) were significantly related to BDS. The desire to change weight accounted for the greatest proportion of the variance explained (.134), weight accounted for less (.051), and race accounted for the least proportion of the variance explained (.021). No interaction was observed among the independent variables of weight, weight change, and race on body dissatisfaction. The absence of interaction indicates that for both black and white women, current weight and the desire to change weight were significantly related to body dissatisfaction. Post hoc comparisons revealed that those in the above-ideal weight category had significantly higher BDS scores than did those in the ideal and below-ideal weight categories. Post hoc comparisons also revealed that those wanting to lose weight had significantly higher BDS scores than did those wanting to gain or neither lose or gain.

EAT-26 means and standard deviations can be seen in Table 3. White women had significantly higher scores than did black women (13.9 vs. 10.6; $F = 10.785$, $p < .05$). EAT-26 means and standard deviations by desired weight change and categorized body dissatisfaction can be seen in Table 4. ANOVA results on the relationship of desired weight change and race and categorized body dissatisfaction on EAT-26 revealed that desired weight change ($F = 7.556$, $p < .05$), race ($F = 5.056$, $p < .05$), and categorized body dissatisfaction ($F = 27.362$, $p < .05$) were significantly related to EAT-26 scores. Body dissatisfaction accounted for the greatest proportion of the variance explained (.094), weight change accounted for less (.025), and race accounted for the least proportion of the variance explained (.008). No interaction was observed among the independent variables of weight change, race, and categorized BDS. The absence of interaction indicates that for both black and white women, the desire to change weight and body dissatisfaction were significantly related to EAT-26 scores. Post hoc comparisons revealed that those wanting to lose weight had significantly higher EAT scores than did those wanting to gain or neither gain nor lose. Post hoc comparisons also revealed that those with high body dissatisfaction had higher EAT-26 scores than those with either moderate or low body dissatisfaction.

Discussion

This study demonstrated a strong relationship between a woman's weight, desire to lose weight, and body dissatisfaction. Although this relationship was significant for both black and white women, black women weighing an average 10 lbs more than their white counterparts did not appear to experience the same level of body dissatisfaction as white women experienced. These results indicate a greater tolerance for higher weights among black women. Further research is needed to determine the factors and influences that exist for black women that foster the development of a more positive body image and prevent the fat phobia and pursuit of thinness that appear to plague white women. In addition, it is impor-

Table 3 EAT -26 Means and Standard Deviations for Black and White Females

	White Females (N=373)	Black Females (N=80)
EAT-26		
Mean	13.9	10.9
SD	10.9	8.5

Note: F = 10.785, p <.05

tant to determine if the more moderate attitudes toward weight held by black women contribute to their risk of obesity and problems associated with obesity.[10] The findings also revealed that factors such as weight category and desire to change weight had a stronger relationship to body dissatisfaction than did race. Women who were above their ideal weight and women who wanted to lose weight (irrespective of their weight category) were dissatisfied with aspects of their bodies.

An important finding of this study is that the desire to lose weight and dissatisfaction with one's body may lead to eating difficulties. Once again, black women did not experience the same level of eating difficulties as did white women. This may indicate that although black women may be overweight, they may not hold pathogenic attitudes or feel compelled to engage in pathogenic weight-loss behaviors to the extent of their white counterparts. Although it is tempting to suggest that a certain cultural protection exists, it may not protect certain vulnerable individuals within that culture.[20] Thus, health promotion professionals planning programs and intervention strategies for weight management or eating disorders prevention should assume that body-image concerns, weight-loss desires, and eating difficulties will be relevant issues for both black and white women. Screening instruments such as the ones used in this study may be used to assess the tendency toward pathogenic weight-loss attitudes and behaviors as well as to detect body dissatisfaction, without regard to race. However, sensitivity to the cultural differences in food selection, food preparation, and exercise patterns should be considered in the planning of educational strategies designed to encourage healthy eating and a healthy, maintainable weight.

The findings of this study were not consistent with the findings of Pumariega et al.[23] in that white women had higher BDS and EAT-26 scores than did blacks (although this study did not compare blacks and whites on these variables). Nonetheless, the conclusions here support the findings of Pumariega et al.[23] in that black and white women face similar issues related to body dissatisfaction and eating difficulties. Sampling differences may account for variations in the findings. Participants in this study were mostly young and middle class women who were not randomly selected. Participants in the abovementioned study were older and also not randomly selected.

In this study, the proportion of the variance explained by the independent variables was modest. Clearly concerns other than one's weight, desire to change one's weight, and body dissatisfaction may also affect eating attitudes and behaviors. Sociocultural, psychological, biological, and developmental factors should be explored for the purposes of prevention and treatment.

Table 4 EAT-26 Means and Standard Deviations by Desired Weight Change and Categorized Body Dissatisfaction

		White			Black		
		N	M	SD	N	M	SD
Desired	Lose	292	15.50	8.31	50	12.92	7.69
Weight	Gain	24	6.95	4.58	13	5.77	3.49
Change	Neither	55	8.29	5.87	17	7.47	4.87
Categorized	Low	161	10.5	7.32	43	7.26	4.49
Body	Moderate	152	5.45	7.93	26	11.88	6.42
Dissatifaction	High	60	19.03	8.63	11	20.64	8.11

References

1. American Psychiatric Association, Diagnostic and Statistical Manual of Mental Disorders, 4th ed., Washington, D.C.: Author, 1994.

2. Fallon A. Culture in the mirror: Sociocultural determinants of body image. In T.F. Cash and T. Pruzinsky (Eds.) Body images: Development, deviance, and change. New York: Guilford Press, 1990: 80-109.

3. Cash TF. The psychology of physical appearance: Aesthetics, attributes, and images. In T.F. Cash, & T. Pruzinsky (Eds.), Body images: Development, deviance, and change. New York: Guilford Press, 1990:51-79.

4. Rosen JC. Body-image disturbances in eating disorders. In T.F. Cash, & T. Pruzinsky (Eds.), Body images: Development, deviance, and change. New York: Guilford Press, 1990:190-214.

5. Cash TF, Brown TA. Gender and body images: stereotypes and realities. *Sex Roles* 1989; 21:357-368.

6. Freedman R. Cognitive-behavioral perspectives on body-image change. In T.F. Cash, & T. Pruzinsky (Eds.), Body images: Development, deviance, and change. New York: Guilford Press, 1990:272-295.

7. Garner DM, Garfinkle PE. Socio-cultural factors in the development of anorexia nervosa. *Psy Med* 1980;10:649-656.

8. Hsu LKG. The gender gap in eating disorders: why are the eating disorders more common among women? *Clin Psychol Rev* 1989; 9:393-407.

9. Rodin J, Silberstein LR, Striegel-Moore RH. Women and weight: a normative discontent. In T.B. Sonderegger (Ed.), Nebraska symposium on motivation: Psychology and gender: Lincoln: University of Nebraska Press, 1985:267-307.

10. Rand CS, Kuldau JM. Epidemiology of bulimia and symptoms in a general population: sex, age, race, and socioeconomic status. *Int J Eat Dis*. 1992;11:37-44.

11. Dolan B. Cross-cultural aspects of anorexia nervosa and bulimia: a review. *Int J Eat Dis* 1991; 10:69-78.

12. Klem ML, Klesges RC, Bene CR, Mellon MW. A psychometric study of restraint: the impact of race, gender, weight and marital status. *Addict Behav* 1990; 15:147-152.

13. Pumariega AJ, Edwards P, Mitchell CB. Anorexia in black adolescents. *J Am Acad Child Psych* 1984;23:111-114.

14. Abrams KK, Allen LR, Gray JJ. Disordered eating attitudes and behaviors, psychological adjustment, and ethnic identity: a comparison of black and white female college students. *Int J Eat Dis* 1993;14:49-57.

15. Gray JJ, Ford K, Kelly LM. The prevalence of bulimia in a black college population. *Int J Eat Dis* 1987;6:733-740.

16. Striegel-Moore RH, Silberstein LR, Rodin J. Toward an understanding of risk factors for bulimia. *Am Psychol* 1986; 41:246-263.

17. Rand CS, Kuldau JM. The epidemiology of obesity and self-identified weight problem in the general population: gender, race, age, and social class. *Int J Eat Dis* 1990;4:329-343.

18. Thomas VG, James MD. Body image, dieting tendencies, and sex role traits in urban black women. *Sex Roles* 1988;18:523-529.

19. Rosen JC, Gross J. Prevalence of weight reducing and weight gaining in adolescent girls and boys. *Health Psychology* 1987;6:131-147.

20. Pyle RL, Mitchell JE, Eckert ED, Halvorsen PA, Newman PA, et al. The incidence of bulimia in freshman college students. *Int J Eat Dis* 1983;2:75-85.

21. Root PP. Disordered eating in women of color. *Sex Roles* 1990;22:525-536.

22. Siber TJ. Anorexia nervosa in blacks and hispanics. *Int J Eat Dis* 1986;5:121-128.

23. Pumariega AJ, Gustavson CR, Gustavson JC, Motes JC, Ayers S. Eating attitudes in African-American Women: The Essence eating disorders survey. *Eating Disorders* 1994;2:5-16.

24. Garner DM, Olmsted MP, Bohr Y. The Eating Attitudes Test: Psychometric features and clinical correlates. *Psychol Med* 1982; 12:871-878.

25. Garner DM, Olmsted MP, Polivy J. Development and validation of a multidimensional eating disorder inventory for anorexia nervosa and bulimia. *Int J Eat Dis* 1983;2:15-34.

26. Zeman FJ. Clinical Nutrition and Dietetics (2nd ed.). New York: Macmillan, 1991.

 Article Review Form at end of book.

How are poor diets associated with the leading causes of death?
In what ways can even small dietary changes yield large benefits?

The American Diet

A costly health problem

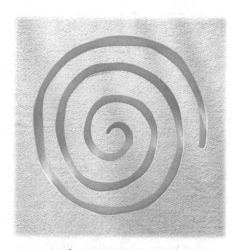

Elizabeth Frazão

The author is an agricultural economist with the Food and Consumer Economics Division, Economic Research Service, USDA.

Scientific evidence increasingly suggests that diet plays an important role in the onset of chronic diseases—contributing to increased illnesses, reduced quality of life, and premature death. Although there is still much that scientists do not know about how diet affects health, there is significant agreement on the components of a healthy diet. In particular, diets high in calories, fat, saturated fat, cholesterol, and salt, and low in fiber-containing foods (such as fruit, vegetables, and whole grain products) are associated with increased risk for coronary heart disease, certain types of cancer, stroke, and diabetes. Diet also plays a role in other health conditions, such as overweight, hypertension, and osteoporosis. And, new research suggests that low intake of folic acid is associated with increased risk of certain birth defects, heart disease, and stroke.

Taken together, these health conditions cost society an estimated $250 billion each year in medical charges and lost productivity. The extent to which these costs might be reduced by an improved diet cannot be calculated precisely, but some researchers estimate that proper diet might forestall at least 20 percent of the annual deaths from heart disease, cancer, stroke, and diabetes.

Poor Diets Associated With Leading Causes of Death...

Of the 10 leading causes of death in the United States, 4—including the top 3—are associated with diets that are too high in calories, fat, saturated fat, cholesterol, and sodium, or too low in fiber-containing foods. These conditions—coronary heart disease, cancer, stroke, and dibetes—account for over half (53.5 percent) of the deaths occurring each year in the United States (table 1).

Coronary heart disease

Coronary heart disease (CHD)-the type of heart disease commonly associated with diet and which ac-

counts for approximately two-thirds of all deaths from heart disease—caused over 480,000 deaths in 1995, second only to cancer. The American Heart Association estimates there are about 1.5 million heart attacks annually, and that CHD costs the United States $56.3 billion each year ($48.3 billion in direct health care costs and $8 billion in lost productivity) (table 2). The major risk factors for CHD which can be modified by an individual are high blood cholesterol levels, hypertension, cigarette smoking, and physical inactivity. Diet—especially intake of saturated fat and cholesterol—can influence blood cholesterol levels in some people, as well as influence other risk factors for CHD, such as obesity and diabetes. In addition, new research suggests that low intake of folic acid—found in many fruits, vegetables, and legumes, as well as in fortified cereals—may increase the risk for heart disease and stroke in adults.

Cancer

Over 500,000 people died of cancer in the United States in 1995—averaging nearly one person

Source: From Elizabeth Frazão, "The American Diet: A Costly Health Problem" in *Food Review*, January-April 1996, Economic Research Service, U.S. Department of Agriculture.

Table 1 Four of the Top 10 Causes of Death in the United States Are Diet-Related

*Heart disease[1]	738,781
*Cancer	537,969
*Stroke	158,061
Chronic obstructive pulmonary diseases	104,756
Accidents and adverse effects	89,703
Pneumonia and influenza	83,528
*Diabetes	59,085
HIV Infections	42,506
Suicide	30,893
Chronic liver disease and cirrhosis	24,848
Other causes	442,073
All causes	2,312,203

Note: *Diet-related diseases. [1]Coronary heart disease, the type of heart disease commonly associated with diet, was responsible for 482,185 deaths in 1995, nearly two-thirds of the deaths from heart disease.
Source: Preliminary estimates from Rosenberg, Harry M., Stephanie J. Ventura, Jeffrey D. Maurer, Robert L. Heuser, and MaryAnne Freedman. "Births and Deaths: United States, 1995." *Monthly Vital Statistics Report*, Vol. 45, No. 3, suppl. 2, Hyattsville, MD: National Center for Health Statistics, Oct. 4, 1996.

every minute. Over 1 million new cases of cancer are diagnosed each year. The American Cancer Society estimates that overall costs for cancer amount to $104 billion each year, with $35 billion in direct medical charges, $12 billion due to lost productivity associated with illness, and $57 billion due to lost productivity associated with premature death. Diets high in fat and low in fiber-containing foods are associated with increased risk of certain types of cancer. Some researchers estimate that about one-third of all cancer deaths could be prevented through dietary changes alone.

Stroke

Strokes affect over 500,000 people each year and killed over 150,000 people in 1995. According to the American Heart Association, stroke is the leading cause of serious disability, and accounts for half of all patients hospitalized for acute neurological disease. More than 3 million people in the United States suffer from stroke-related disabilities, at an annual cost of $19.7 billion ($16.9 billion in direct medical costs and $2.8 billion in lost productivity). Risk factors include a diet high in saturated fat and cholesterol, as well as obesity, diabetes, and hypertension. Some of the observed 57-percent reduction in mortality rates from stroke in the past two decades is likely associated with improvements in the detection and treatment of hypertension (see below).

Diabetes

Diabetes killed nearly 60,000 people in 1995, and is estimated to contribute to an additional 300,000 deaths each year. Diabetes is the single leading cause of kidney disease, and a risk factor for coronary heart disease and stroke. It is also the leading cause of blindness, can cause nerve damage and result in amputations, and can cause birth defects in babies born to diabetic women. Diabetes affects 13-14 million people in the United States, half of whom are not even aware they have it. There are two types of diabetes. Type I, also called insulin-dependent or juvenile-onset diabetes, is characterized by an absolute deficiency of insulin, usually appears well before age 40, and is not diet-related. Type II diabetes, or noninsulin-dependent or adult-onset diabetes, appears in midlife, most often among overweight or obese adults, and can often be controlled by diet and exercise. Of the estimated 7.2 million diagnosed cases of diabetes, 90-95 percent are Type II (undiagnosed cases are likely to be Type II, since the severity of Type I symptoms is likely to lead an individual to a doctor and thus a diagnosis). The total economic costs of diabetes—including direct medical costs and the indirect costs of lost productivity associated with illness and premature death—are estimated at more than $40 billion annually. The maintenance of desirable body weight is the most effective intervention known in the prevention of noninsulin-dependent diabetes. About 80 percent of people with Type II diabetes are overweight, and it is estimated that half of Type II diabetes cases can be prevented by controlling obesity.

...And With Other Health Conditions

Diet also influences other health conditions that, although not listed as a primary cause of death, contribute to premature mortality or reduce the quality of life—in particular, overweight, hypertension, and osteoporosis. New research also suggests that many

Table 2 Costs Associated With Major Diet-Related Health Conditions Add Up

	Million dollars		
Coronary heart disease	56,300	48,300	8,000
Cancer	104,000	35,000	69,000
Stroke	19,700	16,900	2,800
Diabetes	40,000	NA	NA
Obesity	2,400	NA	NA
Hypertension	17,400	14,900	2,500
Osteoporosis	10,000	NA	NA
Neural tube defects	900	NA	NA
Total	250,700	NA	NA

Notes: NA = Not available. [1]In most cases this includes direct health care costs and lost productivity resulting from disability. Sources: For coronary heart disease, stroke, and hypertension: American Heart Association, *Heart and Stroke Facts: 1994 Statistical Supplement,* Dallas, Texas, 1993. For cancer: Brown, Martin L., "The National Economic Burden of Cancer: An Update," Special Report, *Journal of the National Cancer Institute.* Vol. 82, No. 23, pp. 1811-14, Dec. 5, 1990. For diabetes: American Diabetes Association, *Diabetes 1993 Vital Statistics,* Alexandria, VA, 1993. For obesity: Colditz, Graham A., "Economic Costs of Obesity," *American Journal of Clinical Nutrition,* Vol. 55, pp. 503S-507S, 1992. For osteoporosis: National Osteoporosis Foundation, "Fast Facts on Osteoporosis," Washington, DC, 1994. For neural tube defects: adapted from Romano, Patrick S., Norman J. Waitzman, Richard M. Scheffler, and Randy D. Pi, "Folic Acid Fortification of Grain: An Economic Analysis," *American Journal of Public Health.* Vol. 85, No. 5, pp. 667-76, May 1995; National Center for Health Statistics, Public Health Service, "Advance Report of Final Mortality Statistics, 1992," *Monthly Vital Statistics Report,* Vol. 43, No. 6 suppl., Hyattsville, MD, 1995; and Centers for Disease Control, "Recommendations for the use of folic acid to reduce the number of cases of spina bifida and other neural tube defects," *Morbidity and Mortality Weekly Report,* Vol. 41, No. RR-14, Sept. 11, 1992.

cases of neural tube birth defects could potentially be prevented by increased intake of folic acid among women of childbearing age, and that some of the memory loss and confusion associated with aging may stem from small vitamin deficiencies and poor nutrition. Similarly, preliminary studies suggest a role for antioxidants in the prevention of cataracts and senile degeneration of the retina (the leading cause of blindness in the elderly).

Overweight is associated with elevated blood cholesterol levels, high blood pressure, and noninsulin-dependent diabetes. It also increases the risk for some types of cancer and is an independent risk factor for CHD. Recent studies also show that being overweight increases the risk of premature death. Despite growing consumer interest in weight-loss programs, two recent national surveys estimate that one-third of the American population is overweight—up from 25 percent just a decade ago. Among the factors within an individual's control, being overweight is associated with low activity level, excessive intake of calories, and/or high intake of fat.

Hypertension, or high blood pressure, is a common and important risk factor for CHD, stroke, and renal disease, affecting as many as 50 million people over age 6 in the United States. The American Heart Association estimates that more than 33,000 Americans died from high blood pressure in 1991 (58 percent of them women), and that high blood pressure contributed to thousands of additional deaths from other causes. Hypertensive disease costs an estimated $14.9 billion each year in direct medical care charges (with drug costs estimated at about $3.6 billion per year), and $2.5 billion in lost productivity. Age-related increases in blood pressure—as occurs in the United States—are associated with excessive weight and physical inactivity, high sodium and alcohol intakes, and low potassium intake. Although not all people are equally susceptible to the effects of sodium, a low sodium intake might prevent blood pressure from increasing with age. Improvements in the detection, treatment, and control of hypertension are believed to have contributed substantially to the decline in mortality rates from stroke and coronary heart disease in the past two decades.

Osteoporosis affects some 25 million people in the United States—including over half of all women over age 50 and one-third of all men by age 75. Osteoporosis is responsible for 1.5 million bone fractures a year, mostly at the wrist, spine, and hip. Hip fractures alone are estimated to cost $10 billion in medical costs each year. However, this figure does not include productivity losses (see "Osteoporosis-Related Hip Fractures Cost $13 Billion to $18 Billion Yearly," elsewhere in this issue). Low intake of calcium and inadequate physical activity appear to be important risk factors. Recent research suggests that 30-60 percent of fractures in individuals 65 and older could be prevented through improved calcium intake.

Neural tube defects (NTD) occur in approximately 2,500 births each year in the United States as a result of the neural tube failing to close during the first month of pregnancy. Many of these babies are born without a brain (anencephaly) and die shortly after birth; others are born with an exposed spinal cord (spina bifida), and survive, but are handicapped as a result of damage to the exposed spinal cord and many die before adulthood. Medical costs and productivity losses are estimated at over $900 million each year. The Public Health Service estimates that nearly half of all NTD births could be prevented if all women of childbearing age consumed 400 micrograms of folic acid a day—a significant increase from the average of 222 micrograms consumed daily from food sources by females age 12 and older according to USDA's 1989-91 food consumption surveys.

Even Small Dietary Changes May Yield Large Benefits

Because genetic predisposition increases some people's risk for some chronic diseases and health conditions, it is difficult to determine to what extent dietary changes could affect the incidence or mortality rates, by either preventing or delaying the onset of these conditions.

A 1993 article in the *Journal of the American Medical Association* provided the first estimate of the influence of diet on overall mortality, based on the underlying risk factor behind each death—those behaviors which may have been controlled by the individual, such as diet, activity level, and smoking—rather than the official cause of death. Thus, for example, when an obese, inactive, middle-aged person died from a heart attack, the underlying cause of death was attributed to poor diet and inactivity, although the official cause of death was heart dis-

ease. Of the 2.1 million deaths in 1990, the authors estimated that 300,000 (14 percent) could be attributed to poor diet and/or low physical activity level.

From a narrower perspective, researchers at the University of California at San Francisco looked at the lives that could be saved through reduced fat intake alone. They estimated that 42,000 premature deaths from CHD and cancers could be prevented each year—2 percent of all deaths—if all Americans reduced their intakes of total fat, saturated fat, and cholesterol to the recommended levels. Unfortunately, that study looked only at the average effects on mortality, and not at the age distribution of those saved. Yet, CHD and cancer affect not only the elderly, but are also quite high among those aged 40 and over. Data from a longitudinal study suggest, for example, that 40 percent of all heart attacks occur in people aged 40-65.

Both the Food and Drug Administration (FDA) and USDA also estimated the benefits associated with improved diets in their analysis of the impact of the new nutrition labeling regulations that became effective in mid-1994. Looking only at changes in intake of fat, saturated fat, and cholesterol, the agencies estimated that even small average reductions of only about 1 percent in the intake of total fat and saturated fat and 0.1 percent in the intake of cholesterol would prevent over 56,000 cases of CHD and cancer, avoid over 18,000 deaths, and save over 117,000 life-years over 20 years. They further estimated that the medical savings associated with these benefits totaled $ 0.8 billion.

The agencies pointed out, however, that this estimate undervalued the true benefits of improved diets since it did not

include productivity losses or other losses due to pain and suffering. A more inclusive method of valuing such losses is to estimate the amount people are willing to pay to reduce the risk of suffering a heart attack, stroke, or cancer. People routinely make decisions to accept or avoid some incremental amount of risk, such as choosing a high-risk job, or choosing to use a seat belt in the car. A variety of studies have estimated the values that consumers and workers place on risk reduction, including wage differentials between high- and low-risk jobs. The estimates obtained from these studies, which represent people's willingness to pay to reduce the risk of premature death, range between $1.5 million and $8.5 million per life saved.

FDA and USDA estimated the health benefits of mandatory nutrition labeling regulations using two methods and a willingness-to-pay value of $1.5 million per premature death avoided. Approximately a 1-percent reduction in the intake of total fat and saturated fat and a 0.1-percent reduction in the intake of cholesterol resulted in estimated benefits of $5.6 billion to $15.3 billion over 20 years.

In addition, recent research on the role and likely health benefits of increased intake of folic acid suggests significant cost savings from both reduced birth defects and reduced deaths from CHD. The Public Health Service estimates that approximately 1,200 annual cases of neural tube defects in the United States could be prevented if women ingested 400 micrograms of folic acid daily before and during the first 4 weeks of pregnancy. A separate study estimated that if all men increased their intake of folic acid by 350 micrograms per day (280 micrograms for women), this could potentially prevent 9 percent of deaths from coronary heart disease among men 45 years and older—30,500 deaths per year (and 5 percent of deaths among women 45 years and older—19,000 deaths per year).

Although these benefit estimates are relatively crude, they suggest that even small improvements in dietary intake may be associated with large benefits.

Consumers Changing Their Eating Habits

The increasing evidence linking diet and health has not been lost among consumers—92 percent of food shoppers interviewed for the 1995 annual survey by the Food Marketing Institute reported having changed their eating habits to make their diets more healthful. The food industry has also responded actively to consumer demand for foods with improved nutritional profiles. An increasing proportion of new food products carry at least one nutrient content claim—most often claims about reduced fat content—and supermarkets are offering consumers an ever-increasing variety of foods with improved nutritional profiles. The increased availability of lower fat products and lean meats has probably contributed to average fat intake in the United States declining from 40 to 34 percent of calories in the past 20

years. The new nutrition labels, mandated for most processed foods, not only provide an additional incentive for manufacturers to reformulate their products, but should also make it easier for consumers to choose a healthier diet.

However, there is still much room for improvement. Consumption of vegetables, fruits, and dairy products remain below the recommended number of servings (see "Many Americans Are Not Meeting Food Guide Pyramid Dietary Recommendations," elsewhere in this issue). Although fat intake has been declining, consumption is still above the recommended levels, and the prevalence of people classified as overweight has increased.

The difficulty of translating diet and health awareness into effective behavior change is a major challenge to USDA's nutrition education and promotion efforts, since it is well known that dietary advice does not automatically translate into dietary practices. This is particularly true when dietary advice requires large changes in current behavior, or when health problems tend to be concentrated among hard-to-reach populations—those least likely to be aware of the diet-health links or to have adequate nutrition knowledge.

Nutrition education specialists also recognize they must overcome a common belief that the prevention of chronic disease is

beyond one's control, and that a healthy diet is more costly, difficult, time-consuming, and less pleasurable. While motivating consumers to make dietary changes, nutrition education must also provide consumers with the knowledge necessary to make effective dietary changes.

References

Browner, Warren S., Janice Westenhouse, and Jeffrey A. Tice. "What If Americans Ate Less Fat?" *Journal of the American Medical Association,* Vol. 265, No. 24, June 26, 1991, pp. 3285-91.

Doll, Richard, and Richard Peto. "The Causes of Cancer: Quantitative Estimates of Avoidable Risks of Cancer in the United States Today," *Journal of the National Cancer Institute,* Vol. 66, No. 6, June 1981, pp. 1191-1308.

Frazão, E., and J. E. Allshouse. "Sales of Nutritionally Improved Foods Outpace Their Traditional Counterparts," *Food Review,* USDA, Economic Research Service, Vol. 18, No. 3, Sept-Dec 1995.

McGinnis, J. Michael, and William H. Foege. "Actual Causes of Death in the United States," *Journal of the American Medical Association,* Nov. 10, 1993.

U. S. Department of Health and Human Services, Public Health Service, "Recommendations for the Use of Folic Acid to Reduce the Number of Cases of Spina Bifida and Other Neural Tube Defects," *Morbidity and Mortality Weekly Report,* Vol. 41, No. RR-14, Sept. 11, 1992, pp. 1-7.

 Article Review Form at end of book.

What role has the Center Science in the Public Interest taken in changing the nutritional health of Americans?
What are some of the tactics used by the Center for Science in the Public Interest to achieve their goals?

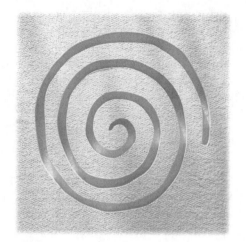

Food Police

In the name of good nutrition, they've busted Chinese food, Italian food, movie popcorn, and now our favorite happy-hour hangouts. Have they gone too far?

Minna Morse

Minna Morse is an assistant editor at Smithsonian *magazine.*

"I'm thinking of having the salad and the baked potato—and the garden burger," the thin man says to his lunch date. "Think that's too much?"

"He eats all the time," she says, talking past him. "Enormous quantities. But healthy food. Only healthy food."

Ordering a meal is a dicey affair when you're known as the country's fussiest eaters—and you're sitting in a restaurant you're about to publicly skewer. The lean and hungry diner is

Michael Jacobson, director of the Center for Science in the Public Interest. Seated at the table with him is dietitian Jayne Hurley, mastermind of a three-year campaign to alert Americans to the dangers of restaurant dining.

These are the folks who slammed Chinese meals, proclaiming kung pao chicken "one of the nastiest dishes" served, "with almost as much fat as four McDonald's Quarter Pounders." They're the ones who denounced fettuccine alfredo as "a heart attack on a plate" and revealed that a large tub of movie popcorn delivers more artery-clogging fat than nine hamburgers.

They've lambasted deli sandwiches, Mexican food, and our favorite sugary snacks. Now, in their latest gambit, they're targeting the upscale burger joints and happy-hour havens—Chili's Houlihan's, Bennigan's, TGI Friday's, Hard Rock Café, Planet Hollywood, Applebee's, and others—that occupy urban corners and riddle suburban malls across the country.

Just a few weeks before, comparable dishes ordered to go at each of these chains had arrived at a lab near Baltimore, shipped overnight in foam ice chests from cities as far-flung as Chicago and Los Angeles, to be weighed, picked apart, ground up, combined, and whirred in a blender into a gray brown goop resembling nothing so much as mud. All simply to peg the dishes' average fat, "artery-clogging fat," calorie, and sodium counts.

The three of us are at a TGIFriday's in downtown Washington, D.C. Nearby are clusters of office workers in dark suits and vacationing families in khaki shorts and denim shirts. They're peering at laminated-plastic menus, munching chips.

What's good? "Let's take a look," Hurley says. It's tough going among the appetizers. You wouldn't want to order the stuffed potato skins, which in CSPI's survey averaged 1,120 calories and 79 grams of fat per basket. That's a whole day's fat for an ordinary woman. Nor would the buffalo wings fly.

"No one thinks of buffalo wings as terribly unhealthy," Hurley says. "I mean, it's chicken, right? But it happens to be the fattiest part of the chicken. Then it's fried. Then it's dipped in blue cheese." The damages: more than 1,000 calories, on average, and around 80 grams of fat, 22 of them saturated.

How about the entrées? Don't pick the mushroom cheeseburger with fries. This dish averaged 1,490 calories, 53 percent from fat—almost 90 grams.

Impatiently, Jacobson and Hurley scan the menu. How about the oriental chicken salad? Their survey results aren't cheerful. "Seven hundred and fifty calories and 49 grams of fat," Hurley says. "We were pretty shocked to learn that this type of salad has twice as much fat as the sirloin steak. Salad dressings can really do you in. Actually, the steak and potato is not that bad a choice. But even better is the grilled chicken and potato."

The results—released in late September—put TGIFriday's and its kin on CSPI's growing roster of eateries where one false move can turn you into a miscreant. At press briefings to trumpet restaurant busts in the past, Jacobson has placed menu items next to big stacks of McDonald's burgers or cylinders full of Crisco to drive home what vast quantities of fat he's talking about.

Jacobson believes the government has not asked Americans to cut back *enough* on the percentage of calories they're getting from fat. "Most experts recommend a 30 percent limit," says a CSPI newsletter. "We say 20 percent." The current average? About 35 percent. Much of that comes from meals eaten in restaurants, Jacobson says, hence the dramatic busts.

"At least 300,000 people a year die from unhealthy diet and sedentary lifestyles," he says. "That's second only to the 400,000 who die from smoking. One in three Americans today is obese. Somebody has to do something."

"We're not out to attack any one chain or restaurant," says Hurley. "We're just trying to provide information on the kinds of selections available on different types of restaurants' menus. We're providing information that cannot be found anywhere else."

"And we're not only trying to change the way people eat," Jacobson says. "We're trying to change an entire industry."

Sure enough, the group's undercover raids convinced movie theaters across the country to switch to unsaturated oils in their popcorn poppers and led Chinese restaurants—where business fell 20 to 35 percent after the exposé—to offer more steamed dishes. But beyond these gains, CSPI's 50 lawyers, scientists, and

policy experts can claim a number of victories.

In the 1980s the group pressured fast-food restaurants like Wendy's, Burger King, and McDonald's into cooking their french fries in vegetable oil instead of beef fat, providing nutrition facts to customers, and offering salads and other light choices. They successfully lobbied the Food and Drug Administration to urge pregnant women to avoid caffeine and won a battle to require that alcohol's health risks be printed on the bottles.

What's more, CSPI is credited with leading a coalition—including the American Heart Association and the American Cancer Society—that fought for detailed nutrition labels on all packaged foods. According to William Schultz, the FDA's deputy commissioner, the 1990 law might never have passed without CSPI. "Government gets a lot of pressure from industry," he says. "Jacobson and CSPI are simply pushing from the other side, in the interests of the consumer."

Not without stiff resistance, however. Jacobson and his colleagues have been called "nutritional terrorists," "puritan deniers," "killjoys," and "gastronomical gestapo," not to mention "anorexic left–wing trust-fund East Coast elitist busybodies." Jeff Nedelman, while a vice president at the Grocery Manufacturers of America, accused Jacobson of single-handedly taking the fun out of eating, suggesting that as proper punishment he be buried up to his neck in sour cream and guacamole.

Complaints have come from other quarters as well: from food writers who object that CSPI looks at food only as fuel, not as a source of pleasure or as a cultural touchstone; from nutritionists who insist there are no bad foods, only bad diets; and from food packagers and restaurateurs who say CSPI has whipped up a tidal wave of fear and confusion.

But is all that true? Is the group defeating its own purposes, scaring us into buying foods that are low in fat but loaded with calories? Or is it actually protecting us from our own harmful habits?

They've turned us into a nation obsessed with fat," says nutritionist Adam Drewnowski, "as if fat were the only message. The message of responsible nutrition should be balance, moderation, and variety, whereas the message of CSPI seems to be 'Eat it and die.' There's no point in demonizing fettuccine alfredo. You just can't eat it all the time."

Drewnowski, who directs the University of Michigan's human nutrition program, points out that CSPI is attempting to treat public health problems—obesity, high cholesterol, and high blood pressure—that don't afflict all Americans. True, Drewnowski says, a meatless diet with 10 percent of its calories from fat, like that advocated by heart specialist Dean Ornish, can help unclog the arteries of individuals who've led unhealthy lives. But there's no evidence that cut-the-fat advice has saved anyone from a heart attack. And it may even be dangerous.

"Adolescent girls are starving themselves of fat and calories," Drewnowski says, "and I'm not talking about girls with eating disorders, just girls concerned about their weight." For them, he says, eating less than 20 percent of their calories as fat can short-change their bones and disturb their reproductive hormones.

"All of us need some fat in our diets," he says. "Beta-carotene, for example, needs to be consumed with fat. Without it, carrots are just roughage. I recently saw a very nice study that made just this point, that blood levels of beta-carotene were much higher after a meal that included fat than after an extremely low-fat meal. The fat-carrier the researchers used happened to be Häagen-Dazs ice cream—one of the foods CSPI says you should never, ever eat.

"We're linear thinkers," Drewnowski continues. "CSPI is telling us that a lot of fat is bad. We assume if a lot is bad, and a little is better, then none is better still. People believe that if something is fat-free, it must be good for you, and they gorge on low-fat, high-calorie foods."

In fact, surveys show that in recent years we've added so many calories that while our percentage of calories from fat has dropped, the actual *amount* of fat we're eating is as high as it's ever been. Apparently, we're simply munching all the new fat-free goodies on top of everything else. Among these are the snacks made with Olestra, the chemical fat substitute developed by Proctor & Gamble.

Jacobson and his colleagues are dead set against it, but not because it's highly processed. Eaten in potato chips and crackers, Olestra can have such unsavory side effects as abdominal cramping, diarrhea, and "anal leakage." It also soaks up antioxidants such as lycopene and beta-carotene and carries them away. The FDA requires Frito-Lay—the company now test-marketing Olean brand chips fried in Olestra—to print warnings on the bags.

Yet despite its tell-us-your-side-effects hotline and a write-your-congressman campaign, and despite vocal support from nutrition scientists across the country, CSPI has failed to convince the government to withdraw its approval of Olestra. There is simply too great a demand for low-fat snacks.

That's not the only trap the group may have laid for itself. According to John Stanton, a professor of food marketing at Saint Joseph's University in Philadelphia, a prime eating trend as we head toward the 21st century is a backlash against nutritionally correct "healthy" foods.

"Hamburger consumption is way up," Stanton says. "Steaks ordered in restaurants are up. Pizza Hut just came out with a triple-decker pizza. And McDonald's recently did a multimillion-dollar study to determine what adults want to eat and found that they want a bigger hamburger with bacon and cheese. Voilà: The same year they pull their McLean burger from the market, they introduce the magnificently unhealthy Arch Deluxe. People like what they like. Just giving them facts doesn't necessarily change their behavior."

The backlash may be building, according to a survey by the Food Marketing Institute. Fifty-five percent of consumers say they're tired of experts telling them which foods are good. And 46 percent say there's so much conflicting news they don't know what to eat anymore.

Those attitudes don't surprise Alan Levy, a social psychologist and the director of consumer studies at the FDA. As a source of facts about food and health, he says, CSPI has had a huge impact.

But sounding too many alarms, he notes, raises questions in the public's mind: Is this for my benefit or for CSPI's?

"The first restaurant studies—the one on Chinese food, the popcorn study—those were great," Levy says. "The information couldn't be found anywhere else, and it was a shock to everyone. But now they've carried it to such an extent that they're seen as the food police. It doesn't do wonders for their credibility—or their ability to change how people eat."

What about the 97 percent of consumers who say they're trying to eat better? Surely the warnings have convinced *some* people. "Actually," says Levy, "the best study I've seen on that was CSPI's own—on their milk campaign in West Virginia. A completely controlled study, showing the impact of their public information campaign on whole, low-fat, and skim milk consumption. Now that was amazing data."

You can't say the citizens of neighboring Bridgeport and Clarksburg, West Virginia, didn't know what hit them. Over a seven-week period in 1995 CSPI bombarded the local airwaves with bluntly worded ads. "A glass of whole milk has the artery-clogging fat of five strips of bacon," says a trustworthy-looking mom standing in front or a supermarket dairy case. "And 2 percent milk isn't much better. But with 1 percent or skim, you get great taste and all the vitamins, with little or no fat."

The group ran taste tests in markets and poster contests in schools; it even prodded local ministers to preach on the links between health and spirituality. Citizens were invited down to the county courthouse to view a 400-pound block of fat—what they would avoid over a lifetime if only they switched from whole milk to skim.

Though many locals were skeptical at first, the campaign quickly struck a nerve. Sales of whole milk fell 20 percent, while sales of skim and 1 percent milk more than doubled. As for any backlash against the message or the methods, it didn't materialize. A year and a half after the last ad ran, the lowest-fat milks continue to hold their gains in the towns' markets.

"We're very pleased with the campaign," says Jacobson, between bites of his garden burger at TGIFriday's. "Hopefully it will serve as a prototype for other, more widespread public information projects. Of course," he adds, "milk is a very important food to change, but it's also an easy switch to make. Switching from buffalo wings to veggie burgers is much harder."

But do we need to make that switch? Can't we be good most of the time and still eat buffalo wings at happy hour?

Not if you're really trying to keep your fat calories down to 20 or even 30 percent, Hurley says. It's just too difficult to keep track of the fat you're eating. You're more likely to stay under the 30 percent mark when you consistently avoid fatty foods.

"This idea that any food can be part of a healthy diet is absurd," says Hurley. "To make fettuccine alfredo part of a healthy diet, you'd have to eat only fruit and vegetables and rice for two and a half days. The problem is, most people who indulge in this kind of food aren't eating that way the rest of the time."

"We're not fanatics," says Jacobson. "We believe in moderation. But we also know that we've got to be heard. So we have become very good at getting our message—however condensed—out through the media. Our whole mission is making this kind of information public."

It's true that despite what hits the headlines, CSPI's message is not all sour grapes and grim statistics. When the restaurant critiques appear in CSPI'S own newsletter, *Nutrition Action*, they're always full of upbeat tips for healthful choices (such as the garden burger and the sirloin steak with baked potato) as well as for improving even the fattiest, saltiest selections (hold the mayo and sour cream).

Besides, the group's boldest moves are made behind the scenes. At the moment it's pressing baby-food makers to stop using starch and sugar as fillers, lobbying against Olestra, and arguing that hydrogenated vegetable oils should be counted with other types of artery-clogging fats on cookie and cracker boxes.

The record speaks loudly. Without CSPI's campaigning, Americans would still be eating cookies laced with cholesterol-raising tropical oils; shoppers would find far fewer low-salt soups and crackers; salad-bar patrons could still be blindsided by greens steeped in sulfites. The words *light* and *lean* would mean whatever food packagers wanted them to mean, and nutrition labels would still be a hodgepodge of meaningless data printed in tiny type. The new labels, installed with the group's blessing, are bold, consistent, and clear. Consumers can decide to read them or not. The important thing, Jacobson says, is that they now have the chance to make smart choices.

Health-minded restaurant diners will be getting better service, too. In July, following a lawsuit by CSPI and the advocacy group Public Citizen, the government issued rules barring restaurants from displaying little heart symbols or calling menu items "guilt-free" or "heart-smart" if they aren't suitably low in fat and saturated fat.

But those buffalo wings and stuffed potato skins in happy-hour joints probably never will come with nutrition data. So Jacobson, Hurley, and their colleagues have taken it upon themselves to crunch the numbers and spread the news. They have no plan to end their surprise raids.

"Before we started these restaurant studies," Hurley says, "there were very few healthy sections on menus. Now most of the chain restaurants have some kind of health-conscious fare. This shows that we're being heard, that consumers are asking for healthier options, and that the industry is responding in kind."

 Article Review Form at end of book.

In what way is physical strength among women a political issue? How does strength training provide an alternative to the fat-versus-thin dichotomy for women?

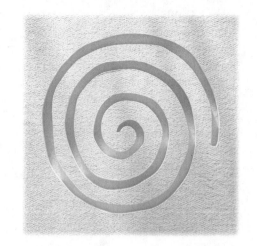

Strong Is Beautiful!

Muscles are feminine. They supply confidence as they increase your physical strength and bolster your political clout.

Gloria Steinem

I come from a generation of women who didn't do sports. Being a cheerleader or a drum majorette was as far as our imaginations or role models could take us. Oh yes, there was also being a strutter—one of a group of girls (and we were "girls" then) who marched and danced and turned cartwheels in front of the high school band at football games. Did you know that big football universities actually gave strutting scholarships? That shouldn't sound any more bizarre than football scholarships, yet somehow it does. Gender politics strikes again.

My sports avoidance contin-

ued into college, where I went through shock about social class and wrongly assumed athletics were only for well-to-do prep school girls like those who brought their own lacrosse sticks and riding horses to school. With no sports training to carry over from childhood—and no place to become childlike, as we must when we belatedly learn basic skills—I clung to my familiar limits. Even years later, at the casual softball games when *Ms.* played the staffs of other magazines, I confined myself to cheering.

When an earlier version of the first interview with the world's strongest woman was pub-

I went out and bought weights. We're talking personal revolution here.

lished in *Ms.* in 1985, it won an Excellence in Women's Sports Journalism Award from the Women's Sports Foundation. The response from my friends and colleagues was not congratulations, but laughter. It was the last award they, or I, ever imagined I would win.

My interest in the politics of strength started from observing the mysterious changes in many women around me. Several of my unathletic friends had deserted me by joining gyms, becoming joggers or discovering the pleasure of learning to yell and kick in self-defense class. Others who had young daughters described the unexpected thrill of seeing them learn to throw a ball or run with a freedom that hadn't been part of our lives in conscious memory. On campuses, I listened to formerly anorexic young women who said their obsession with dieting had diminished when they discovered strength as a third alternative to the usual fat-versus-thin dichotomy. Suddenly, a skinny, androgynous, "boyish" body was no longer the only way to escape the soft, female, "victim" bodies they associated with their mothers' fates.

When I visited other cultures—though the differences were many—I saw political similarities in the way women's bodies were treated. Whether achieved by law and social policy or by way of tribal practice and religious ritual, an individual woman's body was far more subject to other people's rules than that of her male counterpart. Women always seemed to be owned to some degree as the means of reproduction. And as possessions, women's bodies then became symbols of men's status, with a value that was often determined by what was rare. Thus, rich cultures valued thin women and poor cultures valued fat women. Yet all patriarchal cultures valued weakness in women. How else could male dominance survive?

The more I learned, the more I realized that belief in great strength differences between women and men was itself part of the gender mind game. In fact, we can't really know what those differences might be, because they are so enshrined, perpetuated and exaggerated by culture. They seem to be greatest during the childbearing years (when men as a group have more speed and upper-body strength, and women have better balance, endurance and flexibility) but only marginal during early childhood and old age (when females and males seem to have about the same degree of physical strength). Even during those middle years, the range of difference *among* men and *among* women is far greater than the generalized difference *between* males and females as groups. In multiracial societies like ours, where males of some races are smaller than females of others, judgments based on sex make even less sense. Yet we go right on assuming and praising female weakness and male strength.

But there is a problem with keeping women weak, even in a patriarchy. Women are workers, as well as the means of reproduction. Lower-class women are especially likely to do hard physical labor. So the problem becomes: how to make sure female strength is used for work but not for rebellion. The answer is: Make women ashamed of it.

Though hard work requires lower-class women to be stronger than their upper-class sisters, those strong women of the lower class are made to envy and imitate the weakness of women who "belong" to upper-class men. Restrictive dress, from the chadors, or full-body veils, of the Middle East to metal ankle and neck rings in Africa, from nineteenth-century hoopskirts in Europe to corsets and high heels here, started among upper-class women and then sifted downward as poor women were encouraged to envy and imitate them. So did such bodily restrictions as bound feet in China, or clitoridectomies and infibulations in much of the Middle East and Africa, both of which practices gradually became generalized symbols of femininity. In this country the self-starvation known as anorexia nervosa is mostly a white, upper-middle-class, young-female phenomenon, but all women are encouraged to envy a white and impossibly thin ideal.

Sexual politics are also reflected through differing emphases on the reproductive parts of women's bodies. Whenever a patriarchy wants females to populate a new territory or replenish an old one, big breasts and hips become admirable. Think of the bosomy ideal of this country's frontier days, or the zaftig, Marilyn Monroe type of figure that became popular after the population losses of World War II. As soon as increased population wasn't desirable or necessary, hips and breasts were de-emphasized. And the Twiggy look arrived.

Whether bosomy or flat, zaftig or thin, the female ideal remains weak, and it stays that way unless women ourselves organize to change it. Suffragists shed the unhealthy corsets. Instead, they brought in bloomers and bicycling. Feminists of today are struggling against social pressures that exalt siliconed breasts on otherwise stick-thin silhouettes. Introducing health and fitness has already led to a fashion industry effort to reintroduce weakness with the waif look, but at least it's being protested.

For these very political reasons, I've come to believe that society's acceptance of muscular women may be one of the most intimate, visceral measures of change. Yes, we need progress everywhere, but an increase in our physical strength could have more impact on the everyday lives of most women than the occasional role model in the boardroom or in the White House.

Nine years ago, I saw Bev Francis in a screening of *Pumping*

Iron II: The Women. A gentle, intelligent, courageous pioneer who was already a four-time winner of the world's power-lifting championship, a world-class runner, shot-putter, discus and javelin thrower, Bev Francis found fame in bodybuilding. It was only because she had torn her Achilles tendon and had been unable to run or throw that she'd been willing even to consider entering a bodybuilding contest. Once she made the decision, however, she ended up with a body far beyond the limits of imagination for most men and for any women. Pound for pound, she was stronger than Arnold Schwarzenegger.

I've never felt the same about the female body since seeing the strongest woman in the world. Just to give you an idea of the impact: I went out and bought weights. We're talking personal revolution here. Though I wouldn't want to oversell my progress, it was the beginning of my finding a way out of the fat-versus-thin dichotomy this country presents, and also of the patterns inherited from growing up in an overweight family, where strength and physical daring were not alternatives. I wouldn't want to oversell the success of the fitness revolution of the past decade either, but meeting Bev made me understand its source. Bodybuilding and muscles didn't come from upper-class women and anorexic models, for all the political reasons we understand. It was ordinary women who were lifting weights and going to self-defense classes, and who were gradually changing their upper-class sisters.

After seeing Bev Francis, I understood that bodily freedom wouldn't be accomplished solely through reproductive issues. In the future, if we're to seize control of the means of reproduction—which is as radical as it sounds—each of us must have her own strength.

Article Review Form at end of book.

What factors make certain modes of exercise more appropriate than others for some individuals?

Which Indoor Exercise Is Best?

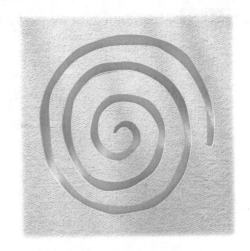

Dr. Hoffman

Dr. Hoffman is Associate Professor of Physical Medicine and Rehabilitation at the Medical College of Wisconsin and Medical Director of the Cardiopulmonary Prevention and Rehabilitation Program at the VA Medical Center in Milwaukee.

Multitude of indoor exercise machines are now available for improving aerobic fitness and controlling body weight. The various manufacturers of these devices seem willing to offer opinions about which machine is best. However, little research has been done to support claims that one machine is better than another. In a study recently published in the Journal of the American Medical Association (vol. 275 [1996]: 1424–27), Anne I. Zeni, D.O., Philip S. Clifford, Ph.D. and I compared the aerobic and caloric demands of six of the most common exercise machines. The comparison was made relative to level of perceived exertion since most people establish exercise intensity by how hard the exercise feels.

The six exercise machines compared were an Airdyne (Schwinn), a cross-country skiing simulator (NordicTrack), a cycle ergometer (Fuji America), a rowing ergometer (Concept II), a stairstepper (Tectrix), and a treadmill (Schwinn). The participants in the study were eight men and five women. They had an average age of 32 years, were healthy and had active lifestyles.

Prior to any testing, we assured that each participant was skilled in the use of each exercise machine. Each participant exercised a minimum of 15 minutes two times per week on each machine during a four-week habitua-tion period. During every 15-minute exercise period, 5 minutes were performed at self-selected work rates corresponding to perceived efforts of "fairly light," "somewhat hard," and "hard," using a standardized scale for assessing perceived exertion. Participants were blinded to the work rate display scales during the last two weeks of the habituation period, yet were very consistent in the selected work rates at each perceived effort with all of the machines. This demonstrated that the participants had mastery of each mode of exercise and were

Table I Mean Rates of Caloric Expenditure at Different Perceived Efforts

Mode	Rate of Caloric Expenditure (calories/hour)		
	Fairly Light	Somewhat Hard	Hard
Treadmill	552	705	865
Stairstepper	505	627	746
Rowing Ergometer	511	606	739
Cross-country Skiing Simulator	507	595	678
Cycle Ergometer	405	498	604
Airdyne	344	509	709

Table 2 Mean Percentages of Oxygen Uptake at Different Perceived Efforts

Mode	Maximal Oxygen Uptake (percent)		
	Fairly Light	Somewhat Hard	Hard
Treadmill	52	57	62
Stairstepper	48	59	70
Rowing Ergometer	50	59	72
Cross-country Skiing Simulator	49	57	65
Cycle Ergometer	40	48	56
Airdyne	34	50	68

Table 3 Mean Percentages of Maximal Heart Rate at Different Perceived Efforts

Mode	Maximal Heart Rate (percent)		
	Fairly Light	Somewhat Hard	Hard
Treadmill	70	80	89
Stairstepper	68	77	85
Rowing Ergometer	69	75	82
Cross-country Skiing Simulator	70	76	80
Cycle Ergometer	62	70	78
Airdyne	56	69	81

consistent in the way perceived effort was determined.

After the habituation period, each participant completed exercise tests on all of the exercise machines. Each test included a brief warm-up, followed by exercise at the participant's self-selected work rates corresponding with the three perceived intensities used during the habituation period. Rates of caloric expenditure were calculated from measurements of oxygen uptake. On a separate day, each subject also performed a maximal exercise test on a treadmill to determine maximal oxygen uptakes and heart rates.

We found substantial differences among exercise machines in the rate of caloric expenditure induced by exercise at a given level of perceived exertion (see Table 1).

The treadmill induced higher metabolic demands than all of the other exercise machines examined. The cycle ergometer and the Airdyne induced the lowest rates of caloric expenditure. As an example, one can see that the participants expended approximately 700 calories per hour on the treadmill at a perceived effort of "somewhat hard," while less than 500 calories per hour were expended at the same perceived effort when using the cycle ergometer. In other words, the rate of caloric expenditure was over 40 percent greater with the treadmill than with the cycle ergometer. Thus, it would appear that if exercise intensity is established by perceived effort, treadmill walking or running is likely to result in the greatest caloric ex-

penditure and cardiorespiratory training stimulus.

While this study provides evidence that the rate of caloric expenditure can be considerably different among modes of exercise, it is important to recognize that all of the exercise devices tested can be used for enhancement of health and cardiorespiratory fitness. Exercise intensity for cardiorespiratory training is generally recommended to be in the range of 60 to 90 percent of maximal heart rate or 50 to 85 percent of maximal oxygen uptake. As displayed in Table 2, exercising at perceived exertions of "somewhat hard" and "hard" elicited mean oxygen uptake values within the recommended intensity range for all the exercise modes examined except the cycle ergometer. The treadmill and the rowing ergometer also elicited mean oxygen uptake values that were within the usual guidelines for enhancing cardiorespiratory fitness at a perceived intensity of "fairly light." Mean heart rates fell within the recommended intensity guidelines for all six modes of exercise at all three perceived exertion levels examined except for the Airdyne at a perceived effort of "fairly light" (see Table 3).

Exercise prescriptions are often based upon heart rate, and many people use heart rate as a monitor for exercise intensity. We found that at a given heart rate, metabolic demand was the same among the different modes of exercise. Therefore, among these types of exercise, a workout performed at a given heart rate will result in a similar caloric expenditure regardless of the exercise machine used. However, the perceived effort at a given heart rate may vary substantially among modes of indoor aerobic exercise. Our study suggests that a specified heart rate could elicit a perceived effort of "fairly light" with one mode of exercise and "somewhat hard" with another mode. Since exercise compliance is associated with the perceived demands of the activity, perceived effort should be considered in exercise prescriptions based on heart rate.

Why are there metabolic differences among exercise modes at a given perceived effort? Part of the explanation has to do with the amount of the exercising muscle mass involved in the exercise. In general, use of a large muscle mass appears to allow a greater metabolic demand of a given perceived effort than exercise with a smaller muscle mass. However, muscle mass does not appear to be the sole factor determining the relationship of metabolic demand with perceived effort. For example, it might be expected that the cross-country skiing simulator and the rowing ergometer would engage a larger muscle mass than the treadmill. Yet the aerobic demands were higher on the treadmill. These findings suggest that factors other than the amount of exercising muscle mass affect this relationship. We speculate that such factors may include the degree to which lengthening and isometric contractions are involved, the incorporation of "programmed" movement patterns, and the familiarity with the movement pattern.

In developing an exercise program, it is important to recognize that individual factors must often be considered. Among these are physical disabilities, existing musculoskeletal disorders, predisposition to develop musculoskeletal overuse injuries, medical conditions affecting balance, accessibility, cost, personal preferences, and training goals. These factors might make certain modes of exercise more appropriate than others for some individuals.

It should also be realized that while the metabolic demands at a given perceived effort may differ among exercise modes, exercise periods of longer duration or at higher perceived efforts can be used to equalize total caloric expenditure during a workout. Each of the exercise machines tested in our study can be used to achieve cardiorespiratory training benefits. To be successful in achieving one's fitness goals, a key element is identifying forms of exercise that are enjoyable enough to perform on a regular basis. No matter how great the exercise machine, it will not improve one's fitness while collecting dust in the attic or basement!

 Article Review Form at end of book.

WiseGuide Wrap-Up

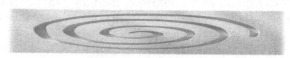

- Good health comes with a balanced and realistic approach to healthy living.

- True healthy living involves celebration and self-acceptance rather than guilt.

- Sound nutrition, tailored physical activity, and appropriate weight management can promote positive health.

R.E.A.L. Sites

The adjacent list provides a print preview of typical **coursewise** R.E.A.L. Sites. (There are over 100 such sites at the **courselinks**™ site.) The danger in printing URLs is that Web sites can change overnight. As we went to press, these sites were functional using the URLs provided. If you come across one that isn't, please let us know via email at webmaster@coursewise.com. Use your Passport to access the most current list of R.E.A.L. sites at the **courselinks**™ site.

Site name: Shape Up America!

URL: http://www.shapeup.org/sua/health-fitness/index.html

Why is it R.E.A.L.? Upbeat and motivational site sponsored by C. Everett Koop designed to promote physical activity.

Key topics: fitness and physical activity, activism and advocacy

Activity: Check your physical activity IQ. Assess your fitness level then find out how long it will take you to get into shape. Find out what is the best physical activity for you.

Site name: American Dietetics Association

URL: http://www.eatright.org

Why is it R.E.A.L.? Web site for the American Dietetics Association, a professional organization for dieticians. Provides information about nutrition resources, job opportunities, frequently asked questions, finding a dietitian, nutrition advocacy, ADA position papers, and hot topics as well as member services.

Key topics: nutrition, professional organization, activism, advocacy

Activity: Try to locate a practicing dietitian who works near you.

Site name: Food Finder

URL: http://www.olen.com/food/

Why is it R.E.A.L.? Provides analysis of food and diet. Highly interactive individual dietary assessment.

Key topics: nutrition, weight management

Activity: Pick your favorite restaurant and food item, then fire up the deep fat fryer to see how many calories, fat, and cholesterol the food item contains.

Site name: FitLife

URL: http://www.fitlife.com/

Why is it R.E.A.L.? Offers information about fitness, health promotion, wellness and lifestyle.

Key topics: fitness, physical activity, general health, wellness

Activity: Click on "Fitness" then find out how to keep from getting bored when you exercise. Try some of the tips. Why do some work and others don't work for you?

Site name: Your Health Daily: New York Times Syndicate
URL: http://nytsyn.com/med/
Why is it R.E.A.L.? Access to the most current health news stories from the New York Times Syndicate.
Key topics: health statistics, news, general health, wellness
Activity: What are the top health news stories today? What direct impact do they have on your life? What would be different if you never read these news stories?

....

Site name: Health A to Z
URL: http://www.HealthAtoZ.com/
Why is it R.E.A.L.? This efficient and searchable database of general health information was catalogued by medical professionals.
Key topics: general health, wellness
Activity: Use this site as a good starting point for researching a term paper. Try to narrow your health topic enough to only generate less than ten websites when you run a search.

....

Site name: Center for Science in the Public Interest
URL: http://www.cspinet.org/
Why is it R.E.A.L.? Promotes a community organization approach to improving the nutrition of Americans. Resource for learning to think critically about nutrition and health activism.
Key topics: nutrition, community organization, health advocacy
Actiivity: Go to "CSPI Nutrition Quizzes" to see what you know about olestra, fat, and your dietary rating.

....

Site name: CyberDiet
URL: http://www.cyberdiet.com/
Why is it R.E.A.L.? Highly interactive and individualized dietary planning available with a searchable database, dietary assessment tools, and food planners.
Key topics: nutrition
Activity: Use CyberDiet's Daily Food Planner to plan your meals for the next week.

....

section 2

Designing Your Own Well-Being

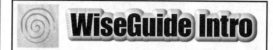

To some degree, we can determine our own health, whether at the personal level or at the societal level. A key to designing you own well-being is gaining the skills to understand and deal with health risk factors. These skills include thinking critically, solving problems, accessing information, and recognizing influences on health decision making.

In the absence of other means to make health decisions, people often rely on their own judgment and experience. Unfortunately, some people tend to misjudge their chances of developing a medical problem. They often base their perception of personal risk on the medical condition's emotional impact or vividness rather than on its actual frequency. This can lead to inappropriate preventive behavior. Accurate and current knowledge of established risk factors and known preventive strategies is essential to establishing and maintaining good health.

In Section 2, the selected readings describe known health risk behaviors and the means to control them. Safe and effective use of over-the-counter and prescription medication is addressed in the next two articles ("OTC Medication Errors" and "Medication Decision-Making and Management: A Client-Centered Model"). The remaining three articles ("Self-Presentation Can Be Hazardous to Your Health: Impression Management and Health Risk," "Addressing Sexual Harassment on Campus," and "Ifs, Ands and Butts") offer various ways to minimize a range of potentially damaging health behaviors including unprotected sex; sun exposure; dieting; alcohol, tobacco, and drug use; physical inactivity; and sexual harassment.

Key Points

- Consumers can protect themselves from making medication errors.

- Concern about one's image can lead to engaging in risky health behaviors.

- Clear definitions of sexual harassment on campus are needed.

- The tobacco settlement represents a turning point in the marketing and distribution of tobacco products.

Questions

R7. What can consumers do to protect themselves from medication errors?

R8. What are the differences between a client-centered model and the medical model in terms of decisions about taking medications? What factors may be related to active client and passive patient roles?

R9. What health risk behaviors seem to be associated with those who have concern about their image?

R10. Why are clear definitions of sexual harassment needed? What is an example of sexual harassment on campus?

R11. How will the tobacco settlement change the marketing of tobacco products?

What can consumers do to protect themselves from medication errors?

OTC Medication Errors

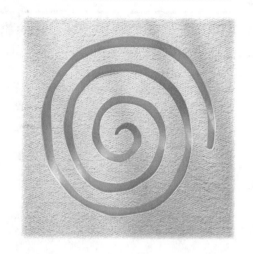

Arthur A. Levin, M.P.H.

A new trend in marketing over-the-counter (OTC) medicines could be causing medication errors that are dangerous for consumers, according to the United States Pharmacopeia (USP). Well-established brand names are being used to market an increased variety of OTC products for different indications. Such products are formulated in new and different strengths, new and different combinations of active ingredients, or different active ingredients altogether.

The USP implicates these products, known as brand name extensions, in the increasing risk of unintentional overdoses, contraindicated use, and adverse interactions with other drugs. In addition, consumers may be not getting either the therapeutic ingredient or the desired outcome that they associate with the brand name. The USP, founded in 1820, is a private not-for-profit organization that establishes and disseminates information on the use of medicines to health professionals and consumers.

Benadryl Combinations

One extension product example is the antihistamine brand Benadryl (generic name: diphenhydramine). For years, while its patent was in effect and its maker protected from competition, Benadryl was available only by prescription. After its patent expired, Benadryl became available as a branded OTC medicine to treat the symptoms of allergy. When *RX News* visited a local chain drugstore recently, the shelves were laden with not only what is now labeled as "Benadryl Allergy" (the original use and containing only diphenhydramine) but "Benadryl Allergy Cold," "Benadryl Allergy Sinus," "Benadryl Sinus Headache," and "Benadryl Allergy Decongestant," each with different active ingredients or combinations of active ingredients.

USP became aware of the problem as a result of reports made to its Practitioner's Reporting Network which collects data on adverse events. One case reported to the USP by a doctor involved a woman with heart disease and high blood pressure who complained of nasal congestion. The doctor advised her to take the OTC medicine Chlor-Trimeton which he assumed contained only a single active ingredient, the antihistamine chlorpheniramine maleate. After taking Chlor-Trimeton, the woman returned to her doctor feeling terrible and found to have very highly elevated blood pressure. The doctor checked the Chlor-Trimeton package and was shocked to discover that it not only contained chlorpheniramine maleate, which is considered safe for use by people with heart disease and high blood pressure, but also pseudoephedrine, which should not be used by people with these conditions.

Drug overdose is another danger for consumers that can result from brand name extension. This is a particular concern with products containing acetaminophen. Overdosing on this analgesic found in Tylenol and many other OTC combination drugs holds risks for young children and the potential for liver toxicity in those with a history of liver disease.

Reprinted from *Healthfacts Newsletter*. Published by The Centers for Medical Consumers.

The recommended dose for children under 12 can be exceeded by parents unaware that they are giving their child more than one acetaminophen-containing OTC product. The same mistake can be made by people with liver disease.

Some makers of OTC medicine, such as Sandoz Consumer Pharmaceuticals, have recognized the danger and taken steps to warn consumers. One extension version of Sandoz's popular cough syrup brand Triaminic is marketed as "Sore Throat Formula." It contains 160 mg of acetaminophen, which is a full-strength dose for children, and does carry a special warning to that effect. Unfortunately, the warning may be easily over-looked by parents who do not read all the information printed on each of the four sides of the product's package.

Another problem identified by USP concerns OTC products that have the same brand name, but are available in different concentrations and strengths. In one such case, compounded by miscommunication between doctor and parents, the doctor recommended an appropriate pediatric dose of acetaminophen *elixir*, but the parents purchased and gave their child acetaminophen *suspension drops*, which contain more than two and one-half times the concentration of acetaminophen. As a result of the acetaminophen overdose, their two year old child had to undergo a liver transplant.

Since manufacturers invest considerable resources in creating brand name recognition to inspire consumer loyalty, the trend towards extension OTC products is likely to continue. The more pharmacy shelf space products under a single brand name occupy, the better the sales and the less competition.

Consumers can protect themselves from medication errors by carefully reading the OTC label before purchasing a product and by avoiding OTC medicines containing combinations of active ingredients.

 Article Review Form at end of book.

What are the differences between a client-centered model and the medical model in terms of decisions about taking medications? What factors may be related to active client and passive patient roles?

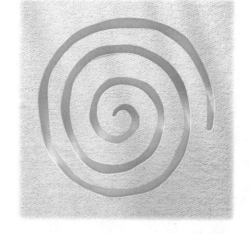

Medication Decision-Making and Management

A client-centered model

**Betty Chewning[1] and
Betsy Sleath[2]**

[1]Sonderegger Research Center, School of Pharmacy, University of Wisconsin, 425 N. Charter St., Madison, WI 53706, U.S.A. and [2]College of Pharmacy, University of New Mexico, Albuquerque, NM 87131, U.S.A.

Abstract—Although the traditional medical model dominates how 'provider-patient' roles are viewed, research has documented that client medication behavior strongly influences health outcomes, health care utilization, and ultimately health care costs. This paper explores the position that medication management outcomes can be improved by adopting more client-centered approaches. To examine the implications of a client-centered relationship this paper reviews research regarding client involvement in: (1) identifying treatment goals; (2) choosing from regimen options; (3) monitoring symptoms and evaluating regimens; and (4) self care with nonprescription pharmaceutical products. Based on this literature review, a collaborative client-centered model of medication consultation is examined, and implications for health care provider roles and public policy in pharmaceutical care are discussed.

Key words—patient-centered care, medication management, patient provider relationship, pharmaceutical care, collaborative medical decision-making

Introduction

Traditionally the medical model has dominated the manner in which the "provider-patient" relationship is conceptualized and conducted. However, as more research documents the client's critical role in health care outcomes, it is time to re-examine assumptions underlying the medical model, especially as they relate to medication decision-making and management. In this era of increased outpatient medication therapy for even the most serious conditions, training and policy frameworks have not evolved at the same speed as the health care system's unacknowledged reliance on patients to manage their medication regimens. This paper explores the position that the medical model is outdated as a basic framework for medication management. Research on the outcomes and process of provider-client decision-making is presented, a client-centered vs medical model of medication consultation is examined, and implications for health care provider roles and public policy in pharmaceutical care are discussed. Specifically, we propose a more participatory model of medication management which acknowledges the decision-making responsibility and power of the client in partnership with health care providers. Particularly at this time when public policy is shaping the health system, it is useful to re-examine the role of the client as the most critical and yet under-

Reprinted with the permission from Betty Chewning and Betsy Sleath, "Medication Decision-Making and Management" in *Social Science and Medicine*, 42(3), 389-398. February 1996, Elsevier Science, Ltd, Oxford, England.

used resource for improved health care outcomes and cost control.

Client Medication Management Outcomes

The need to re-examine the medical model arises in part from growing documentation of negative health outcomes and increased health care utilization associated with poor medication management by clients. In a study of 315 elderly patients admitted consecutively to an acute care hospital, Col *et al.* [1] found that 28% of the admissions were drug-related, 36 due to noncompliance (11.4%) and 53 due to adverse drug reactions (16.8%). One hundred three patients had a history of noncompliance (32.7%). Sullivan *et al.* [2] conducted a meta-analysis of the extent and direct cost of hospital admission related to drug therapy noncompliance. Applying a strict protocol for study inclusion, seven studies were selected for the meta-analysis. The seven contained a total of 2942 admissions with comparable methodologies for evaluation. Analysis revealed that 5.5% of the admissions could be attributed to drug therapy noncompliance. Using annual U.S. hospital admission rates and inpatient hospitalization costs, the authors estimate that in 1986 over 1.94 million admissions were due to drug therapy noncompliance, representing about $8.5 billion in hospital expenditures. In one of the larger studies of medication problems and ensuing hospital admissions, Grymonpre *et al.* [3] studied 863 admissions of patients aged 50 or older to a Canadian health sciences hospital. The four-month study found 162 admissions were

related to one or more adverse drug reactions. Sixty-two hospital admissions (8.6%) were a direct result of noncompliance with drug therapy. Similarly, McKenney and Harrison [4] and Bergman and Wiholm [5] found significant hospital admissions due to clients' drug-related errors and adverse drug effects.

This line of research offers evidence that clients' medication management patterns can either decrease or increase their risk of serious health outcomes and subsequent hospitalization at considerable cost. The question is not whether clients should manage their medication regimens since they do so immediately upon leaving the interaction with the health care provider. Rather the question is how can a health system support this client function more effectively?

Medical vs Client-Centered Models

To examine this question, we will compare assumptions underlying the medical model to those from a client-centered model and then relate research on medication management issues that clarify implications of one model vs the other. It is important to note that in reality provider–patient interactions fall along a continuum of these models. However, in order to clarify the distinctions between either end of the spectrum and stimulate discussion, the following table summarizes the purest form of each of these models as though they are dichotomous.

The client role in the medical model is more receptive, compliant and passive while in a client-centered model, the client actively

collaborates in the medication decision-making process. For the purposes of this paper we define a client-centered model as one where the client collaborates with the provider in helping to:

(1) identify treatment goals

(2) choose from regimen options

(3) monitor symptoms and evaluate regimens and

(4) revise regimens if problems occur.

The provider's role is to be active as a partner in the decision process influenced by the client's desires and abilities, generating options based on these desires as well as expertise. While the medical model enhances the control and status of the provider, the client-centered model enhances the control and status of the client. How active a role health care providers want for patients strongly influences the nature of their client assessment, regimen planning, education, and monitoring. Likewise, how active a role clients want also influences this process.

Traditionally, clients were viewed as rather passive and dependent, needing and following the expert instructions of the clinician in a compliant fashion. This perspective was derived from work examining patients in hospital settings, where more severe symptoms and dependence would encourage a passive role [6, 7]. Later work began to differentiate types of patient–provider interactions in ambulatory settings. As self-care and social science research began to interact with the medical model, other theorists identified important ways that clients are active, evaluating their symptoms, regimens, and their health care providers [8–15]. Several researchers interested in nonadherence urged a more client-centered approach [16–23]. Trostle [24] argued that the term "medical compliance" itself perpetuated the notion that therapeutic recommendations should be dictated to patients by physicians. Research on adherence supported the importance of patient-centered interactions with health care providers where the patient's point of view is actively sought by the physician [25, 26]. In summary, as research turned to investigating patient-provider interaction and to examining patient medication behaviors in ambulatory settings, the value of a more participatory relationship with clients emerged.

Factors Related to Active vs Passive Client Roles

A client's level of involvement in decision-making during provider-patient interactions varies on a continuum ranging from a totally passive patient [6, 7] to an extremely active consumerist who challenges the provider's ability to make unilateral decisions and demands a share in reaching closure on diagnosis and treatment plans [8, 9, 16]. Both clients and providers can assume roles at different points along the continuum depending on the individual's health status, nature of the medical decision and the setting.

Several factors are thought to influence the client's level of participation during provider-client interactions. Several studies suggest that younger clients prefer to be more involved in medical decision-making [27–31]. Additionally, in some studies clients with higher incomes, higher educational levels, and higher occupational levels

also report a greater desire for active participation in decision-making processes about their health care than do patients with lower incomes, lower educational levels, and lower occupational levels [27, 28, 30, 31]. In another study of Canadian patients, however, sociodemographic variables accounted for only 15% of the variance in how active a role patients wanted in cancer treatment decisions [35]. It is important therefore to consider both the nature of the medical decision and patient condition as additional influences.

How involved clients want to be in a decision depends on the specific topic of the medical decision. When clients believe their expertise or preferences are relevant to the decision, they are more likely to want to participate in selecting one drug from two equally effective drugs which otherwise differ only in lifestyle or side effect implications [27, 32–34]. In contrast clients are less likely to want to collaborate around emergency or diagnostic test decisions [27].

Some studies suggest that the client's condition affects both client and provider perspectives on patient roles, with a few suggesting that clients prefer their health care provider to take a stronger role in decision-making as their condition worsens [28, 35]. Other research documented that breast cancer patients wanted input into selecting between the options of radical mastectomy vs lumpectomy, which the women felt had strong quality of life implications [32]. A patient's condition may also influence how actively the provider wants to involve a patient. Providers may have a more client-centered interaction style with patients who have chronic diseases as com-

pared to clients seeking care for more acute or life-threatening conditions [6, 8, 36]. Taken together this research suggests that client and provider judgements about the relevance of client expertise and health status can influence how collaboratively a medical decision is made.

The type of ambulatory setting in which a client receives care may also influence the type of provider-patient interaction that takes place. Callahan and Bertakis [37] found that physician-patient interactions in a Health Maintenance (HMO) setting were longer and included significantly more patient questions, preventive services, and treatment planning than interactions in fee-for-service settings. Freidson [38] has suggested that more client-centered interactions may occur in HMO's in part because this group of clients may need to be assertive since they cannot easily switch health plans and providers.

In summary, these findings suggest that demographic characteristics, health status, setting, and nature of the decision may all influence how client-centered an interaction is. The reality is that health care providers face a full array of situations and clients with different expectations and preferences regarding their involvement in decision-making, making provider assessment of patient preferences and potential for participation all the more important. This variation gives rise to the question, how feasible is it for providers to incorporate flexible client-centered relationships into practice. The following sections examine research related to this question with respect to each of the collaborative client-centered consultation steps outlined in Table 1.

Table 1 Medical vs collaborative client-centered model

Dimension	Medical model	Client-centered collaborative model
Definition of regimen goals	Emphasizes clinical status	Emphasizes client priorities, quality of life and clinical status
Regimen selection	Provider defines	Client co-defines from options
Patient education focus	Increases regimen compliance	Increases client's ability to manage and monitor regimen
Drug monitoring and regimen evaluation	Provider evaluates clinical outcomes and patient compliance	Client and provider evaluate clinical outcomes and regimen problems/options
Self-care by client	Largely ignored	Integrated in consultation
Control and status	Provider control and status enhanced	Client control and status enhanced

Defining Regimen Goals

Defining regimen goals is a key step in selecting a therapeutic strategy. From a client-centered approach, each ensuing consultation step depends on having accurately identified the client's most desired outcomes. The medical model assumes that the provider's expertise about clinical symptoms and clinical outcomes should be the foundation of diagnosis and treatment decisions. Signs and symptoms of clinical significance dominate the provider's assessment of client needs, therapy selection, and ensuing regimen monitoring and evaluation process. As a result there is a danger that providers may underattend to client concerns at each of these steps unless they have clinical significance. The medical model de-emphasizes the psychological and behavioral dimensions of illness and therapy which the client is experiencing [39, 40].

Recently, health outcomes researchers have argued that providers should expand their focus beyond clinical outcomes and symptoms [41–44]. They suggest that functional status and well-being defined from the patient perspective are as important as more clinical outcomes of care.

Anderson [43] argues that health care practitioners are focusing too much on diagnoses, specific interventions and outcomes (the trees) rather than on a patient's quality of life (the forest). Others point out that for years patients have said that they have been noncompliant because of drug-induced changes in their quality of life [44]. There is growing recognition that patient priorities for treatment outcomes and quality of life should influence therapeutic goals and treatment approaches, particularly for patients with chronic conditions. Because most interventions affect a patient's quality of life, asking for their priorities and treatment goals could alter both the regimen selection and evaluation of subsequent regimen outcomes [45].

Regimen Selection as a Collaborative Process

Fink [46] argues "there is no such thing as a standard regimen for a standard patient." Rather, there is a need to tailor regimens to patient beliefs, personality, lifestyle, and priorities [47, 48]. This implies that not only is client-centered interaction needed to gather key information, but this information is then used to design regimens responsive to the unique client. An example of one collaborative approach implemented in practice is the PREPARED Checklist [49]. This checklist for patients and providers is intended to aid health care decision-making when there is more than one treatment option. Together client and provider discuss the recommended (P) prescription or procedure, (R) reason or indication for prescription, (E) expectation or patient-focused benefit, (P) probability benefit will occur compared to the (A) alternatives, (R) risks involved and (E) expenses including direct and indirect costs [49]. A (D) decision is then based on the discussion. Using this framework with employees of a large corporation, clients exhibited significant increases in their self-efficacy for making health care decisions [45].

Other providers have evaluated giving clients their choice of different types of interventions and medications to reduce cardiovascular risk and control blood pressure [50, 51]. Clients try out two medication options and based on their experience choose their preferred medication. Ongoing drug monitoring is conducted at return visits in terms of clients' somatic experiences, evaluation of the regimen, and home blood pressure measurement [51]. The studies report improved pill counts and appointment keeping. Decision analysis schema have been developed for clients with arthritis to help them interpret changing symptoms and modify their exercise programs, recognize symptoms of drug toxicities and manage their side effects [52]. While more work is needed with representative samples to evaluate the impact of such interventions on health outcomes, the first question of whether a client-centered approach can be operationalized in practice appears to have been answered affirmatively.

From the medical model perspective, medication prescribing is the domain of the health care provider. However, as health care provision incorporates a client-centered model, the provider could act as an expert consultant to the client. Client preferences could be assessed, acknowledged and incorporated into drug selection and regimen design (dose and schedule). Several parameters are relevant in the drug regimen selection:

(1) modality (injection, liquid, pill form)

(2) drug product (choosing among several brands)

(3) regimen (schedule, number of doses per day).

Especially with the expanded pharmaceutical product options today, clients have the opportunity to select a modality, product, and regimen which is sensitive to their preferences and draws upon their experience unless insurance and drug formulary restrictions limit choice.

Client perceptions and preferences regarding characteristics of the medication represent an additional area for assessment. As Buckalew and Sallis [53] have argued, a medication's perceptual properties may have important and specific meaning to patients that may support or detract from adherence. For example, Hussain [54] noted that shape, size, color, and taste of medications have been neglected in studies of patient perception of medications. Several researchers have pointed out the importance of patient input into clinical decision-making [55–57] and provider prescribing of medications [58–61]. Yet few researchers have examined the prescribing process using observational techniques [59, 62–65]. Most of the observational studies that exist have relied on small samples, have focused primarily on the discourse and language used during the prescribing process [63, 65], and have not examined how the client influences the prescribing process [59, 63–65]. However, Sleath et al. [62], who examined psychotropic prescribing during 508 primary care physician-client interactions, found that patients initiated the psychotropic prescribing process in 42% of the interactions where psychotropic medications were prescribed. This line of research suggests that some clients already influence prescribing of psychotropic drugs. Thus incorporating clients consciously into the selection process may not be as foreign as it might seem.

Providers have been asked about their prescribing behavior and the factors that influence it. Findings suggest providers attribute prescribing decisions to control of the disease state and side effect profile more than to patient demand [66–68]. However, Avorn et al. [69] suggest that physician assessment of factors influencing their prescribing may not be reliable. While only 2% of physicians rated patient preference as very important in influencing their prescribing decisions, when asked specifically about analgesics, 84% said they often or occasionally prescribed Darvon because patients were not satisfied with over-the-counter products like aspirin [69]. We find it interesting that, although physicians report patients are not an important influence on their *appropriate* prescribing, physicians do cite patient demand as a reason for *inappropriate* prescribing. Schwartz et al. [70] found that physicians cited patient demand most often as the reason for their inappropriate prescribing of the medications.

In order to move toward a more effective and planned, collaborative process of regimen selection, there is a need to:

(1) better understand how patients unconsciously influence the medication prescribing process

(2) identify how patients can best help with regimen selection in a conscious manner, and

(3) teach health care providers to be more accepting of patients' opinions when designing and monitoring a medication treatment regimen.

Drug Monitoring

Drug monitoring is an important function of the health care provider team—physician, pharmacist, and nurse. However, it is an equally important function for clients. There is evidence of a parallel, private process of drug monitoring performed by clients, often using different criteria than those of the provider. The self-regulation framework posits that clients naturally attempt to understand and evaluate their somatic experience [71–76]. This framework views individuals as active problem solvers whose actions are the result of their perception and emotional response to a perceived health threat. From this theory, individuals translate symptoms or other stimuli into a threat with perceived causes, consequences, and expected duration. An individual interprets the symptoms and then adopts coping procedures to deal with the perceived threat. Lastly, the individual appraises or evaluates the outcomes of their coping action [13, 14, 71–83].

Whether right or wrong, clients often believe they can tell when a medication regimen benefits their previously diagnosed chronic illness. In interviews with individuals diagnosed with hypertension, 88% reported that they could tell when their blood pressure was up through symptoms such as headaches, warm face, heart beating [14]. The number of patients who reported nonadherence and had poor blood pressure control was significantly higher among patients who thought their medication had no effect on the symptoms they were monitoring. Similarly, Enlund [83] found that 60% of their sample thought they felt symptoms of high blood pressure.

Leventhal [76] argues that patients' self generated theories about their illnesses and treatment are not "oddities," but conceptual systems that should be incorporated into the theories devised by providers. Without identifying how a client conceptualizes or monitors a condition, the provider is at a disadvantage for understanding patient judgements and medication decisions. From a client-centered model, the drug monitoring step would follow from earlier client involvement in selecting a regimen responsive to clients' desired out-

comes. By then preparing clients to monitor the regimens they helped shape, it is hoped that clients' natural desire to evaluate symptoms can help to refine or modify the regimen as needed in subsequent visits.

Patient involvement in drug monitoring needs to be done thoughtfully with respect to interaction style of the provider using tools to assist patients in their monitoring task. In research on the impact of a clinician's interaction style at follow-up visits, client openness regarding regimen problems was extinguished if a provider ignored or negatively evaluated client admissions that they departed from the regimen [26]. A provider's reaction to a client's concerns regarding side effects, inconvenience of the regimen, and adherence problems has considerable influence on how likely the client will continue in a problem-solving mode in future visits. Further, there is a need to train clients to monitor their regimens with specific diaries or summary sheets. Simply informing clients of the inaccuracy of their symptom monitoring to evaluate hypertensive drug regimens has been shown to be insufficient to change client beliefs about inaccurate monitoring strategies they already use [73].

More research is needed on how clients can be taught effectively to monitor both benefits and side effects so that regimen tradeoffs can be reassessed and options openly discussed between client and provider. Although attention is starting to be given to how providers can inform patients about the risks involved in various treatment options, much less has gone into identifying how clients can inform providers about their experience with regimens [84]. One example of the latter is a

client-centered approach to drug monitoring, in which decision analysis schema have been developed for clients with arthritis to help them interpret changing symptoms and modify their exercise programs, recognize symptoms of drug toxicities and manage their side effects [52]. The first refill or return visit may be particularly important as a time for careful client-provider consultation regarding drug monitoring. Recent research in community pharmacies identified a greater number of client questions and concerns voiced at the first refill visit than at the time of initial prescription was filled [85, 86]. At such visits the client can use the provider as a consultant to answer questions and concerns, interpret symptoms noticed, tailor or simplify regimens, generate therapy alternatives or revisit the tradeoffs involved in the regimen prior to a possible discontinuation decision.

Self-Care Choices

The inadequacy of the medical model for describing the client role with respect to medication management is nowhere more evident than in clients' self-care. Self-care is defined by Dean [87] as the range of behavior undertaken by individuals to promote or restore their health. Clients frequently engage in considerable self-care for symptom relief prior to and simultaneous with seeking care from the formal health care system [87–96]. Self-medication, one of the most frequent first responses to illness [92, 93], occurs across age, education and income groups, with better educated and more knowledgeable consumers using more OTC drugs and spending more of their drug budget on OTC products [96].

Dean notes that health professionals view lay care as supplemental to professional care in spite of the fact that, ". . . professional care is the supplemental form of care" [95, p. 275]. Although professionals often discuss self-care in terms of its potential dangers [95], Verbrugge and Ascione [93] found that people are both parsimonious and rational in caring for their symptoms. For acute problems, decisions about care are made in the short run and hinge mostly on symptoms. For chronic symptoms, people apply strategies during flare-ups which they have devised over months and years [93].

Ultimately, the intersection between self-care and medical care reveals the starkest conflict of assumptions regarding client roles in terms of self-sufficiency in over-the-counter medication decision-making vs a more passive role around prescription medication decision-making. Although over-the-counter medications prescription medications are the most frequently reported self-care strategies [92, 93], providers typically do not record a complete profile of patients' over-the-counter and prescription medications. While Canada and European countries have developed categories of over-the-counter drugs which require distribution through pharmacies and/or pharmacists, the United States population can select and buy nonprescription drug without health provider consultation. The separation between the self-care and medical care worlds need not persist as modelled by collaborative projects between health professionals and community educators promoting self-care in Scandinavia [97, 98]. Given the self-monitoring and decision-making done by clients, the question is how health care providers can best integrate the self-care roles their patients have taken and will continue to take.

Shared vs Exclusive Power in Patient-Provider Relationship

All of the assumptions addressed in this paper up to this point rest fundamentally on a central difference between the medical model vs client-centered model—the issue of control and power in the patient-provider relationship. In the extreme, the medical model retains the view that the provider's expertise justifies exclusive control over health-related decisions regarding medication regimens. This view overlooks the fact that clients exercise control over medication management as soon as they leave a visit. Many do not fill a prescription [99], let alone follow the prescribed regimen [1, 2, 11, 13, 14, 19–26, 46, 48]. It underestimates the extent to which self-care [87–96] and monitoring [13, 14, 71–83] precede and follow the visit. The challenge is to affirm and incorporate into the relationship the shared expertise and power of providers and clients. While health care providers' expertise is central for the diagnostic step in medication selection, the subsequent steps of setting goals, product selection, adapting the regimen to the client's lifestyle, implementing the regimen, monitoring and revising the regimen depend on client participation and openness as much as the diagnostic step, if not more so. As Charles and DeMaio [55] describe in their review of Canadian efforts for greater lay participation, these efforts break down the traditional asymmetry of knowledge between providers and patients. As that asymmetry is lessened so is the asymmetry of control.

We need a clear delineation of rights and responsibilities of both patients and providers for models of shared power to be effective. Meyer [100] suggests that patient responsibilities are derivable from the same idea which typically grounds the idea of patient rights—patient autonomy. He suggests that patient duties include, but are not limited to:

- a duty to be honest about why the patient seeks care

- a duty to collect information on available treatments and likely side-effects

- a duty for a patient who has an infectious condition to act on that information which can best prevent further transmission.

We suggest that additional responsibilities include:

- a duty to communicate preferences for health and quality of life outcomes and treatments

- a duty to share openly their full range of self-care

- a duty to monitor, evaluate and communicate the outcomes of care and

- a duty to share insights and concerns about the regimen.

In conceptualizing the responsibilities of health care providers in a model of shared power around medication management, it may be useful to draw upon the pharmaceutical care framework introduced over twenty years ago and recently reintroduced by Hepler and Strand. It has stimulated interest in the field of pharmacy and may have usefulness for broader segments of the health professions [101–107]. The framework has the potential to elevate the participation of clients or to continue the medical model. As defined by Hepler and Strand, pharmaceutical care is defined as: "the responsible provision of drug therapy for the purpose of achieving definite outcomes that improve a patient's quality of life." [101, p. 539]. A focus on quality of life implies a more client-centered approach to select goals and judge regimen progress based on the client's perceptions. However, lists of provider responsibilities for pharmaceutical care omit overt reference to the collaborative nature of the client-provider relationship for several responsibilities. We suggest that the simple addition of one term "in collaboration with patients" to the delineation of each of the following responsibilities allows the pharmaceutical care model to generate meaningful guidelines for collaborative medication management in the following wording:

It is the provider's responsibility to assess the patient's drug-related problems after receiving the patient's permission to do so and then, *in collaboration with the patient:* "prioritize actual and potential drug-related problems; . . . establish a desired pharmacotherapeutic outcome; . . . devise the best drug, dose, formulation, regimen, schedule; . . . . design a therapeutic drug-monitoring plan; . . . .implement the individualized regimen and monitoring plan; . . . and measure its success" [106, p. 15].

From this perspective of mutual responsibility the provider is responsible to, but not for, the patient.

Implications For Policy

Recommendations for altering client-provider roles often focus on individual behavior and train-ing. While this is important, external forces shape much of what happens in the health care system, particularly where a shift in roles is being proposed. Four types of policy issues could be critical in determining whether a collaborative client-centered model is adopted widely and effectively:

(1) reimbursement policies

(2) regulatory policies

(3) policies protecting patients' privacy and

(4) professional societies' policies.

Recommendations regarding each will be briefly discussed.

International concern about the cost, efficacy and necessity of medical interventions is high. The resulting growth of drug formularies and health maintenance organizations has led to restricted reimbursement for specific prescription drugs and decreased prescribing options. Thus, drug reimbursement policy has decreased rather than expanded client choice of prescription medications. In addition, rarely does one hear about governmental reimbursement policy to increase patient education and consultation for medication management. In a few countries such as the Netherlands, government funding has supported patient education, but this has been more the exception than the rule [108]. The question is whether third party reimbursement will acknowledge the significance of client medication behavior on cost and outcomes by reimbursing the full range of providers (physicians, pharmacists, nurses) for collaborative medication consultation services with patients. A recommendation we would propose is that reimbursement policies be evaluated as to whether they promote effective client involvement and choice in medication management. Recognizing that short term cost concerns will never be absent, we propose that reimbursement policy take a longer term view of cost and quality in judging how best to foster effective client medication management.

Regulation offers a second type of policy initiative that could influence the adoption of more client-centered models. As part of the recent United States Omnibus Budget Reconciliation Act of 1990 (OBRA '90), the Medicaid Drug Utilization Review provision was adopted and went into effect on 1 January 1993. This provision mandates drug utilization review, patient counseling (including techniques for self-monitoring drug therapy), and other cognitive services involved in recording and maintaining an up-to-date patient record relevant to his or her drug therapy. Although these regulations are insufficient by themselves to change provider behaviors, they express support for valued behavior. If third party reimbursement were contingent upon such services being performed, an obvious incentive would be introduced into the health care system. Technological advancements in computerized record-keeping can facilitate the type of consultative relationship described. Our second recommendation would be to combine regulatory with reimbursement policies to reinforce effective client preparation for medication management and its documentation.

The same advancements in computerized communication and documentation unfortunately raises a third issue regarding a client's right to control access to medical information and decisions. To the extent that third party payers, physicians, pharmacists and employers begin to request information about client medication compliance or health status from each other, a basic patient right to privacy must be protected. Just how this right can be protected has yet to be clearly delineated and as the electronic communication and compliance monitoring systems expand so do the possibilities for release of medical information without client knowledge or desire. Hence, societies need to examine and reinforce individual rights for privacy and intentional noncompliance such that no employer or insurance company could impose restrictions or reduce benefits as a result of information from an individual's medical or pharmacy records. Our third recommendation is that health professional organizations examine how the covenant of patient privacy can be protected as electronic documentation of patient health behavior increases.

Lastly, professional role identity must be addressed for widespread adoption of client-centered models regardless of which health profession is being discussed. One can hope that the past twenty years of social science research on medication use [109] will be translated into behavioral science curricula in the health sciences to foster both attitudes and skills by health professionals for collaborative relationships with patients. As DiMatteo states, these relationships require: "a recognition of the need for effective communication, a conscious approach to the therapeutic relationship as a collaboration, and a recognition of the patient's right to choose her own course of action" [45, p. 64].

Until health professional societies and educational programs endorse such a goal, it appears unlikely that major shifts in roles will occur. Dole [107] points out

that of some 140 recommendations in the proceedings of the conference on implementing pharmaceutical care conducted by the Association for Society of Hospital Pharmacists Research and Education Foundation, only 10 contain any mention of patients. No recommendations mention patient participation in the development of their medication regimens. Thus, our final proposal is that professional health organizations address what the most basic contract is between client and health provider. Is the health care provider responsible 'for' or 'to' the client?

We have suggested that national health care policy makers, as well as providers, should encourage a more patient-centered approach to medication management from both a cost control and efficacy perspective. The health care system's dependence on clients to manage their regimens has forced the question. No matter how sophisticated our medication technology becomes, ultimately, their success depends on the client's motivation and behavior. We need to lay a foundation for informed patient–provider partnerships by consciously avoiding regulation and finance systems which undercut patients' taking active roles with respect to medication management. Over the past twenty years, the gap has widened between policy makers who acknowledge the centrality of an individual's health behavior to the health of a country [110] vs policy makers who focus steadfastly on short term cost control as though clients are an irrelevant resource. The net result has been policy which works against a client-centered model in some health domains, but works for it in others. The challenge now

within health care reform is to identify areas of agreement and examine how drug and provider reimbursement and regulatory systems can promote active, well informed client partners in medication management. The alternative is to continue underusing perhaps the most critical resource for reducing unnecessary and costly health care utilization—clients.

References

1. Col N., Fanale J. and Kronholm P. The role of medication noncompliance and adverse drug reactions in hospitalizations of the elderly. *Arch. Int. Med.* **150**, 841, 1990.
2. Sullivan S. D., Kreling D. H. and Hazlet T. K. Noncompliance with medication regimens and subsequent hospitalizations: A literature analysis and cost of hospitalization estimate. *J. Res. Pharm. Econ.* **2**, 12, 1990.
3. Grymonpre R. B., Mitenko P. A. and Sitar D. S. Drug-associated hospital admissions in older medical patients. *J. Am. Geriat. Soc.* **36**, 1092, 1988.
4. McKenney J. M. and Harrison W. L. Drug-related hospital admissions. *Am. J. Hosp. Pharm.* **22**, 792, 1976.
5. Bergman U. and Wiholm B. E. Patient medication on admission to a medical clinic. *Europ. J. clin. Pharmacol.* **20**, 1, 1981.
6. Szasz T. S. and Hollander M. H. A contribution to the philosophy of medicine. The basic models of the doctor-patient relationship. *Arch. Int. Med.* **97**, 585, 1956.
7. Parsons T. *The Social System.* The Free Press, Glencoe, Ill., 1951.
8. Haug M. R. and Lavin B. *Consumerism In Medicine: Challenging Physician Authority.* Sage Publications, Beverly Hills, CA, 1983.
9. Freidson E. *Profession Of Medicine.* Dodd, Mead, New York, 1970.
10. Haug M. R. Deprofessionalization: An alternative hypothesis for the future. *Social Rev. Monographs,* **20**, 195, 1973.
11. Hulka B. S. Patient-clinician interactions and compliance. In *Compliance in Health Care* (Edited by Haynes R. B., Taylor D. W. and

Sackett D. L.). Johns Hopkins University Press, Baltimore, 1979.

12. Korsch B. and Negrete V. Doctor-patient communication. *Scient. Am.* **227**, 66, 1972.

13. Leventhal H. and Cameron L. Behavioral theories and the problem of compliance. *Patient Educ. Counseling* **10**, 117, 1987.

14. Meyer D., Leventhal H. and Gutmann M. Commonsense models of illness: the example of hypertension. *Hlth Psychol.* **4**, 115, 1985.

15. Rimer B. K. Perspectives on intrapersonal theories in health education and health behavior. In *Health Behavior and Health Education: Theory, Research and Practice* (Edited by Glanz K., Lewis F. M. and Rimer B. K.). Jossey-Bass, San Francisco, 1991.

16. Roter D. L. and Hall J. A. *Doctors Talking with Patients, Patients Talking With Doctors: Improving Communication In Medical Visits.* Auburn House, Westport, CT, 1992.

17. Fallsberg M. Reflections on medicines and medication: a qualitative analysis among people on long-term drug regimens. Linkping studies in dissertations. No. 31. Linkping University, Sweden, 1991.

18. Friedman H. S. and DiMatteo M. R. *Health Psychology.* Prentice Hall, Englewood Cliffs, NJ, 1989.

19. Conrad P. The meaning of medications: another look at compliance. *Soc. Sci. Med.* **20**, 29, 1985.

20. Zola I. Structural constraints in the doctor-patient relationship: the case of non-compliance. In *The Relevance Of Social Science For Medicine* (Edited by Eisenberg L. and Kleinman A.), pp. 241-252. D. Reidel, Dordrecht, 1981.

21. Arluke A. Judging drugs: patients' conceptions of therapeutic efficacy in the treatment of arthritis. *Human Organization* **39**, 84, 1980.

22. Hayes-Bautista D. E. Modifying the treatment: patient compliance, patient control and medical care. *Soc. Sci. Med.* **10**, 233, 1976.

23. Stimson G. V. Obeying doctor's orders: a view from the other side. *Soc. Sci. Med.* **8**, 97, 1975.

24. Trostle J. A. Medical compliance as an ideology. *Soc. Sci. Med.* **27**, 1299, 1988.

25. Stewart M. A. What is a successful doctor-patient interview? A study of interactions and outcomes. *Soc. Sci. Med.* **19**, 167, 1984.

26. Svarstad B. L. Patient-practitioner relationships and compliance with prescribed medication regimens. In *Applications Of Social Science To Clinical Medicine and Health Policy* (Edited by Aiken L. H. and Mechanic D.). Rutgers University Press, New Brunswick, 1986.

27. Thompson S. C., Pitts J. S. and Schwankovsky L. Preferences for involvement in medical decision-making: situational and demographic influences. *Patient Educ. Counseling* **22**, 133, 1993.

28. Ende J., Kazis L., Ash A. and Moskowitz M. A. Measuring patients' desire for autonomy: decision-making and information-seeking preferences among medical patients. *J. gen internal Med.* **4**, 23, 1989.

29. Haug M. and Lavin B. Practitioner or patient who's in charge? *J. Hlth Soc. Behav.* **22**, 212, 1981.

30. Haug M. and Lavin B. *Consumerism in Medicine: Challenging Physician Authority.* Sage Publications, Beverly Hills, CA, 1983.

31. Hibbard J. H. and Weeks E. C. Consumerism in health care: prevalence and predictors. *Medical Care* **25**, 1019, 1987.

32. Morris J. and Royle G. T. Cancer: Pre- and post-operative levels of clinical anxiety and depression in patients and their husbands. *Br. J. Surg.* **74**, 1017, 1987.

33. Strull W. M., Lo B. and Charles G. Do patients want to participate in medical decision-making? *J. Am. Med. Assoc.* **252**, 2990, 1984.

34. Biley F. C. Some determinants that effect patient participation in decision-making about nursing care. *J. Adv. Nursing* **17**, 414, 1992.

35. Degner L. P. and Sloan J. A. Decision-making during serious illness: what role do patients really want to play? *J. clin. Epidemiol.* **45**, 941, 1992.

36. Reeder L. G. The patient-client as a consumer: some observations on the changing professional-client relationship. *J. Hlth Soc. Behav.* **13**, 406, 1972.

37. Callahan E. J. and Bertakis K. D. A comparison of physician-patient interaction as fee-for-service and HMO sites. *Family Practice Res. J.* **13**, 171, 1993.

38. Freidson E. *Medical Work in America: Essays on Health Care.* Yale University Press, New Haven, CT, 1989.

39. Ben-Sira Z. Primary care practitioners' likelihood to engage in a bio-psychosocial approach: an additional perspective on the doctor patient relationship. *Soc. Sci. Med.* **31**, 565, 1990.

40. Engel G. L. The need for a new medical model: a challenge for biomedicine. *Science* **196**, 129, 1977.

41. Schipper H., Clinch J. and Powell V. Definitions and conceptual issues. In *Quality of Life Assessments in Clinical Trials* (Edited by Spilker B.), pp. 11-24. Raven Press, New York, 1990.

42. Stewart A. L., Greenfield S., Hays R. D. and Wells K. Functional status and well-being of patients with chronic conditions. *J. Am. Med. Assoc.* **262**, 907, 1989.

43. Anderson O. and Morrison E. Worth of medical care: a critical review. *Med. Care Rev.* **46**, 121, 1989.

44. Angaran D. M. Quality assurance to quality improvement: measuring and monitoring pharmaceutical care. *Am. J. Hosp. Pharm.* **48**, 1901, 1991.

45. DiMatteo M. R. The physician-patient relationship: effects on the quality of health care. *Clin. Obstet. Gynecol.* **37**, 149, 1994.

46. Fink D. L. Tailoring the consensual regimen. In *Compliance With Therapeutic Regimens* (Edited by Sackett D. L. and Haynes R. B.). Johns Hopkins University Press, Baltimore, 1976.

47. Best J. A. Tailoring smoking withdrawal procedures to personality and motivational differences. *J. Consult. Clin. Psych.* **43**, 1, 1975.

48. Haynes R. B., Taylor D. W. and Sackett D. L. *Compliance in Health Care.* Johns Hopkins University Press, Baltimore, 1979.

49. Gambone J. C.. Reiter R. C. and DiMatteo M. R. Putting risk into perspective by a process of informed collaborative choice. The PREPARED checklist. Paper presented at the Open Conference, Communicating Risk To Patients, U.S. Pharmocopeial Convention, Reston, VA, September 1994.

50. England S. L. and Evans J. Patients' choices and perceptions after an invitation to participate in treatment decisions. *Soc. Sci. Med.* **34**, 1217, 1992.

51. Pfeiffer C. S. and Walker M. Enhancing achievement of therapeutic goals through drug choice. *Cardiovascular Nursing* **26**, 19, 1990.

52. Mahowald M. L., Steveken M. E., Young M. and Ytterberg S. R. The Minnesota arthritis training program: emphasis on self-management, not compliance. *Patient Educ. Counseling*, **11**, 235, 1988.

53. Buckalew L. W. and Sallis R. E. Patient compliance and medication perception. *J. clin. Psych.* **42**, 49, 1986.

54. Hussain M. Z. Effect of shape of medication in treatment of anxiety states. *Br. J. Psych.* **120**, 507, 1972.

55. Charles C. and DeMaio S. Lay participation in health care decision making: a conceptual framework. *J. Hlth Politics, Policy Law*, **18**, 881, 1992.

56. Clark J. A., Potter D. A. and McKinlay J. B. Bringing social structure back into clinical decision-making. *Soc. Sci. Med.* **32**, 853, 1991.

57. Eisenberg J. M. Sociologic influences on decision-making by clinicians. *Ann. Internal Med.* **90**, 957, 1979.

58. Gabe J. Towards a sociology of tranquilizer prescribing. *Br. J. Addict.* **85**, 41, 1990.

59. Raynes N. Factors affecting the prescribing of psychotropic drugs in general practice consultation. *Psychol. Med.* **9**, 671, 1979.

60. Hall D. Prescribing as social exchange. In *Prescribing Practice and Drug Usage* (Edited by Mapes R.), pp. 39-57. Croom Helm, London, 1980.

61. Hemminki E. Review of the literature on the factors affecting drug prescribing. *Soc. Sci. Med.* **9**, 111, 1975.

62. Sleath B., Svarstad B. and Roter D. Physician versus patient initiation of psychotropic prescribing: an exploration of the prescribing process during the physician-patient interaction. Paper presented at *Eighth International Social Pharmacy Workshop*, Berlin, 1994.

63. Todd A. A diagnosis of doctor-patient discourse in the prescription of contraception. In *The Social Organization of Doctor-patient Communication* (Edited by Todd A. and Fisher S.), pp. 183-212. Ablex Publishing Corporation, Norwood, NJ, 1993.

64. Cockburn J., Reid A. L. and Sanson-Fisher R. W. The process and content of general-practice consultations that involve prescription of antibiotic agents. *Med. J. Australia* **147**, 321, 1987.

65. Heath C. On prescription-writing in social interaction. In *Prescribing Practice and Drug Usage* (Edited by Mapes R.), pp. 58-72. Croom Helm, London, 1980.

66. Denig P., Haaijer-Ruskamp F. M. and Zijsling D. H. How physicians choose drugs. *Soc. Sci. Med.* **27**, 1381, 1988.

67. Segal R. and Hepler C. D. Drug choice as a problem-solving process. *Medical Care* **23**, 967, 1985.

68. Segal R. and Hepler C. D. Prescribers' beliefs and values as predictors of drug choices. *Am. J. Hospital Pharmacy* **39**, 1891, 1982.

69. Avorn J., Chen M. and Hartley R. Scientific versus commercial sources of influence on the prescribing behavior of physicians. *Am. J. Med.* **73**, 4, 1982.

70. Schwartz R. K., Soumerai S. B. and Avorn J. Physician motivation for nonscientific drug prescribing. *Soc. Sci. Med.* **28**, 577, 1989.

71. Baumann L. J., Cameron L. D., Zimmerman R. S. and Leventhal H. Illness representations and matching labels with symptoms. *Hlth Psych.* **8**, 449, 1989.

72. Baumann, L. J. and Keller M. L. Responses to threat information. *Image: J. Nurs. Scholarship* **23**, 13, 1991.

73. Baumann, L. J., Zimmerman R. and Leventhal H. An experiment in common sense: education at blood pressure screening. *Patient Educ. Counseling* **12**, 53, 1989.

74. Baumann L. J. and Leventhal H. "I can tell when my blood pressure is up: can't I?" *Hlth Psych.* **4**, 203, 1985.

75. Leventhal H., Leventhal, E. and Schaefer P. Vigilant coping and health behavior. In *Aging, Health, and Behavior* (Edited by Ory M. and Abeles R.). Johns Hopkins, Baltimore, 1991.

76. Leventhal H. Common-sense theory and the practice of health psychology. In *Advances in Theory and Practice in Behavior Therapy* (Edited by Emmelkamp P. M. G., Everserd W. T. A. M., Krasimast F. and van Son M. J. M.). Annual Series of European Research in Behavior Therapy. Swets & Zeitlinger, Amsterdam, 1988.

77. Morris L. S. and Schulz R. M. Medication compliance: the patient's perspective. *Clin. Therap.* **15**, 593, 1993.

78. Arluke A. Judging drugs: patients' conceptions of therapeutic efficacy in the treatment of arthritis. *Human Organization* **39**, 84, 1980.

79. Chubon S. J. Personal descriptions of compliance by rural southern blacks: an exploratory study. *J. Compliance Hlth Care* **4**, 23, 1989.

80. Cooper J. K., Love D. W. and Raffoul P. R. Intentional prescription nonadherence (noncompliance) by the elderly. *J. Am. Geriatric Soc.* **30**, 329, 1982.

81. Conrad P. The meaning of medications: another look at compliance. *Soc. Sci. Med.* **20**, 29, 1985.

82. Hunt L. M., Jordan B., Irwin S. and Browner C. H. Compliance and the patient's perspective: controlling symptoms in everyday life. *Cult. Med. Psychiat.* **13**, 315, 1989.

83. Enlund H., Vainio K., Wallenius S. and Poston J. W. Adverse drug effects and the need for drug information. *Med. Care.* **29**, 558, 1991.

84. U.S Pharmacopeial Convention. Communicating Risk To Patients. Open Conference. Reston, VA, September, 1994.

85. Schommer J. C. and Wiederholt J. B. The influence of prescription question asking on pharmacist-patient communication. Presented at the Economic, Social and Administrative Science Section of the *Annual Meeting of the Academy of Pharmaceutical Research and Science,* American Pharmaceutical Association, Seattle WA, March 1994.

86. Wiederholt J. B., Clarridge B. R. and Svarstad B. L. Verbal consultation regarding prescription drugs: findings from a statewide study. *Med. Care* **30**, 159, 1992.

87. Dean K. Conceptual, theoretical, and methodological issues in self-care research. *Soc. Sci. Med.* **29**, 117, 1989.

88. Segall A. A community survey of self-medication activities. *Medical Care* **28**, 301, 1990.

89. Stoller E. P. Prescribed and over-the-counter medicine use by the ambulatory elderly. *Med Care* **26**, 1149, 1988.

90. Hickey T. and Dean K. Emerging trends in gerontology and geriatrics: implications for the self-care of the elderly. *Soc. Sci. Med.* **23**, 1363, 1986.

91. Haire-Joshu D., Fisher E. B., Munro J. and Wedner H. J. A comparison of patient attitudes toward asthma self-management among acute and preventive care settings. *J. Asthma* **30**, 359, 1993.

92. Stroller P. E., Forster E. L. and Portugal S. Self-care responses to symptoms by older people: a health diary study of illness behavior. *Med. Care* **31**, 24, 1993.

93. Verbrugge L. M. and Ascione F. J. Exploring the iceberg: common symptoms and how people care for them. *Med. Care* **25**, 539, 1987.

94. Dean K. Self-care components of lifestyles: the importance of gender, attitudes and the social situation. *Soc. Sci. Med.* **29**, 137, 1989.

95. Dean K. Lay care in illness. *Soc. Sci. Med.* **22**, 275, 1986.

96. Liebowitz A. Substitution between prescribed and over-the-counter medications. *Med. Care* **27**, 85, 1989.

97. Launso L. *A Registration of Alternative Therapists in the Municipality of Hralso and Development of a Cooperation with Alternative Therapists, Physicians, and Pharmacists in Hralso.* Royal Danish Institute of Pharmacy, Copenhagen, Denmark, 1993.

98. Launso L. and Brendstrup E. Evaluation of a non-drug intervention program for younger seniors. *J. Soc. Admin. Pharm.* **10**, 23, 1993.

99. Whitney H. A., Bloss J. L., Cotting C. M., Jaworski P. G., Myers S. L. and Thordsen D. J. Medication compliance: a health care problem. *Ann. Pharmacother.* **27**, 5, 1993.

100. Meyer M. J. Patients' duties. *J. Med. Phil.* **17**, 541, 1992.

101. Hepler C. D. and Strand L. M. Opportunities and responsibilities in pharmaceutical care. *Am. J. Hosp. Pharm.* **47**, 533, 1990.

102. Strand L. M., Cipolle R. J., Morley P. C. and Perrier D. G. Levels of pharmaceutical care: a needs-based approach. *Am. J. Hosp. Pharm.* **48**, 547, 1991.

103. Brodie D. C., McGhan W. F. and Lindon J. The theoretical base of pharmacy. *Am. J. Hosp. Pharm.* **48**, 536, 1991.

104. Smith W. E. and Benderev K. Levels of pharmaceutical care: a theoretical model. *Am. J. Hosp. Pharm.* **48**, 540, 1991.

105. Penna R. P. Pharmaceutical care: pharmacy's mission for the 1990's. *Am. J. Hosp. Pharm.* **47**, 543, 1990.

106. Strand L. M., Cipolle R. J. and Morley P. C. *Pharmaceutical care: An Introduction. Current Concepts.* Upjohn Co., Kalamazoo MI, 1992.

107. Dole E. J. Beyond pharmaceutical care. *Am. J. Hosp. Pharmacists* **51**, 2183, 1994.

108. Bartlett E. E. Patient-centered health care: desideratum for medical care reform. *Patient Educ. Counseling* **19**, 237, 1992.

109. Svarstad B. Development of behavioral science curricula and faculty in pharmacy: some issues requiring attention. *Am. J. Pharmaceut. Educ.* **58**, 177, 1994.

110. *Healthy People 2000: National Health Promotion and Disease Prevention Objectives.* U.S. Department of Health and Human Services, Public Health Service, 1990.

 Article Review Form at end of book.

What health risk behaviors seem to be associated with those who have concern about their image?

Self-Presentation Can Be Hazardous to Your Health

Impression management and health risk

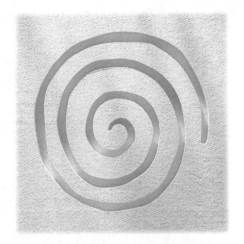

Mark R. Leary, Lydia R. Tchividjian, and Brook E. Kraxberger

Mark R. Leary, Lydia R. Tchividjian, and Brook E. Kraxberger, Department of Psychology, Wake Forest University

We thank Robin Kowalski for her helpful comments on an earlier draft of this article.

People's concerns with how others perceive and evaluate them can lead to behaviors that increase the risk of illness and injury. This article reviews evidence that self-presentational motives play a role in several health problems, including HIV infection; skin cancer; malnutrition and eating disorders; alcohol, tobacco, and drug use; injuries and accidental death; failure to exercise; and acne. The implications of a self-presentational perspective for research in health psychology, the promotion of healthful behaviors, and health care delivery are discussed.

Key words: self-presentation, impression management, health promotion, illness prevention, health motivation

The first step in promoting healthy behavior is to understand why people do not take adequate care of their health. Most research on this question has focused on people's health-relevant cognitions, such as their estimates of the likelihood that they will experience a certain medical problem, their perceptions of the severity of the problem, and their expectations regarding whether behavioral change will improve their health (e.g., DiClemente, 1986; Janz & Becker, 1984; Rosenstock, 1974).

In contrast, relatively little attention has been devoted to interpersonal motives that affect health-related behaviors. Such processes are sometimes included in cognitively oriented models of health behavior as factors related to health values, outcomes, or barriers, but their role in health has rarely been studied in its own right. The focus of this article is on the role of self-presentational motives in health-relevant behaviors. The premise is that several patterns of behavior that increase the risk of illness and injury arise from people's concerns with how they are regarded by others.

Self-Presentation: An Overview

Self-presentation (also called *impression management*) refers to the processes by which people control how they are perceived and evaluated by others (Goffman, 1959; Leary, 1994; Leary & Kowalski, 1990; Schlenker, 1980). Because many of people's material, social, and personal outcomes in life depend in part on how others regard them, people are understandably concerned that others perceive them in desired ways. The impressions others form have implications for their friendships and social lives, job success, romantic involvements, and casual interactions, as well as for their self-evaluations and mood (Baumeister, 1982; Schellenker, 1980).

Although the notion of self-presentation sometimes evokes images of Machiavellian deceit, most self-presentational behaviors are not deceptive. Rather, people tactically control the inferences that others draw about them by selectively presenting sides of themselves that will result in the outcomes they desire while concealing information that is inconsistent with the impressions they want others to form (Schlenker & Weigold, 1992). Of course, people sometimes do lie about themselves, presenting images that they know are not accurate, but self-presentational dissimulation is the exception rather than the rule (Leary, 1993). Not only do most people view self-presentational deceit as wrong, but fabrication carries interpersonal risks (Baumeister & Jones, 1978; Goffman, 1959; Schlenker, 1980).

Although the impressions people try to make are often positive and socially desirable, self-presentation is motivated by more than pure approval seeking. People sometimes present undesirable images of themselves and sacrifice others' good will when they think negative self-presentations will help them achieve important social goals (E. E. Jones & Pittman, 1982).

Regardless of how hard people try to enhance and protect their public images, self-presentational failures inevitably befall them. Projecting undesired impressions results in aversive feelings that people typically call *embarrassment* and in behavioral efforts to repair the damage to one's social image (R. S. Miller, 1986; R. S. Miller & Leary, 1992). Because embarrassment is distressing, people try to avoid self-presentational failures; some health-relevant behaviors discussed below involve attempts to avoid embarrassment.

Self-presentation is essential for smooth interpersonal relations

and for the accomplishment of people's social goals (Goffman, 1959; Schlenker, 1980). People would have much difficulty negotiating social encounters if others did not purposefully convey information regarding their personal characteristics, attitudes, preferences, emotional states, and intentions. Likewise, people would find it difficult to pursue their social goals without regulating the amount and type of information others have about them. Unfortunately, the motive to convey certain social images can lead to behaviors that are deleterious for the individual, if not for others as well. Self-presentational motives are often so strong that they lead people to engage in impression-creating behaviors that are, in the long term, dangerous to themselves or to others.

The focus in this article is on ways in which self-presentational processes affect health-related behaviors. People's concerns with their social images can increase health risks as diverse as cancer, HIV infection, and substance abuse. It must be emphasized that this does not suggest that the health-related behaviors described in this article arise solely from people's concerns with others' impressions. Yet research evidence suggests that self-presentational motives play an important role in these behaviors and that the self-presentational perspective has implications for understanding, preventing, and treating a diverse array of health problems.

Condom Use and the Risk of AIDS

Although health professionals have long advocated using condoms to prevent pregnancy and sexually transmitted diseases

(STDs), the impetus for condom use increased markedly with the spread of AIDS during the past 10 years. Recent data suggest, however, that many people continue to take inadequate precautions against pregnancy and STDs. Approximately 1 million teenage girls in the United States become pregnant each year (Fielding & Williams, 1991), and over 12 million Americans contract some form of STD ("Sexually Transmitted Diseases Up", 1993). Less than 20% of the sexually active college students surveyed in one American study reported using condoms regularly ("Safer Sex", 1991; see also Hanna, 1989).

Although younger teens might not fully understand the implications of sexual behavior for pregnancy and health, for most people the failure to use condoms is not due to lack of information about pregnancy, STDs, or condoms (M. A. Bruch & Hynes, 1987; Markova, Wilkie, Naji, & Forbes, 1990; "Safer Sex", 1991). Rather, one primary reason people fail to use condoms seems self-presentational: People are concerned about how they will be perceived by others if they obtain condoms or discuss condoms with their sexual partners.

Self-presentational concern about obtaining condoms seems a primary barrier to their use. Studies have shown that between 30% and 63% of sexually active respondents reported being embarrassed when buying condoms (Hanna, 1989; Herold, 1981). Teenagers in particular are deterred from obtaining condoms and other forms of contraception by concerns about others' perceptions of them (Clinkscales & Gallo, 1977; Herold, 1981; Sorenson, 1973; Zabin, Stark, & Emerson, 1991).

One study of embarrassment arising from obtaining contraception from a physician or pharmacist showed that young women were more embarrassed about getting condoms than other forms of contraception such as contraceptive pills or foam, which, of course, do not protect against AIDS and other STDs (Herold, 1981). This may be because they think that others view it as more acceptable for women to purchase oral contraceptives or contraceptive foam than condoms. Not only do many people associate condoms with casual sex, STDs, and promiscuity (Lees, 1986), but, unlike using condoms, being on the pill does not necessarily imply that a woman is sexually active (e.g., she may be taking the pill because of menstrual problems; Herold, 1981).

Even if a person acquires condoms, self-presentational concerns may deter him or her from using them in a sexual encounter (Herold, 1981). Leary has talked to college students who had unprotected sexual intercourse even though they had a condom in their possession at the time. With a new sexual partner, people may worry that having a condom will imply that they had anticipated having sex, or worse, had actively worked to seduce the other person. In a study of adolescents in five American cities, teenagers of both sexes indicated that making plans to use a contraceptive would be perceived as too calculating unless they were involved in a stable, ongoing relationship (Kisker, 1985). Similarly, a recent study of Scottish teenagers concluded that "perceived barriers, particularly awareness of impression-management processes, were important predictors of teenagers' endorsement of HIV-preventive intentions" (Abraham,

Sheeran, Spears, & Abrams, 1992, p. 369). Women in particular may be reluctant to carry condoms because they are afraid that their partners will perceive them as very sexually experienced (if not promiscuous) and as too bold (Abraham et al., 1992; Lees, 1986).

Among gay men, a primary justification for having unprotected anal intercourse was a fear of making a negative impression on one's partner (e.g., "He'll think I'm a wimp. Real men should be willing to take a risk") (Gold, Skinner, Grant, & Plummer, 1991). Over one third of the respondents indicated that concerns with their partners' impressions of them had led them to have unprotected anal intercourse (see Catania et al., 1991).

Other people seem to think that insisting on using a condom will lead sexual partners to conclude that they have an STD. This is a particular concern for people who do, in fact, have an STD. In one study of hemophiliacs, the primary reason for not using a condom was anxiety about being rejected if others learned they were HIV positive. Thus, those who have the greatest need to use a condom may not do so because they fear that insisting on a condom will cause their STD to be detected (Markova et al., 1990)!

Given the effects of self-presentational worries on condom use, one might expect people who are highly concerned about others' impressions of them to be particularly unlikely to discuss safe sex with their partners. One study showed that socially anxious women, who are more concerned about others' impressions of them (Schlenker & Leary, 1982), were less likely to discuss contraception with their partners before having intercourse (M. A. Bruch & Hynes, 1987; see also Leary &

Dobbins, 1983). In contrast, high self-esteem, which is associated with self-presentational confidence and low need for social approval, is associated with more effective contraceptive use (Herold, Goodwin, & Lero, 1979).

The effects of self-presentational concerns on condoms use are perhaps the most important discussed in this article. Not only is the potential risk involved with failure to use a condom exceptionally serious, but the failure to use a condom poses a health risk not only for oneself but for others as well.

Sunbathing and Skin Cancer

The incidence of skin cancer has increased markedly in the United States during the past 30 years. The risk of basal cell carcinoma (the most common but least dangerous form) has been increasing at a rate of about 3% per year, whereas malignant melanoma (which is most likely to be fatal) has quadrupled since 1960 (Fears & Scotto, 1982). This increase is due to the convergence of several factors, including increased time spent sunbathing, increased vacationing in southern latitudes, and the popularity of tanning salons (Elwood, Whitehead, & Gallagher, 1989). Whatever the specific cause, the predominant cause of skin cancer is excessive exposure to ultraviolet radiation.

Sometimes people receive excessive exposure to the sun incidentally while engaging in outdoor work or recreational activities. However, many people purposefully expose themselves to the sun to obtain a tan. Because people tend to judge tanned people more positively than untanned people (Broadstock, Borland, & Gason, 1992; A. G.

Miller, Ashton, McHoskey, & Gimbel, 1990), many people think (perhaps correctly) that being tanned will help them make a better impression.

To the extent that this is true, people who are most interested in enhancing others' impressions of them may be at an increased risk for skin cancer. Leary and Jones (1993) found that the best predictors of engaging in behaviors that increase one's risk for skin cancer involve concerns with others' impressions generally or with one's appearance specifically. The best single predictor of risk behaviors was the belief that being tan enhanced one's physical appearance. Similarly, people who scored high in public and body self-consciousness, characteristics associated with a concern about others' impressions, were more likely to engage in behaviors that put them at risk for skin cancer (see also Mermelstein & Riesenberg, 1992).

Given that much tanning behavior is motivated by a desire to make better impressions on others, J. L. Jones and Leary (1994) reasoned that messages that emphasize the negative effects of tanning on appearance (e.g., wrinkling, aging, and scarring) might be more effective in promoting safe sun attitudes than messages that emphasize the cancer risk. Their findings showed that overall this was true, although appearance-based warnings were less effective for people high in appearance motivation.

A self-presentational approach suggests that the most direct way to deter voluntary tanning is to alter the positive stereotype of the tanned individual (A. G. Miller et al., 1990). During the 19th century, pale skin was prized because being tanned was associated with manual out-door labor. Only after the industrial revolution, when much of the working class began to work indoors, did being tan become associated with leisure and healthfulness (Keesling & Friedman, 1987). Efforts could be made to change contemporary American stereotypes of tanned people. For example, undermining the image that tanned people are healthier (Broadstock et al., 1992) may stigmatize tanning in much the same way that stressing the negative effects of smoking has led many to view smoking as a stigma (Jeffrey, 1989). Well-regarded celebrities who are seen as attractive and fashionable without being tan would further reinforce a more positive stereotype of untanned people (see Borland, Hill, & Noy, 1990).

Nutrition, Weight, and Eating Disorders

People tend to draw more favorable inferences about attractive people than unattractive people, inferring that attractive people are more sociable, warm, intelligent, socially skilled, and so on (Feingold, 1992). In light of this, people are understandably concerned with maintaining an attractive appearance or at least with not being perceived as unattractive.

In contemporary America, physical attractiveness involves not only facial appearance but also having an appropriate body weight and, often, being in good physical shape (Hayes & Ross, 1987). Besides the fact that being overweight is generally viewed as aesthetically unappealing, people tend to draw negative inferences about overweight people—that they are lazy and self-indulgent and lack self-control. Put simply, being fat is a stigma (Allon, 1982; Crocker, Cornwell, & Major, 1993; Millman, 1980). In contrast, being thin is viewed as a sign of status, discipline, and healthfulness. As Brownell (1991b) observed, "the body therefore becomes a visible means to project these qualities for all to see" (p. 307). In short, people may regulate their weight as a self-presentational strategy.

Self-presentational concerns involving weight can have both positive and negative effects on health. On the one hand, people try to eat nutritionally and to control their weight as much out of a concern for their appearance to others as for healthfulness per se (Hayes & Ross, 1987). If everyone suddenly lost their motivation to be regarded positively, most people might soon gain weight.

On the negative side, excessive concerns with weight can lead to a range of unhealthy behaviors. At the mild end, over twice as many people diet as need to diet for health reasons (see Brownell, 1991b). This excessive rate of dieting is fueled by the fact that Americans' perceptions of the ideal weight is actually below the average weight for healthy, normal-weight individuals (Brownell, 1991a). Rather than improving health, unnecessary dieting leads to problems including mild malnutrition, lowered resistance to illness and infection, insufficient energy, and decreased performance.

Furthermore, certain kinds of diet regimens are hazardous to one's health. People, particularly women, may come to rely on diet pills, amphetamines, and even cigarette smoking to control their weight (e.g., Camp, Klesges, & Relyea, 1993; Gritz and Crane, 1991). In more extreme cases, the excessive use of laxatives or purposeful vomiting to control weight can affect one's digestive system and heart.

Furthermore, yo-yo dieting (also called *weight cycling*) can have negative implications for health. Chronic on-again–off-again dieters develop an increasing preference for fat and sugar (Drewnowski, Kurth, & Rahaim, 1990), and recent research also suggests a link between yo-yo dieting and the risk of coronary heart disease (Hamm, Shekelle, & Stameller, 1989; Lissner et al., 1991).

The most serious consequences of insufficient eating are life-threatening eating disorders. Eating disorders represent a diverse set of problems with a variety of antecedents, some of which have little to do with self-presentation. Nevertheless, excessive concerns about one's social image lead certain people, particularly women, to starve or to purge themselves in an attempt to be thin (Hayes & Ross, 1987). Women with eating disorders tend to have a high need for social approval and an intense fear of rejection, particularly by men (Dunn & Ondercin, 1981; Katzman & Wolchik, 1984; Weinstein & Richman, 1984). Anorexics, for example, have been described as highly motivated to fulfill others' expectations (H. Bruch, 1978), and bulimics indicate that they "live to please others—family, friends, even strangers" (Weinstein & Richman, 1984, p. 211).

One experimental study showed that women with anorexic tendencies reduced how much they ate when they were unsuccessful at controlling how much attention another person paid to them (Rezek & Leary, 1991). Although this research did not study self-presentation directly, its results are consistent with the idea that perceived self-presentational failures can affect the eating behavior of women predisposed to eating disorders. Women with eating disorders also tend to have lower self-esteem and higher social anxiety than women of normal weight (Gross & Rosen, 1988; Katzman & Wolchik, 1984), factors associated with self-presentational concerns (Leary, 1983).

It is interesting that women with eating disorders often manifest a discrepancy between how they think they truly are and their public presentation. For the most part, for example, bulimics are as successful, attractive, and socially active as anyone else, and they are often regarded quite favorably by other people. Yet they believe that their public persona is but a ruse to hide their true, inner selves from others. Because of their concerns with others' reactions, bulimics are often dutifully good, passive, and nonassertive (Weinstein & Richman, 1984).

Direct evidence for the role of self-presentational factors in eating was provided by the finding that female subjects ate less with a socially desirable male confederate than with a less desirable man or with a woman (Mori, Chaiken, & Pliner, 1987; Pliner & Chaiken, 1990). Women also ate less when they were motivated to convey an impression of being feminine to the male confederate (Mori et al., 1987).

The fact that eating disorders are far more common among women than among men may reflect the fact that appearance, eating behaviors, and body weight are more important in others' impressions of women than of men (Freedman, 1984; Hayes & Ross, 1987; Nasser, 1988; Rodin, Silberstein, & Striegel-Moore, 1985; Rolls, Fedoroff, & Guthrie, 1991). Studies showed that subjects' perceptions of women were affected by how much they ate (women who ate less were viewed as more feminine and less masculine), whereas perceptions of men were not affected by their eating (Chaiken & Pliner, 1987; Pliner & Chaiken, 1990). Furthermore, Guy, Rankin, and Norvell (1980) found that subjects judged unusually thin female silhouettes as *most feminine* but judged normal-weight male silhouettes as *most masculine*. These findings suggest that cultural views of femininity may contribute to eating disorders in women by prescribing unrealistically thin body shapes and sizes (Brownell, 1991a). Even among women without eating disorders, feeling that oneself is fat is associated with perceiving that friends and family exert pressure for one to be thin (Striegel-Moore, McAvay, & Rodin, 1986), and decisions to lose weight are often based on perceived social pressure to be thin and the stigma of obesity (Rosen, Gross, & Vara, 1987).

Although cultural standards for men's weight are more lenient than standards for women's weight, men also experience pressure to be fit and trim. In one study, 17% of male college students indicated that their greatest fear in life was becoming fat (Collier, Stallings, Wolman, & Cullen, 1990), suggesting that researchers should pay greater attention to the weight concerns of men.

Some researchers have suggested that the increase in anorexia nervosa and bulimia in the past 30 years has resulted from the idealization of thinness in American culture (Nasser, 1988). Eating disorders of the sort common in the United States are almost nonexistent in cultures that prize plumpness (Nasser,

1988). As other cultures adopt American values about weight, dieting, and their implications for others' impressions of the individual, an increase in eating disorders would be observed.

Alcohol, Tobacco, and Illegal Drug Use

The cumulative effects of excessive alcohol, tobacco, and illegal drug use are staggering. Hundreds of thousands of people die of illnesses and injuries each year as a result of alcohol, tobacco, and other drugs. Tobacco use alone is the single most preventable cause of death in the United States; approximately 500,000 people die of smoking-related illnesses each year in the United States (U.S. Department of Health and Human Services, 1990). In this section we examine evidence that drug use and abuse is initiated and maintained in part by self-presentational processes.

Self-presentational motives are strongly involved in the decision to use alcohol, tobacco, and illicit drugs. Few people sneak off alone for their first experiences with any of these substances. Indeed, one study found that only 11% of adolescents reported that they first smoked cigarettes alone (L. S. Friedman, Lichtenstein, & Biglan, 1985). Rather, most people first try alcohol, tobacco, and other drugs in an interpersonal context in which they want others to perceive them as adventuresome, sociable, or unrepressed.

Although laypeople often speak of adolescents succumbing to peer pressure in such contexts, the so-called pressure is typically implied rather than explicit. Adolescents and young adults often believe, sometimes correctly, that the use of alcohol and other drugs can facilitate their social image and, thus, peer acceptance (Kandel, 1980). As Shute (1975) noted,

the influences of peers related to the individual's felt needs to be "cool," to respond to challenges or dares, to prove one's openness and flexibility, and to demonstrate one's maturity and emotional depth are thought to be quite powerful motivators toward (or away from) experimentation with drugs. (p. 233)

The use of alcohol, tobacco, and other drugs depends in part on the belief that such behavior is tolerated, if not condoned, by important reference groups. People are unlikely to drink, smoke, or use drugs when they know that such behaviors seriously undermine the impressions that important people in their lives have of them. For example, boys who smoke indicate that smoking "makes you feel part of the gang" (Clayton, 1991, p. 119), presumably because one has conveyed the impression of being the right kind of person for group membership. Adolescents associate images of toughness, independence, and maturity with cigarette smoking (Camp et al., 1993; Chassin, Presson, Sherman, Corty, & Olshavsky, 1981; Covington & Omelich, 1988).

In addition, a study of the reasons why people drink alcohol revealed two primary factors, one of which involved drinking as a means toward attaining goals such as peer acceptance and social approval (Farber, Khavari, & Douglass, 1980). Among adolescents, those who drink are perceived as tougher, more precocious, and more rebellious than those who do not drink. Furthermore, many adolescent boys believe that their peers admire the attributes that characterize one who drinks alcohol and aspire to that image (Chassin, Tetzloff, & Hershey, 1985).

The effect of image concerns on substance abuse is also seen in the case of smokeless tobacco. Smokeless tobacco (oral snuff and chewing tobacco) is currently quite popular among adolescent and young adult males. Risks associated with smokeless tobacco include cancer of the mouth, noncancerous oral pathologies (recession of the gums, dental carries, and leukoplakia—white lesions of the oral mucosa), loss of bone mass in the jaw, and nicotine dependence (Boyd & Glover, 1989; White, 1990). The current popularity of smokeless tobacco can be traced in part to the fact that it is associated with a professional athlete image (Strauss, 1991). In one survey of over 1,000 minor- and major-league baseball players and coaches, 39% reported that they had used smokeless tobacco in the week before the study (White, 1990)! Apparently some boys and men begin using smokeless tobacco as a self-presentational tactic so they will be seen as athletic and tough.

Studies of personality predictors of drug and alcohol use also support the role of self-presentation in these behaviors. Wolfe, Lennox, and Cutler (1986) showed that college students who scored high on a measure of concern for appropriateness reported that they used drugs because of the influence of other people. In addition, drug abusers tend to score higher on measures related to self-presentational concern, such as social anxiety, than nonabusers (Lindquist, Lindsay, & White, 1979).

In addition to serving as a means of conveying desired images of oneself to one's peers, drug use can serve self-presentational goals in at least four other ways. First, adolescents may use alcohol, tobacco, or drugs as a means of conveying their autonomy or rebelliousness to parents and other adults (see Clayton, 1991). Second, people who are socially insecure may use alcohol or other drugs to reduce their anxiety in interpersonal contexts or because they think doing so will produce positive changes in their social behavior (Leonard & Blane, 1988).

Third, people may use alcohol or other drugs as self-handicapping strategies. By getting drunk or stoned before important evaluative events (e.g., tests), people who doubt their ability to perform well can create a viable excuse for poor performance (Berglas, 1986; E. E. Jones & Berglas, 1978). Although self-handicapping has sometimes been described as a tactic for preserving one's self-esteem, research shows clearly that it is also used for self-presentational purposes (Kolditz & Arkin, 1982).

Finally, some substances may be used because they have a secondary effect on a person's image. For example, many adolescent girls and adult women say they smoke because it is a good way to control their weight (Charlton, 1984; Gritz & Crane, 1991; Page & Gold, 1983; Pirie, Murray, & Leupker, 1991). Such people smoke not because they think smoking per se projects a desired image but because smoking has other self-presentational benefits.

Although to our knowledge no controlled studies have been conducted on the effects of self-presentational processes on actual tobacco, alcohol, or drug use, Shute (1975) demonstrated that college students readily conform to the expressed attitudes of their peers regarding drugs in laboratory group discussions. This occurred even when the peers were strangers with whom the subject had no previous contact. Clearly, subjects were motivated to convey an accepting attitude toward drugs to others whom they thought were in favor of drugs. If such effects occurred with complete strangers, one can only imagine the power of natural peer groups to induce self-presentational compliance.

Self-presentational motives can also facilitate and impede people's attempts to stop their use of alcohol, tobacco, and other drugs. On the positive side, people often decide to stop unhealthy habits because of what other people think. The stigmatization of smoking in the United States during the past 25 years has been credited with the steadily decreasing number of adult smokers (Jeffrey, 1989).

On the other hand, self-presentational concerns can interfere with people's willingness to stop using certain substances. The most clear-cut example involves people who are unwilling to stop smoking because they are afraid they will gain weight (Klesges & Klesges, 1988). Such concerns are not unfounded; smokers have been found to gain an average of 4.5 to 7.5 lb after they stop smoking (e.g., Klesges, Meyers, Klesges, & LaVasque, 1989). That people are willing to risk very serious health consequences (such as cardiovascular disease, emphysema, and lung cancer) because they fear gaining 5 or 6 lb demonstrates the potency of the self-presentational motive.

As evaluation of one school-based drug prevention program showed that the most potent mediator of the program's effects involved perceived changes in friends' tolerance of drug use (MacKinnon et al., 1991). Analyses showed that 66% of the program's effect on drug use and 45% of its effect on smoking was explained by changes in friends' reactions to drug use. Although this is but a single study, it suggests that large-scale efforts to reduce alcohol, tobacco, or drug use should include a component that attempts to change the prevailing impressions of people who use such substances.

Accidental Injury and Death

Although data on this point do not exist, we suspect that a high percentage of injuries and accidental deaths result from self-presentational motives. Many injuries result from reckless behaviors that are performed primarily, if not solely, for self-presentational reasons. Because the image of being fearless and risk taking is often valued (Finney, 1978; Hong, 1978), people sometimes engage in dangerous behaviors to convey an impression of being brave or adventuresome (or, conversely, so as not to be regarded as a wimp). For instance, many people (adolescents and young adults in particular) drive at excessive and unsafe speeds to convey an impression of bravery or recklessness. In the extreme case, the game of "chicken"—in which two drivers speed toward one another to see who swerves first—is essentially a self-presentational game in which the competitors play for the right to claim certain social identities (i.e., brave vs. cowardly). Russian roulette is a similar example. People sometimes try risky activities that they do not have the experience or ability to perform safely (e.g., spelunking, white water canoeing, and repelling) because they do not want to be perceived as cowardly or as a poor sport. Adolescents appear particularly prone to engage in dangerous activities because of concerns with what other people think (H. L. Friedman, 1989; Jonah, 1990).

In addition, injuries sometimes occur when people do not take adequate precautions with everyday activities. Although some such injuries occur because of pure carelessness or misfortune, others happen because the person did not want others to perceive him or her as too careful. For example, many people seem to avoid wearing seat belts in automobiles, helmets on bicycles and motorcycles, and life preservers in boats because such devices convey an impression of excessive cautiousness. In addition, many people seem reluctant to wear protective gear (e.g., safety goggles, gloves, and helmets) when operating power tools or dangerous machinery because they will be viewed as neurotic or extremely careful. This concern emerges at a young age; anecdotally, children as young as 6 or 7 years old are sometimes reluctant to wear knee pads and helmets when rollerskating because of what other children will think of them.

We know of no research that has investigated the role of self-presentational motives in accidental injury and death. If our theory is correct, such motives are a leading cause of injuries and deserve greater research attention. We also suspect that men are more likely than women to suffer self-presentationally caused injuries because men are more motivated to be perceived as brave, adventuresome, and reckless than women (Doyle, 1989).

Steroid Use

Steroids cause a number of health problems including acne, early balding, changes in the reproductive organs, stunted growth, heart problems, and possibly brain cancer. Undesirable behavioral changes, including aggressiveness and depression, are also common. Unfortunately, black market steroid use is increasing in the United States. It is estimated that 1 million Americans use steroids, one-half of whom are adolescents. Although steroid use is often associated with competitive athletes, such as weight lifters and football players, approximately one third of the male adolescents who use steroids are not involved in competitive athletics (Schrof, 1992). For these young men, the motivation is primarily self-presentational—to have a muscular physique that will enhance their social image and bring about desired rewards such as attention, respect, romantic involvements, and increased self-esteem.[1]

Failure to Exercise

Similar to weight control, physical exercise is sometimes motivated by self-presentation. People often get in and stay in shape not to be healthier but to make better impressions on other people. In this regard, self-presentational motives can facilitate good health.

Yet we suspect that there are certain people who need and want to exercise but do not do so because of concerns with the impressions they make while exer-

[1]The self-presentational benefits of being heavily muscled are easily seen on the covers of many bodybuilding magazines. For example, the cover of *Muscle and Fitness* typically features a very well-built man surrounded by one or more adoring, beautiful (and often scantily clad) women.

cising. People who perceive themselves to be overweight, scrawny, or disproportioned may be reluctant to be seen bouncing around in an aerobics class, swimming at the local pool, jogging in public, or lifting weights. Such concerns are likely to be particularly acute among those who are high in physique anxiety (Hart, Leary, & Rejeski, 1989).

A study of overweight women's reactions to exercise programs showed that self-presentational concerns were quite salient. "Although factors such as safety, comfort, and quality of instruction affected the women's exercise behaviors, the most powerful influences seemed to be the social circumstances of the exercise setting, especially concerns about visibility, embarrassment, and judgment by others" (Bain, Wilson, & Chaikind, 1989, p. 139). For example, these women reported that they preferred exercise classes that included only overweight women. Sport psychologists and fitness professionals should begin to pay increased attention to the effects of self-presentational concerns on people's willingness to exercise (Leary, 1992).

Acne

In American culture, many girls and women use makeup as a way of enhancing others' impressions of them. Furthermore, those most attuned to others' impressions are more likely to wear makeup to enhance their appearance (L. C. Miller & Cox, 1982). Unfortunately, frequent use of cosmetics can have negative consequences for health. It is estimated that one third of adolescent girls who regularly use cosmetics develop facial blemishes caused solely by the cosmetics, and this can occur even in girls who are not otherwise prone to acne (Freedman, 1984). This problem can become cyclical when women apply additional makeup to cover their blemishes, which further exacerbates the skin problem, leading to more covering makeup, then to more acne, and so on.

Although admittedly a minor affliction compared with AIDS, drug abuse, or skin cancer, acne creates a great deal of distress for many people. *Acne cosmetica* is an example of a condition for which people seek medical attention that is precipitated solely by attempts to manage one's impressions.

Cosmetic Surgery

When people think of medicine, they generally think of a field that deals with illness and injury. However, at least one medical specialty provides services that are primarily self-presentational rather than medical. Over 1.5 million people underwent cosmetic surgery in 1988 (Findlay, 1989), a substantial increase during the past decade. Between 1981 and 1989, the number of face lifts increased from 39,000 to 75,000, breast augmentation from 72,000 to 100,000, and liposuction from 1,000 to 250,000. Historically, women have sought cosmetic surgery at a higher rate than men, but an increasing number of men are now seeking plastic surgery (Yoffe, 1990).

Although some cosmetic surgery is conducted to repair disfigurements resulting from birth defects, accidents, or disease, the majority involves elective surgery intended to enhance appearance (Schouten, 1991). For example, the primary reason women give for seeking breast augmentation is to reduce their self-consciousness and embarrassment over the size of their breasts, a purely self-presentational motive (Birtchnell, Whitfield, & Lacey, 1990). Similarly, 80% of people who seek orthodontic treatment do so solely for cosmetic reasons (Giddon, 1983). Permanent modification of the body for self-presentational purposes is by no means new. Cultures throughout history have relied on various methods of mutilation (e.g., scarring, piercing, and stretching) to achieve cultural standards of beauty (Freedman, 1984).

Although safer than ever, cosmetic surgery is not risk free. Infection, abnormal bleeding, and pain are risks with all types of cosmetic surgery, and more serious consequences, including muscle damage, blood and fat clots, and death, can result (Findlay, 1989; Yoffe, 1990). The serious problems associated with silicone breast implants have recently become well-known (Podolsky, 1991). Breast augmentation carries the additional risk of obscuring breast tissue on standard mammograms, thereby reducing the early detection of breast cancer (Podolsky, 1991). Complications of liposuction occur in roughly 10% of patients (Henig, 1989).

Given the degree to which others' impressions are influenced by physical appearance, the desire to use surgical procedures to enhance one's appearance is understandable, and we should not be interpreted as criticizing cosmetic surgery. Yet these procedures, which are most often performed for self-presentational rather than for medical reasons, can constitute a health risk.

Implications of the Self-Presentation Perspective

We have reviewed several ways in which people's self-presentational motives can be hazardous to their health. In some cases, such as with sun-induced skin cancer or *acne cosmetica*, self-presentation may be the most important factor that places the person at risk. In other instances, such as contracting HIV through unsafe sex or using steroids, self-presentation is but one of many factors that lead to unhealthy behaviors. In either case, our review suggests that interpersonal motives, which have been largely neglected by health researchers and practitioners, deserve greater attention.[2]

Traditionally, health educators have tried to promote healthy lifestyles by warning people of the unhealthy consequences of certain behaviors. Our review suggests that, for certain health problems, increased attention should be devoted to the self-presentational motives that maintain unhealthy patterns of behavior. For example, one way to promote safe sex practices is to destigmatize condom use. If people come to believe that not using a condom will make a bad

[2]In addition to contributing to unhealthy behaviors, self-presentational concerns can interfere with obtaining adequate medical care. For example, self-presentational concerns regarding the nature of one's problem (as in the case of STDs or alcoholism) or about the medical exam itself (as in the case of cervical screening or mammograms; e.g., Kowalski & Brown, in press) may deter people from seeking treatment. Furthermore, people may fail to disclose medically relevant information to medical practitioners if they believe they will convey an undesired image by doing so. People may even hesitate to follow prescribed medical regimens if doing so may affect others' impressions of them. Leary and Kowalski (in press) discuss ways in which self-presentation may interfere with health care.

impression—connoting to a sexual partner that the individual is irresponsible, immature, or sexually repressed—condom use should increase. Similarly, getting people to regard a suntan as a sign of poor health should reduce purposeful tanning, and changing attitudes about the attractiveness of excessive thinness should reduce the prevalence of eating disorders. In each case, widespread changes in behavior are unlikely as long as people believe that their pubic images (and others' reactions to them) are enhanced by unhealthy behaviors.

Furthermore, people may be induced to behave more healthfully if they see the negative consequences of doing so for the impressions others form. For example, Klohn and Rogers (1991) showed that stressing the visibility of osteoporosis strengthened women's intentions to engage in behaviors that prevent the disorder. Similarly, stressing the negative effects of tanning on appearance increased safe sun intentions (J. L. Jones & Leary, 1994). In particular, when problems have consequences for both health and physical appearance, people may be more likely to be persuaded to change unhealthy behaviors when the risks to appearance are emphasized.

Unfortunately, efforts to minimize the unhealthy effects of self-presentational motives on health wrestle against two facts of interpersonal life: (a) The impressions that people make often do have important consequences for their relationships with others, and (b) people's assumptions about how others will regard them if they engage in certain unhealthy behaviors are often correct. At the present time, there are many people who really do frown on women who carry condoms,

rate tanned individuals positively, view extreme thinness as attractive, advocate that women use cosmetics, reward risky behaviors, and so forth. The big question for health researchers and professionals is how to lead people to pay more attention to their health and less attention to their public image when health and self-presentation collide.

References

Abraham, C., Sheeran, P., Spears, R., & Abrams, D. (1992). Health beliefs and promotion of HIV-preventive intentions among teenagers: A Scottish perspective. *Health Psychology, 11,* 363–370.

Allon, N. (1982). The stigma of overweight in everyday life. In B. B. Wolman (Ed.), *Psychological aspects of obesity* (pp. 130–174). New York: Van Nostrand Reinhold.

Bain, L. L., Wilson, T., & Chaikind, E. (1989). Participant perceptions of exercise programs for overweight women. *Research Quarterly for Exercise and Sport, 60,* 134–143.

Baumeister, R. F. (1982). A self-presentational view of social phenomena, *Psychological Bulletin, 91,* 3–26.

Baumeister, R. F., & Jones, E. E. (1978). When self-presentation is constrained by the target's knowledge: Consistency and compensation. *Journal of Personality and Social Psychology, 36,* 608–618.

Berglas, S. (1986). A typology of self-handicapping alcohol abusers. In M. J. Saks & L. Saxe (Eds.). *Advances in applied social psychology* (Vol. 3, pp. 29–56). Hillsdale, NJ: Erlbaum.

Birtchnell, S., Whitfield, P., & Lacey, J. H. (1990). Motivational factors in women requesting augmentation and reduction mammaplasty. *Journal of Psychosomatic Research, 34,* 509–514.

Borland, R., Hill, D., & Noy, S. (1990). Being Sun Smart: Changes in community awareness and reported behavior following a primary prevention program for skin cancer control. *Behavior. Change, 7,* 126–135.

Boyd, G. M., & Glover, E. D. (1989). Smokeless tobacco use by youth in the U.S. *Journal of School Health, 59,* 189–194.

Broadstock, M., Borland, R., & Gason, R. (1992). Effects of suntan on

judgments of healthiness and attractiveness by adolescents. *Journal of Applied Social Psychology, 22* 157–172.

Brownell, K. D. (1991a). Dieting and the search for the perfect body: Where physiology and culture collide. *Behavior Therapy, 22,* 1–12.

Brownell, K. D. (1991b). Personal responsibility and control over our bodies: When expectation exceeds reality. *Health Psychology, 10,* 303–310.

Bruch, H. (1978). *The golden cage: The enigma of anorexia nervosa.* New York: Vintage.

Bruch, M. A., & Hynes, M. J. (1987). Heterosexual anxiety and contraceptive use. *Journal of Research in Personality, 21,* 343–360.

Camp, D. E., Klesges, R. C., & Relyea, G. (1993). The relationship between body weight concerns and adolescent smoking. *Health Psychology, 12,* 24–32.

Catania, J. A., Coates, T. J., Stall, R., Bye, L., Kegeles, S. M., Capell, F., Henne, J., McKusick, L., Morin, S., Turner, H., & Pollack, L. (1991). Changes in condom use among homosexual men in San Francisco. *Health Psychology, 10,* 190–199.

Chaiken, S., & Pliner, P. (1987). Women, but not men, are what they eat: The effect of meal size and gender on perceived femininity and masculinity. *Personality and Social Psychology Bulletin, 13.* 166–176.

Charlton, A. (1984). Smoking and weight control in teenagers. *Public Health, 98,* 277–281.

Chassin, L., Presson, C. C., Sherman, S. J., Corty, E., & Olshavsky, R. W. (1981). Self-images and cigarette smoking in adolescence. *Personality and Social Psychology Bulletin, 7,* 670–676.

Chassin, L., Tetzloff, C., & Herskey, M. (1985). Self-image and social-image factors in adolescent alcohol use. *Journal of Studies on Alcohol, 46,* 39–47.

Clayton, S. (1991). Gender differences in psychosocial determinants of adolescent smoking. *Journal of School Health, 61,* 115–120.

Clinkscales, K., & Gallo, J. (1977). How teens see it. In D. J. Bogue (Ed.). *Adolescent fertility* (pp. 134–134). Chicago: University of Chicago Press.

Collier, S. N. Stallings, S. F., Wolman, P. G., & Cullen, R. W. (1990). Assessment of attitudes about weight and dieting among college-aged individuals. *Journal of the*

American Dietetic Association, 90, 276–279.

Covington, M. V., & Omelich, C. L. (1988). I can resist anything but temptation: Adolescent expectations for smoking cigarettes. *Journal of Applied Social Psychology, 18,* 203–227.

Crocker, J., Cornwell, B., & Major, B. (1993). The stigma of overweight: Affective consequences of attributional ambiguity. *Journal of Personality and Social Psychology, 64,* 60–70.

DiClemente, C. C. (1986). Self-efficacy and the addictive behaviors. *Journal of Social and Clinical Psychology, 4,* 302–315.

Doyle, J. A. (1989). *The male experience* (2nd ed.). Dubuque, IA: Wm. C. Brown.

Drewnowski, A., Kurth, C. L., & Rahaim, J. (1990). *Human obesity and sensory preferences for sugar and fat: Age at onset and history of weight cycling.* Unpublished manuscript.

Dunn, P. K., & Ondercin, P. (1981). Personality variables related to compulsive eating in college women. *Journal of Clinical Psychology, 37,* 43–49.

Elwood, J. M., Whitehead, S. M., & Gallagher, R. P. (1989). Epidemiology of human malignant skin tumors with special reference to natural and artificial ultraviolet radiation exposures. In C. J. Conti, T. J. Slaga, & A. J. P. Klein-Szanto (Eds.), *Skin rumors: Experimental and clinical aspects* (pp. 55–84). New York: Raven Press.

Farber, P. D., Khavari, K. A., & Douglass, F. M., IV. (1980). A factor analytic study of reasons for drinking: Empirical validation of positive and negative reinforcement dimensions. *Journal of Consulting and Clinical Psychology, 48,* 780–781.

Fears, T. R., & Scotto, J. (1982). Changes in skin cancer morbidity between 1971–72 and 1977–78. *Journal of the National Cancer Institute, 69,* 365–370.

Feingold, A. (1992). Good-looking people are not what we think. *Psychological Bulletin, 111,* 304–341.

Fielding, J. E., & Williams, C. A. (1991). Adolescent pregnancy in the United States: A review and recommendations for clinicians and research needs. *American Journal of Preventive Medicine, 7,* 47–52.

Findlay, S. (1989, May 1). Buying the perfect body. *U.S. News and World Report,* pp. 68–75.

Finney, P. D. (1978). Personality traits attributed to risky and conservative decision-makers: Culture values more than risk. *Journal of Psychology, 99,* 187–197.

Freedman, R. J. (1984). Reflections on beauty as it relates to health in adolescent females. *Women and Health, 9,* 29–45.

Friedman, H. L. (1989). The health of adolescents: Beliefs and behavior. *Social Science and Medicine, 29,* 309–315.

Friedman, L. S., Lichtenstein, E., & Biglan, A. (1985). Smoking onset among teens: An empirical analysis of initial situations. *Addictive Behaviors, 10,* 1–13.

Giddon, D. B. (1983). Through the looking glasses of physicians, dentists, and patients. *Perspectives in Biology and Medicine, 26,* 451–458.

Goffman, E. (1959). *The presentation of self in everyday life.* New York: Doubleday.

Gold, R. S., Skinner, M. J., Grant, P. J., & Plummer, D. C. (1991). Situational factors and thought processes associated with unprotected intercourse in gay men. *Psychology and Health, 5,* 259–278.

Gritz, E. R., & Crane, L. A. (1991). Use of diet pills and ampethamines to lose weight among smoking and nonsmoking high school seniors. *Health Psychology, 10,* 330–335.

Gross, J., & Rosen, J. C. (1988). Bulimia in adolescents: Prevalence and psychological correlates. *International Journal of Eating Disorders, 7,* 51–61.

Guy, F., Rankin, B., & Norvell, M. (1980). The relation of sex-role stereotyping to body image. *Journal of Psychology, 105,* 167–173.

Hamm, P., Shekelle, R. B., & Stamler, J. (1989). Large fluctuations in body weight during young adulthood and twenty-five-year risk of coronary death in men. *American Journal of Epidemiology, 129,* 312–318.

Hanna, J. (1989, September 25). Sexual abandon: The condom is unpopular on the campus. *Maclean's.* p. 48.

Hart, E. A., Leary, M. R., & Rejeski, W. J. (1989). The measurement of social physique anxiety. *Journal of Sport and Exercise Psychology, 11,* 94–104.

Hayes, D., & Ross, C. E. (1987). Concern with appearance, health beliefs, and eating habits. *Journal of Health and Social Behavior, 28,* 120–130.

Henig, R. M. (1989, October). Health. *Vogue, 179,* p. 294.

Herold, E. S. (1981). Contraceptive embarrassment and contraceptive behavior among young single women. *Journal of Youth and Adolescence, 10,* 233–242.

Herold, E. S., Goodwin, M. S., & Lero, D. S. (1979). Self-esteem, locus of control, and adolescent contraception. *Journal of Psychology, 101,* 83–88.

Hong, L. K. (1978). Risky shift and cautious shift: Some direct evidence on the culture-value theory. *Journal of Social Psychology, 41,* 342–346.

Janz, N. K., & Becker, H. M. (1984). The health belief model: A decade later. *Health Education Quarterly, 11,* 1–47.

Jeffrey, R. W. (1989). Risk behaviors and health: Contrasting individual and population perspectives. *American Psychologist, 44,* 1194–1202.

Jonah, B. A. (1990). Age differences in risky driving. *Health Education Research, 5,* 139–149.

Jones, E. E., & Berglas, S. (1978). Control of attributions about the self through self-handicapping strategies: The appeal of alcohol and the role of underachievement. *Personality and Social Psychology Bulletin, 4,* 200–206.

Jones, E. E., & Pittman, T. S. (1982). Toward a general theory of strategic self-presentation. In J. Suls (Ed.), *Psychological perspectives on the self* (Vol. 1, pp. 231–262). Hillsdale, NJ: Erlbaum.

Jones, J. L., & Leary, M. R. (1994). Effects of appearance-based admonitions against sun exposure on tanning intentions in young adults. *Health Psychology, 13,* 86–90.

Kandel, D. B. (1980). Drug and drinking behavior among youth. *Annual Review of Sociology, 6,* 235–285.

Katzman, M. A., & Wolchik, S. A. (1984). Bulimia and binge eating in college women: A comparison of personality and behavioral characteristics. *Journal of Consulting and Clinical Psychology, 52,* 423–428.

Keesling, B., & Friedman, H. S. (1987). Psychosocial factors in sunbathing and sunscreen use. *Health Psychology, 6,* 427–428.

Kisker, E. E. (1985). Teenagers talk about sex, pregnancy, and contraception. *Family Planning Perspectives, 17,* 83–90.

Klesges, R. C., & Klesges, L. M. (1988). Cigarette smoking as a dietary strategy in a university population. *International Journal of Eating Disorders, 7,* 413–417.

Klesges, R. C., Meyers, A. W., Klesges, L. M., & LaVasque, M. E. (1989). Smoking, body weight, and their effects on smoking behavior: A comprehensive review of the literature. *Psychological Bulletin, 106,* 204–230.

Klohn, L. S., & Rogers, R. W. (1991). Dimensions of the severity of a health threat: The persuasive effects of visibility, time of onset, and rate of onset on young women's intentions to prevent osteoporosis. *Health Psychology, 10*, 323–329.

Kolditz, T. A., & Arkin, R. M. (1982). An impression management interpretation of the self-handicapping strategy. *Journal of Applied Social Psychology, 43.*

Kowalski, R. M., & Brown, K. (in press). Psychosocial barriers to cervical cancer screening. *Journal of Applied Social Psychology.*

Leary, M. R. (1983). *Understanding social anxiety: Social, personality, and clinical perspectives.* Beverly Hills, CA: Sage.

Leary, M. R. (1992). Self-presentational processes in exercise and sport. *Journal of Sport and Exercise Psychology, 14*, 339–351.

Leary, M. R. (1993). The interplay of private self-processes and interpersonal factors in self-presentation. In J. Suls (Ed.). *Psychological perspectives on the self* (Vol. 4. pp. 127–155). Hillsdale, NJ: Erlbaum.

Leary, M. R. (1994). *Self-presentation: Impression management and social behavior.* Dubuque, IA: Brown & Benchmark.

Leary, M. R., & Dobbins, S. E. (1983). Social anxiety, sexual behavior, and contraceptive use. *Journal of Personality and Social Psychology, 45*, 1347–1354.

Leary, M. R., & Jones, J. L. (1993). The social psychology of tanning and sunscreen use: Self-presentational motives as a predictor of health risk. *Journal of Applied Social Psychology, 23*, 1390–1406.

Leary, M. R., & Kowalski, R. M. (1990). Impression management: A literature review and two-component model. *Psychological Bulletin, 107*, 34–47.

Leary, M. R., & Kowalski, R. M. (in press). *Butterflies, blushes, and bashfulness: Social anxiety and interpersonal behavior.* New York: Guilford Press.

Lees, S. (1986). *Losing out: Sexuality and adolescent girls.* London: Hutchinson.

Leonard, K. E., & Blane, H. T. (1988). Alcohol expectancies and personality characteristics in young men. *Addictive Behaviors, 13*, 353–357.

Lindquist, C. U., Lindsay, J. S., & White, G. D. (1979). Assessment of assertiveness in drug abusers. *Journal of Clinical Psychology, 35*, 676–679.

Lissner, L., Odell, P. M., D'Agostino, R. B., Stokes, J., Kreger, B. E., Belanger, A. J., & Brownell, K. D. (1991). Variability in body weight and health outcomes in the Framingham population. *New England Journal of Medicine, 324*, 1839–1844.

MacKinnon, D. P., Johnson, C. A., Pentz, M. A., Dwyer, J. H., Hansen, W. B., Flay, B. R., & Wang, E. Y. (1991). Mediating mechanisms in a school-based drug prevention program: First-year effects of the Midwestern Prevention Project. *Health Psychology, 10*,164–172.

Markova, I., Wilkie, P. A., Naji, S. A., & Forbes, C. D. (1990). Knowledge of HIV/AIDS and behavioural change of people with haemophilia. *Psychology and Health, 4*, 125–133.

Mermelstein, R. J., & Riesenberg, L. A. (1992). Changing knowledge and attitudes about skin cancer risk factors in adolescents. *Health Psychology, 11*, 371–376.

Miller, A. G., Ashton, W. A., McHoskey, J. W., & Gimbel, J. (1990). What price attractiveness? Stereotype and risk factors in suntanning behavior. *Journal of Applied Social Psychology, 20*, 1272–1300.

Miller, L. C., & Cox, C. L. (1982). For appearances' sake Public self-consciousness and make-up use. *Personality and Social Psychology Bulletin, 8*, 748–751.

Miller, R. S. (1986). Embarrassment: Causes and consequences. In W. H. Jones, J. M. Cheek, & S. R. Briggs (Eds.). *Shyness: Perspectives on research and treatment* (pp. 295–311). New York: Plenum Press.

Miller, R. S., & Leary, M. R. (1992). Social sources and interaction functions of emotion: The case of embarrassment. In M. S. Clark (Ed.). *Emotion and social behavior* (pp. 202–221). Beverly Hills, CA: Sage.

Millman, M. (1980). *Such a pretty face: Being fat in America.* New York: Berkley Press.

Mori, D., Chaiken, S., & Pliner, P. (1987). "Eating lightly" and the self-presentation of femininity. *Journal of Personality and Social Psychology, 53*, 693–702.

Nasser, M. (1988). Eating disorders: The cultural dimension. *Social Psychiatry and Psychiatric Epidemiology, 23*, 184–187.

Page, R. M., & Gold, R. S. (1983). Assessing gender differences in college cigarette smoking intenders and nonintenders. *Journal of School Health, 53*, 531–535.

 Article Review Form at end of book.

Why are clear definitions of sexual harassment needed?
What is an example of sexual harassment on campus?

Addressing Sexual Harassment on Campus

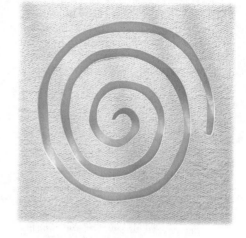

Jonathan Holub

ERIC Clearinghouse for Community Colleges
Los Angeles, California

Although statistical data on the incidence of sexual harassment at community colleges are limited, two things are clear. First, sexual harassment does occur on community college campuses. Second, it is obviously in serious conflict with the college's educational mission, and must be addressed and eliminated.

A definition of sexual harassment varies depending on context. Ethical perspectives can dictate a definition that is somewhat broader than a legal definition. However, legal and ethical definitions overlap and are constantly evolving pursuant to current developments on campuses, in industry, and in the courts. This Digest examines the need for clear definitions in order to address the problem of sexual harassment and discusses some of the remedies being implemented to create and maintain an hospitable educational community for all students.

Community colleges, as integral members of the higher education system, must address the realities of sexual harassment with the utmost seriousness, or they will face the inevitable consequences of costly litigation, public embarrassment, and the unacceptable degradation of students, staff, and faculty.

What Constitutes Sexual Harassment?

One important definition of sexual harassment is provided by the Equal Employment Opportunity Commission "sexual harassment consists of verbal or physical conduct of a sexual nature, imposed on the basis of sex . . . that denies, limits, or provides different . . . treatment." (Dey, Korn, and Sax, 1996). An example of what is considered sexual harassment at institutions of higher learning comes from this excerpt from the University of Iowa's Sexual Harassment Policy:

- Physical assault: physical touching of any kind that is sexual in nature.

- Direct or implied threats that submission to sexual advances may favorably affect employment, work status, promotion, grades, or letters of recommendation, or that rejection of sexual advances may produce a negative effect.

- Direct propositions of a sexual nature.

- Subtle pressure for sexual activity, one element of which may be conduct such as repeated or unwanted staring.

- A pattern of conduct that tends to bring discomfort and/or humiliation, which may include comments of a sexual nature, or sexually explicit jokes, statements, questions, or anecdotes.

- A pattern of conduct that would tend to bring discomfort or humiliation to a reasonable person at whom the conduct was directed, which may include unnecessary touching, patting, hugging, or brushing against a person's clothing or body, or remarks about sexual activity or speculations about previous sexual experience.

Source: From Jonathan Holub, "Addressing Sexual Harassment on Campus", in *ERIC DIGEST*, June 1996, ERIC Clearinghouse for Community Colleges, Los Angeles, CA.

Some of these acts are offenses punishable by law. Others relate to ethical considerations of the academic workplace. All behaviors mentioned can result in costly civil action.

In the legal arena, recent developments have dictated that colleges and universities create clear policies to deal with alleged incidents of sexual harassment. Title IX of the Educational Amendments of 1972 requires institutions to establish documents that enumerate the policies and procedures to be followed in cases of alleged sexual harassment of students.

A range of behaviors can lead to sexual harassment, especially where issues of power held by virtue of gender, rank (i.e., interaction between senior faculty and administrative staff), or role (i.e., faculty and student) create an unequal relationship. Harassment occurs when behavior is based on a quid pro quo relationship—for example, a professor promises a better grade to a student in return for an intimate or sexual relationship. Another category of harassment behavior creates a hostile environment for an individual. The Supreme Court, in a 1986 case (Meriter Savings Bank, FSB v. Vinson) defined sexual harassment as "unwelcome sexual advances, requests for sexual favors, and other verbal or physical conduct of a sexual nature . . . when (1) submission to or rejection of such conduct is made explicitly a term or condition of an individual's employment, (2) submission to or rejection of such conduct by an individual is used as the basis of employment decisions affecting such individual, or (3) such conduct has the purpose or effect of unreasonably interfering with an individual's work performance or creating an intimidating or offensive working environment." This definition, when applied to the academic realm, has obvious and powerful implications for many types of relationships within academia.

Harassment can result from both welcome and unwelcome acts and can involve persons in both lateral and vertical professional relationships. For example, a professor and an adult student may have a consensual sexual relationship. Despite the fact that the relationship is legal in the eyes of the law by virtue of its consensual nature, many colleges are adopting the stance that it is nonetheless unethical behavior on the part of the professor, given the inequity of power in the relationship.

Remedies

The American Council on Education (ACE) has stated that each "institution has the obligation for moral as well as legal reasons, to develop policies, procedures, and programs that protect students and employees from sexual harassment and to establish an environment in which such unacceptable behavior will not be tolerated" (p. 2). ACE endorses the following five elements as potentially beneficial when creating effective sexual harassment policies and procedures:

1. A definition of sexual harassment.

2. A strong policy statement indicating intolerance of sexual harassment.

3. Effective communication with those involved or with those subject to the provisions.

4. Education for everyone.

5. An accessible grievance procedure (Dozier, 1990; Wagner, 1990)

There is evidence to indicate that the implementation of a policy which integrates the above elements will have a noticeable effect on the incidence of sexual harassment on campus. A study conducted by Williams, Lam, and Shivery at the University of Massachusetts at Amherst (1992) states: ". . . the evidence suggests that the [decline in] reports of sexual harassment of women students by University faculty and staff represents a real change in the behavior of University employees, and this change most likely occurred in response to the University's sexual harassment policy and grievance procedure" (p. 61). The study indicates that those schools that report decreased incidents of sexual harassment have made creating awareness of the problem a top priority. The change in behavior occurring "in response" to the University of Massachusetts at Amherst's policy, for example, is possible only when people in the academic community are made aware that policies and procedures exist.

Conclusion

Recent developments in addressing the issue of sexual harassment makes two things very clear for colleges and universities: neither society at large, nor the legal system, will tolerate a passive approach to curbing sexual harassment on campus. It is imperative that community colleges make concerted efforts to address and remedy sexual harassment within their classrooms and offices—not just to avoid the threat of social stigma or legal proceedings, but to protect the integrity of the institution and the well-being of its students, faculty, and staff. Experience suggests that the best method for approaching the issue of sexual harassment at community colleges is to develop clear and respected policies for dealing with complaints and, most importantly, educating the entire campus community about sexual harassment and its consequences.

References

Most of the material for the Digest was drawn from "Sexual Harassment in Higher Education: From Conflict to Community." ASHE-ERIC Higher Education Reports—Report Two by Robert O. Riggs, Patricia H. Murrell, and Joann C. Cutting, 1993.
Other sources cited:

Dey, E. L., J. Korn, and L. Sax. "Betrayed by the Academy: The Sexual Harassment of Women College Faculty." *Journal of Higher Education 67* (2): 1996.

Dozier, J. "Sexual Harassment: It Can Happen Here." *AGB Reports 32* (1): 1990, 15–20.

Meriter Savings Bank FSB v. Vinson. 477 U.S. 57, 106 S. Ct. 2399 (1986).

University of Iowa. *The University of Iowa Policy on Sexual Harassment and Consensual Relationships.* Iowa City: University of Iowa, 1991.

Wagner, K. "Prevention and Intervention: Developing Campus Policies and Procedures." *Initiatives: Journal of the National Association for Women Deans, Administrators, and Counselors 52* (4): 1990, 37–45.

Williams, E. A., J. A. Lam and M. Shivley. "The Impact of a University Policy on the Sexual Harassment of Female Students." *Journal of Higher Education 63*(1): 1992.

 Article Review Form at end of book.

How will the tobacco settlement change the marketing of tobacco products?

Ifs, Ands and Butts

Anti-tobacco forces have achieved a huge victory. But is it enough to stub out smoking in America?

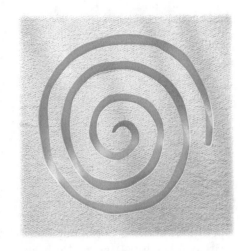

Matthew Cooper

Spread out in their pastel-toned conference rooms at a Washington Park Hyatt hotel last week, the tobacco lobbyists were grumpy. As they negotiated with state attorneys general, they'd already had to swallow a thick cloud of concessions. A so-called global settlement would force them to shell out $368 billion for the medical ravages of smoking, bid farewell to Joe Camel, slap warning labels the size of Texas on their products and accept more speech restrictions than Howard Stern. Adding insult to injury was the room-service crisis. The chocolate torte and grilled chicken that tobacco-company lobbyists had arrayed for themselves were getting nibbled away by the opposing attorneys general. "One more price to pay," sighed a tobacco ally.

By the time they emerged, the anti-tobacco forces seemed to have had their torte and eaten it, too. The deal struck last week between 40 state attorneys general and the tobacco industry marked

an American *pere-stroika*, not a complete collapse of the smoking industry but a historic turning point. The tobacco companies agreed to pony up $368 billion to defray the smoking-related medical costs shouldered by states. They'd stomach a new culture of marketing: no ads with pictures, no vending machines, no sports promotion. In exchange, the tobacco companies would get limited immunity from lawsuits and, above all, the state A.G.s would remove their 40 pending suits. We "have changed the world," said Matt Myers of the Campaign for Tobacco-Free Kids, perhaps America's leading anti-smoking advocate.

Not yet, of course: Congress must sign on to this Rube Goldberg contraption. And that is no sure thing. Congressional liberals are eager to get out their "editing pencils," says Sen. Ron Wyden, an Oregon Democrat. On the right, Newt Gingrich scolded that the settlement is a Marshall Plan for Democratic-leaning trial

lawyers. (Hard to argue with that: lots of lawyers will get rich off the deal.) And the anti-smoking community is divided on the agreement, sometimes to comic effect. While the American Heart Association said it was "encouraged" by the agreement, the American Lung Association trashed it. Still, no one could deny the agreement's magnitude. Some 32 years after the surgeon general slapped warnings on cigarette packs, anti-tobacco forces had achieved their greatest victory. "The Marlboro Man," said Florida Attorney General Bob Butterworth, "will be riding into the sunset on Joe Camel." Indeed, if there was any romance left to tobacco, it was, on a June day, snuffed out.

If the deal survives congressional scrutiny, the fallout will affect all Americans—whether they light up or not. The nation's 45 million smokers can expect higher prices—up to a buck a pack, more than $500 annually for a carton-a-week habit. Taxpayers will see billions flow into state coffers—money to defray the medical costs of treating smokers. Another proviso, albeit a shaky one: tobacco companies will provide money for health insurance for children who now lack it. Philip Morris meets Ira Magaziner.

Despite the monumental deal, the impact on the nation's businesses is likely to be limited. Tobacco ads account for about 1 percent of the nation's advertising spending, and the companies can still pitch cigarettes as long as they avoid models or gimmicks like Joe Camel. Some outlets will suffer. Since the agreement bans tobacco billboards, the outdoor-advertising industry takes a disproportionate hit. And sporting events like auto and boat racing will lose reliable sponsors. (What now? "The Charmin 500"?) Since convenience stores get 26 percent of their revenue from tobacco, they're nervously watching the deal, hoping there's no drop in cigarette sales. It won't help them that all "points of sale" advertising will go. Cigarettes will be sold a bit like condoms were 20 years ago—a bit hard to find, and if the activists prevail, embarrassing to ask for.

Still, to the chagrin of some activists, much will not change. This is hardly Prohibition. Multinational tobacco will still be in business, free to peddle its wares in the United States and overseas, where billions of virgin lungs await. (Caps, knapsacks, billboards, vending machines and sexy models will be banished in America but can stay abroad.) "It's immoral to call this a 'global settlement'," says perennial activist Ralph Nader, "when these companies can continue their brutal marketing and advertising to hundreds of millions of teenagers and young people around the world." And

their profits may not even be affected that much. The deal is estimated to cost the tobacco companies close to $15 billion annually for 25 years, about twice their domestic profits last year. Yet tobacco stocks rose as the agreement approached, dipping only modestly after the ink was dry.

How did all this come to pass? It's the stuff of a John Grisham screenplay. For years, tobacco was Goliath. Sure, smoking had steadily declined since World War II, falling from half of American adults in the 1950s to a quarter today. Still, tobacco remained largely unfettered. While regulatory agencies took occasional slaps, like the Federal Communications Commission's 1971 ban on TV tobacco ads, elected officials mostly kept hands off Big Tobacco. And in the courts, the tobacco companies seemed to have it all over any "My Cousin Vinny" litigator who took them on. In 1988 the industry lost a rare one—the case of Rose Cipollone, a smoker who died of cancer. But the $400,000 settlement granted her estate was overturned.

That all changed with the arrival of the Mississippi crusaders. The very idea of a Mississippi anti-smoking movement seemed about as likely as an anti-bourbon crusade in Kentucky. But in 1994 Michael Moore, the state's attorney general, teamed with his law-school classmate, Dick Scruggs, a rangy Mississippi trial lawyer. This time, instead of suing just on behalf of individual plaintiffs, they championed taxpayers who had lost billions paying for Medicare and Medicaid treatments for smokers. The distinction was crucial. While juries were tempted to blame individual smokers when they went to trial—*after all, they chose to smoke!*—they tended to be much more sympa-

thetic to cases brought by a state. The jurors were, after all, taxpayers themselves. Among those helping the legal team: the ubiquitous Dick Morris, the erstwhile political consultant. Morris's polling showed that potential jurors had much more empathy when the case was about damages done to a state. What now seems brilliant, of course, seemed kooky at the time—akin to taking on the candy industry for a state's dental bills. Most Mississippi pols thought Moore was a nut; the governor denounced him. Notably, one pol didn't criticize Moore: Mississippi Sen. Trent Lott, Scrugg's brother-in-law and, at the time, Morris's client.

As they now readily acknowledge, circumstances helped Scruggs and Moore. The crusading of public officials like former Food and Drug Administration head David Kessler and ex-surgeon general C. Everett Koop scared the tobacco companies. The FDA made moves to regulate tobacco and, incredibly, a supposedly tobacco-friendly judge in North Carolina upheld the agency—a move that could allow the Feds to force disclosure of cigarette ingredients or even ban them altogether. Suddenly the courts weren't such a friendly forum for Big Tobacco. Not surprisingly, other state attorneys general caught the wave. (Most have higher aspirations; Bill Clinton was once an attorney general.) Massachusetts' Scott Harshbarger, who will run for governor in a heated primary against Joe Kennedy, joined the suit. When Dan Lungren, California's attorney general and an aspiring gubernatorial candidate, dithered about climbing aboard, he was lambasted at home. He signed on. Suddenly, by the summer of 1996, Goliath wanted to settle.

The $368 Billion Deal

It was years in the making , and its fate is far from certain, but the settlement reached by American's tobacco manufacturers and 40 states would affect everything from how cigarettes are advertised to how they are sold. A look at the plan's highlights:

Punitive Damages

The companies would pay $50 billion, and in return further punitive-damage awards would be barred. Much of the money would probably go to health programs, such as insurance for children in need. And although individuals would still be able to sue the companies for compensatory damages, class-action lawsuits for past tobacco-company actions would be banned.

Other Annual Payments

After smaller payments in the first years of the settlement, the companies would pay an average of $15 billion a year until 2022—and possibly beyond—to help pay for treatment of illnesses and fight smoking . The money would roughly break down like this:

- $5 billion a year available for smokers who have sued for illness, death and legal fees. Each individual smoker could receive no more than $1 million a year.
- $5 billion for the 40 states that brought the lawsuit against the tobacco industry, to cover Medicaid costs
- $1.5 billion to fund state and federal anti-smoking campaigns and research into addiction, and to compensate sports events that lose tobacco sponsors
- $1.5 billion for programs to help smokers kick the habit

Advertising and Education

The companies would have to pay for anti-tobacco advertising and would have no control over the campaigns' content. In addition:

- Cigarette-vending machines would be banned
- Tobacco products would have to be placed behind store counters
- Advertisements would have to be in black and white and would have to be text only—except in adult establishments and publications
- All tobacco billboards, store signs that face the outside, and outdoor signs, including those in enclosed stadiums, would be eliminated
- All human images and cartoon characters (like the Marlboro Man and Joe Camel) on advertising and packaging would be eliminated
- All Internet ads, product placement in movies and merchandise with brand names and logos would be eliminated

Regulation

- The agreement would formally give the Food and Drug Administration regulatory authority over tobacco products. The FDA could recognize nicotine as a drug, reduce the amount of it in cigarettes and completely ban it in 2009. Cigarettes would come with tough new warnings such as SMOKING CAN KILL YOU and SMOKING CAUSES CANCER. Smoking in public places, workplaces and fast-food restaurants would be banned. In addition, cigarette makers would have to disclose ingredients and additives. And the companies would have to reveal past and future data an health effects, toxicity and addiction.

Reaching Out to Kids

The proposal demands that tobacco companies play a role in cutting smoking among youths and identifies specific targets for reductions. Within five years the number of youths smoking would have to drop by 30 percent. In seven years it would have to fall 50 percent. And in 10 years after the agreement is signed, the number would have to fall by 60 percent. Failure to meet these targets would result in fines starting in 2002, with companies paying $80 million for each percentage point they are off target.

Enforcement

Tobacco companies would be responsible for funding enforcement costs for both the FDA and state authorities. And any tobacco company that violated FDA rules would face penalties 10 times higher than the FDA fines other companies now face. The proposal demands that states meet strict numerical criteria in terms of cutting cigarette sales to minors. In addition, states would have the authority to adopt laws that are tougher than the federal standard.

The first efforts at a deal ended with the two sides wide apart. But earlier this year the talks began in earnest behind closed doors in Dallas, New York, Washington and Chicago. The attorneys general had the upper hand. A telling moment: after one meeting in New York, when tobacco companies offered a particularly puny settlement offer, Arizona A. G. Grant Woods stood up and said: "It's been nice working with you." The tobacco companies backed down and the negotiations resumed.

The decisive talks came last week, as negotiators gathered in two Washington hotels on opposite sides of the street. To tobacco companies made concession after concession in talks that ran from 9 p.m. to 3 a.m. At one point, Moore was so tired that he could barely push open the plate-glass door to his hotel's entrance. An aide had to help him. A cultural barometer: in the ultimate back-room deal, no one smoked.

On Friday, the deal was almost at hand when the two sides hit a snag: what about Jeffrey Wigand? The whistle-blower was responsible for exposing evidence showing that tobacco companies knew about the addictive nature of their wares. Brown & Williamson, Wigand's former employer, wanted to continue its prosecution of Wigand for exposing company materials. The state attorneys general, motivated by sympathy and politics—how could they abandon a martyr?—demanded amnesty for Wigand. After about an hour, Ron Motley, an anti-tobacco lawyer, formed the language to absolve Wigand. Applause went up. The deal was done.

Now the action moves from the hotel to the Hill. Can this deal get past a skeptical Congress? The odds are pretty good that it can, in some form. Despite the huffing and puffing of liberals, they're un-

likely to get a better deal. And while Big Tobacco still has political muscle, it's better off with the settlement than without it. "A bitter pill," said one Philip Morris executive, but one worth taking. Interestingly, one of the key players on Capitol Hill expressed cautious optimism about the deal. Thomas Bliley, the head of the House Commerce Committee, who represents Philip Morris's Richmond, Va., expressed openness to the deal. Insiders think Lott will embrace the deal too. And while the White House will scrutinize the pact—Donna Shalala, whose Health and Human Services was cut out of the entire process, is said to be eager to make her mark—can anyone imagine a lip-biting Bill Clinton resisting a Rose Garden ceremony declaring the end of the Tobacco Cold War?

Real questions about the impact of the agreement remain. Will the tobacco companies find loopholes? One of the provisions demands steady reductions in youth smoking but threatens "lookback" penalties that may be too small to do any good. The extent of the FDA's jurisdiction over tobacco

and nicotine content are sketchy. Even the attorneys general acknowledge that the proof will be in the numbers of lives saved. Still, they defend the deal, insisting it was better than slogging along in the courts. "If the lawsuits kept going," Moore told NEWSWEEK, "the companies would have gone Chapter 11 but come back clean as Clorox. Those who say you should never deal with the Devil have their heads in the sand."

It's ironic that the tobacco deal comes in the age of William Rehnquist (and even Ruth Ginsburg), when courts aren't supposed to be legislating policy. And yet, it was the courts that forced this change. That it began with a few Mississippi lawyers makes it still more improbable. And it's fitting that this deal comes at the end of the century. The cigarette belongs to the 20th century, popularized by World War I, billed as a modern, convenient way for doughboys to light up in the trenches. By 2000, that image may seem a distant memory.

 Article Review Form at end of book.

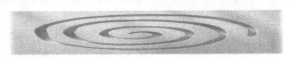

WiseGuide Wrap-Up

- Knowing your ethnic background and personal family health history and other health information can alert you to take appropriate preventive health measures.

- Protect yourself from making medication errors and inappropriate health behavior decisions by being an active and informed partner with your healthcare professional.

- You can foster positive well-being by examining and rejecting factors that influence risky health behaviors.

R.E.A.L. Sites

The adjacent list provides a print preview of typical **coursewise** R.E.A.L. Sites. (There are over 100 such sites at the **courselinks**™ site.) The danger in printing URLs is that web sites can change overnight. As we went to press, these sites were functional using the URLs provided. If you come across one that isn't, please let us know via email at webmaster@coursewise.com. Use your Passport to access the most current list of R.E.A.L. sites at the **courselinks**™ site.

Site name: The Web as a Research Tool: Evaluation Techniques
URL: http://www.science.widener.edu/~withers/evalout.htm
Why is it R.E.A.L.? Provides opportunities to critique the WWW as a source of information. Fosters critical thinking skills with online instruction on how to evaluate.
Key topics: activism and advocacy, evaluation
Activity: Critique one of the websites listed in this book according to the criteria set forth.

Site name: healthfinder
URL: http://www.healthfinder.gov
Why is it R.E.A.L.? Extensive searchable database of reliable online health publications, clearinghouses, web sites, self-help groups, government agencies, and nonprofit agencies. A gateway site on consumer health information with links to over 550 web sites and 500 selected documents as well as frequently asked health questions. Developed by DHHS Office of Disease Prevention and Health Promotion.
Key topics: consumer health, general health and well-being, self-help
Activity: Take a tour of the website then send your feedback to the website developers. Also, use this site to narrow your health topic for a term paper.

Site name: You First
URL: http://www.youfirst.com/
Why is it R.E.A.L.? Highly personalized, confidential and interactive opportunity to determine your health risks with free online health risk appraisal. Links to seasonal health tips, America's health risks, top 10 causes of death, and frequently asked questions.
Key topics: risk factors, self-assessment
Activity: Find out what a health risk appraisal is and what it can be used for. What are your personal health risks?

Site name: Action on Smoking and Health
URL: http://ash.org
Why is it R.E.A.L.? Anti-smoking activist web site that provides specific strategies for decreasing smoking behavior in America and protecting the rights of nonsmokers.
Key topics: tobacco, community agency, activism, advocacy
Activity: Gather enough information to be able to debate either pro or con for a ban on all advertising of tobacco.

Site name: Prevline: Prevention Hotline and National Clearinghouse for Alcohol and Drug Information
URL: http://www.health.org/
Why is it R.E.A.L.? Provides a comprehensive database of alcohol and drug information and links.
Key topics: alcohol and drugs, governmental agency, health statistics
Activity: Use this site to begin your research for term papers on alcohol and drug topics.

....

Site name: Facts about Sexual Harassment
URL: http://www.feminist.org/911/sexharfacts.html
Why is it R.E.A.L.? Practical information for those dealing with sexual harassment issues.
Key topics: sexual harassment
Activity: What should you do if you are sexually harassed according to "911"?

....

Site name: National Library of Medicine
URL: http://www.nlm.nih.gov
Why is it R.E.A.L.? Comprehensive medical information available along with free access to the Medline literature search engine.
Key topics: medicine, governmental agency
Activity: Use Medline to conduct a literature search on a fitness or nutrition topic.

....

Site name: National Center for Health Statistics
URL: http://www.cdc.gov/nchswww/nchshome.htm
Why is it R.E.A.L.? Searchable database of health data, charts, tables, and statistics. Includes answers to frequently asked questions about the health status of Americans.
Key topics: governmental agency, health statistics
Activity: Go to "Frequently Asked Questions" to find out what percentage of adults engage in smoking, experience stress, and excercise regularly.

....

Site name: The Longevity Game
URL: http://www.northwesternmutual.com/games/longevity/
Why is it R.E.A.L.? The Northwestern Mutual Insurance Company sponsors this highly interactive opportunity for self-discovery related to health risk factors.
Key topics: health insurance, health statistics, risk factors
Activity: Play the Longevity Game and find out your estimated longevity. What insights do the results give you about your health status and behavior?

....

Site name: Guide to Locating Health Statistics
URL: http://www.hsls.pitt.edu/intres/guides/statcbw.html
Why is it R.E.A.L.? Provides a gateway to sites on health statistics.
Key topics: health statistics
Activity: Find and print the census data for your zip code. What does the data tell you about the health status of people who live near you?

....

Site name: American Psychological Association
URL: http://www.apa.org/pubinfo/
Why is it R.E.A.L.? The American Psychological Association is a professional organization for those working in the mental health field. Reliable source of mental health information.
Key topics: professional organization, mental health, self-assessment
Activity: Use one of the many self-assessment tools available to find out more about yourself. What will you do with this information?

....

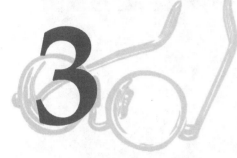

section 3

Key Points

- Various health conditions and emotional circumstances may threaten your sexual well-being.

- Your choice of contraceptive method needs to be reconsidered whenever changes occur in your life.

- Women with unplanned pregnancy tend to have more health problems related to pregnancy than women do with planned pregnancy.

- Safer sex practices are not always well understood by those at increased risk of contracting a sexually transmitted disease.

- Few health differences have been established between circumcised and uncircumcised men.

- Over-the-counter feminine products may harm women.

- Negative attitudes toward homosexuals can impact the health of gays and lesbians.

Sexual and Reproductive Health

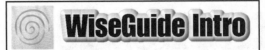 **WiseGuide Intro**

Maintaining healthy sexuality in the United States today is complicated and challenging. With the decline of adherence to traditional sex roles associated with contemporary social norms, clear guidelines for appropriate and acceptable sexual behavior no longer exist. With sexual freedom comes increased individual responsibility for health decision making and problem solving.

Your sexual health is best served by knowing how to differentiate established threats to sexual health, such as unsafe sex, unplanned pregnancy, and misuse of over-the-counter feminine hygiene products, from unsubstantiated risks, such as circumcision. An acceptance of your own sexuality and the sexuality of others can also contribute to well-being.

The articles in Section 3 were selected to highlight specific threats to sexual and reproductive health and the information needed to combat these threats. The first article ("Your Sexual Health in the 90s") identifies a number of common sexual health issues along with basic information about solutions. The next two articles ("Rethinking Birth Control" and "It's Not Only Mammographies and Menopause") address family planning difficulties, reminding us that, while these choices are hard to make, they are necessary to good reproductive health. Two other articles ("Misunderstanding of Safer Sex by Heterosexually Active Adults" and "Circumcision in the United States") report on studies that demonstrate that common perceptions of sexual health risk, whether regarding safer sex or circumcision, may not be accurate. The remaining two articles ("Feminine Needs" and "Homophobia Is a Health Hazard") describe how misperceptions can have health consequences.

Questions

R12. What is one of the most common sexual complaints today? What are some threats to sexual well-being?

R13. What are six reasons to switch contraceptive methods? Which group has a higher rate of unplanned pregnancies: women in their 20s or 40s?

R14. What are some of the repercussions of unplanned pregnancy?

R15. What does the term "safer sex" refer to, according to Wenger, Kusseling, and

Shapiro? How does a misunderstanding of the term "safer sex" place people at increased risk of contracting a sexually transmitted disease?

R16. Which group of men is more likely to contract sexually transmitted diseases: circumcised or uncircumcised?

R17. How can the use of over-the-counter feminine products harm women?

R18. What is homophobia? How is homophobia harmful to the health of gays and lesbians?

What is one of the most common sexual complaints today?
What are some threats to sexual well-being?

Your Sexual Health in the '90s

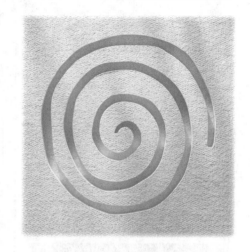

Derek C. Polonsky, M.D.

Dr. Polonsky is a psychiatrist at Boston's Beth Israel Hospital. He is on the faculty at Harvard Medical School and has a private practice in Brookline, Massachusetts. His most recent book, TALKING ABOUT SEX (Washington, D.C.: American Psychiatric Press, 1996), was reviewed in the December 1996 issue of HEALTHLINE.

The seamless sexual progression shown in the movies—where both people know automatically what to do, experience no uncertainty or worry, and never have any difficulties—rarely happens in real life. And yet for many people, this has become the unrealistic standard by which they measure themselves. Unrealistic expectations and performance anxiety, sexually transmitted diseases, and a variety of other physical and emotional problems may threaten your sexual well-being in the '90s.

People today must be more circumspect in their choices of partners and their behaviors than they were during the '60s and '70s. They need to be direct in discussing their sexual histories with prospective sexual partners. Each partner in a new relationship needs to know what risky behaviors the other has engaged in previously. Risky behaviors include having multiple sexual partners or unprotected oral, anal, or vaginal sex. The AIDS epidemic has made the use of latex condoms an essential precaution, and many couples today get tested for HIV before they have sex. These actions not only protect your health, but may lead to more rewarding relationships. Frank discussions can provide the opportunity to get to know your partner better before the relationship becomes sexual.

About half of all couples experience serious, long-term sexual difficulties at some point in their marriages. One of the most common sexual complaints today is inhibited sexual desire. In addition, 30 to 40 percent of women do not have orgasm with intercourse, and about 10 percent do not experience orgasm at all. Roughly 5 percent of women suffer with vaginismus (the involuntary contraction of the muscles around the vagina). Among men,

> **People today must be more circumspect in their choices of partners and their behaviors than they were during the '60s and '70s.**

almost 25 percent suffer with premature ejaculation and about 10 percent have erectile difficulties.

A history of childhood sexual abuse can cause sexual problems in adulthood. An estimated 20 to 25 percent of women and 10 to 15 percent of men were sexually abused as children. This prevalence of sexual abuse is well documented, and the aftermath in adulthood in terms of sexual difficulties can be profound. For survivors of childhood sexual abuse, treatment aims at helping people to reclaim their sexuality through the use of supportive and behavioral techniques. Antidepressant medication such as Prozac or Zoloft is sometimes helpful as well.

I frequently see couples with unconsummated marriages due to vaginismus, often stemming from early childhood sexual trauma. Behavioral techniques, relaxation approaches, and vaginal dilators have brought relief to many women with this problem. The behavioral approach to treating sexual difficulties, pioneered by Masters and Johnson, has proved to be extremely helpful for a variety of problems, including those caused by sexual trauma.

Many medications can have powerful effects on sexual functioning. Anyone who notices any change in sexual functioning that follows the use of a prescribed medication should ask a physician about the drug's known sexual side effects. Often, a change in medication can solve the problem.

Hormone imbalances are at the root of many sexual problems, and can be detected through a medical evaluation. It was long believed that arousal and erection problems were always psychological in nature, but it is clear now that hormonal imbalances can affect sexual performance. An endocrinologist, a physician who specializes in hormones, can assess and treat such problems.

For men with erectile difficulties, a number of possible medical problems need to be addressed. Smoking does major damage to blood vessels, and this affects the blood supply to the penis. (I have often thought that a warning on cigarette packages stating that "smoking can damage your penis" would have more impact than current warning labels.) Heavy drinking affects many organ systems, and may lead to diminished desire and erectile dysfunction. Erectile problems also can result when the penile valves are unable to hold an erection (venous leak syndrome). Sufferers appear to have performance anxiety (the man develops an erection, but loses it after intercourse begins), but the cause is physical. Such cases should be evaluated by a urologist.

Intrapenile injections have been helpful for many men with erectile problems, particularly older men. Although it sounds awful, injecting medication directly into the penis is not painful, and can produce a reliable erection that frees men and their partners from worries about "failure." Penile implants are a final option when other methods of treatment do not work.

Getting information can be an important part of changing sexual behavior. A number of books offer sound, commonsense approaches. My favorites are: *The New Male Sexuality*, by Bernie Zilbergeld (Bantam Press, 1992); *Male Sexual Awareness and Female Sexual Awareness,* by Emily and Barry McCarthy (Carol and Graff Publishers, 1988); *The Family Book About Sexuality*, by Mary S. Calderone and Eric Johnson (Harper & Row, 1990); and, of course, *On Sex and Human Loving,* by Masters and Johnson (Little, Brown & Co., 1988). A final book, *The Potent Male,* by Goldstein and Rothstein (The Body Press, 1990), is an excellent source of information about urological difficulties from a medical, surgical, and psychological perspective.

Self-help videos can be another good source of information, but be forewarned that many titles in this genre are merely pornographic films masquerading as "legitimate" teaching aids. Focus International has a collection of excellent teaching tapes that address such subjects as touching techniques, impotence, vaginismus, premature ejaculation, and approaches for women who are anorgasmic. Their catalog is available by calling (800) 843-0305.

Our sexual health is vital to our well-being. If you are worried about a sexual problem, help and information are available. Your family doctor, a trained sex therapist—and even the self-help section of your neighborhood bookstore—are all good places to start.

 Article Review Form at end of book.

What are six reasons to switch contraceptive methods?
Which group has a higher rate of unplanned pregnancies: women in
their 20's or 40's?

Rethinking Birth Control

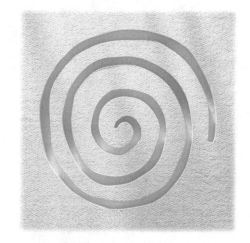

Julia Califano

Julia Califano is a writer in Hoboken, NJ.

If you still believe the IUD is dangerous and the Pill is for women under 35, you may be stuck in a contraception rut. Here's a roundup of the most effective methods for midlife women.

Through two years of dating, 10 years of marriage and two kids, Chris, a college professor in Syracuse, NY, relied almost exclusively on a diaphragm for birth control. Indeed, this 40-year-old would still be putting up with the hassle and mess if, at her last checkup, her doctor hadn't suggested she try an intrauterine device (IUD). Persuaded by his argument that it was highly effective, long-lasting and, for most women, nearly free of side effects, she switched. She hasn't regretted her decision. "It's such a pleasure not to have to plan ahead or get out of bed in the heat of passion," she says. "We don't even think about birth control anymore."

By the time a woman turns 35, she's moved an average of eight times, switched jobs seven times and had two children, yet there's only a 50-50 chance that she has ever thought about changing her method of birth control, according to a survey by Ortho Pharmaceutical. But the truth is she should. "A woman's contraceptive needs change as her life changes," says Anita Nelson, M.D., medical director of the Woman's Health Care Clinic at Harbor UCLA Medical Center in Los Angeles. "A barrier method may be great when you're 21 and concerned about AIDS and other sexually transmitted diseases [STD's], but it's probably not ideal when you're 35 and married with kids."

Perhaps more surprising is the staggering rate of unplanned pregnancies among women in their 40s: According to the Alan Guttmacher Institute in New York City, eight out of 10 pregnancies in this age group are unintended—the same rate as for women under age 20.

How can you tell if your current choice is still your best choice? Reassess your birth control periodically, taking your lifestyle, health, sex life and desire for children into consideration. Here's a guide to the options, plus expert advice on what to use when.

The IUD: Unfounded Fear

What it is: The current IUD of choice is ParaGard, a piece of plastic with copper inside it that's put into the uterus to stop sperm from reaching eggs for up to 10 years. Another IUD called Progestasert contains hormones; it works for one year.

Benefits: Long-term, reversible, worry-free protection, and an insertion process that's only slightly more involved than a Pap smear. Progestasert also reduces menstrual cramps and the flow of monthly bleeding.

Drawbacks: The copper IUD can cause heavier than usual periods, won't protect you from STD's and shouldn't be used if you're not in a mutually monogamous relationship. Users with multiple partners are at increased risk for pelvic inflammatory disease (PID), an infection that can cause infertility.

What you may not know: Though most people still associate this device with the dreaded Dalkon Shield (an IUD that caused infection and infertility in thousands of women, along with a few deaths, in the '70s),

ParaGard is considered one of the best and safest birth control options. In fact, it's the most popular form of reversible contraception outside the U.S., with 85 million users worldwide.

When to consider it: If you're in a mutually monogamous, long-term relationship and have had at least one child (for childless women there's a small risk that the device will be expelled). "An ideal time to switch to the IUD is when you've completed your family but don't want to take the irreversible step of sterilization," says nurse practitioner Kara Anderson, a medical consultant to the Planned Parenthood Federation of America in New York City.

The Pill: Now for Older Women

What it is: This oral contraceptive is a combination of two hormones, progestin and estrogen, that suppresses ovulation.

Benefits: Easy, reliable and offers a wealth of health benefits. After five years the Pill halves your risk of endometrial and ovarian cancers, an effect that, for endometrial cancer, may last as long as 15 years after you stop using it. [Experts aren't sure how long the protective effects last for ovarian cancer.] It also reduces the risk of benign breast lumps, ovarian cysts, iron-deficiency anemia and PID.

Drawbacks: Side effects include breast tenderness, nausea, weight gain and headaches (though these usually clear up after two to three months). The Pill must be taken every day, and it doesn't protect against STD's. In addition, studies show it increases the risk of heart attack and blood

Contraception 911

Condoms break, diaphragms slip and even the most responsible woman sometimes misses a Pill. The good news is that postcoital contraceptive options are expanding. An FDA advisory panel recently agreed unanimously that the Pill can safely be used as a morning-after contraceptive. The procedure—taking two doses of two or four pills each, depending on the brand, within 72 hours of unprotected sex—reduces the risk of pregnancy by 75%, though nausea and vomiting are common side effects. Several different Pill brands can be used; check with your doctor for specifics. Note: Don't try this on your own.

An emergency IUD insertion can also be done within five to seven days of unprotected sex and is more than 99% effective. Contact your doctor or Planned Parenthood, or call the new 24-hour Emergency Contraception Hotline (800-584-9911) for a list of doctors who provide emergency contraception in your area. You'll also find a list of local providers on the Internet at http://opr.princeton.edu/ec/.

Alternatives to surgical abortion are on the way. The long-awaited French abortion drug mifepristone, better known as RU 486, is expected to be available in this country later this year. The drug blocks progesterone and causes the uterus to discard its lining along with the implanted egg. It can be used up to nine weeks into pregnancy and may also be used as emergency birth control up to three days after unprotected sex, with fewer side effects than oral contraceptives.

On the horizon: Two FDA-approved drugs already on the market, methotrexate (a chemotherapy drug) and misoprostol (used to prevent stomach bleeding), induce abortion when combined. Since research is still limited on this method, few doctors use it, but that may soon change. Planned Parenthood has received FDA clearance for a large-scale clinical trial to test the technique's safety and effectiveness.

clots in women over 35 who smoke. Some studies have also shown that the Pill increases breast cancer risk, though a recent analysis of 150,000 users found this risk to be negligible. In most cases, say experts, the health benefits far outweigh the risks.

What you may not know: A study at San Francisco State University found that women who use triphasic pills such as Orthonovum 7/7/7 (in which hormone levels vary throughout the course of the month) experience heightened sex drive compared with women on other types of pills.

When to consider it: If you're in a committed relationship and want a highly effective form of contraception. Contrary to what many believe, the Pill can be ideal for fortysomething non-smoking women. It eases the transition to menopause, says David Grimes, M.D., vice chairman of the department of obstetrics and gynecology at the University of California at San Francisco. "The Pill helps regulate periods, prevent hot flashes and protect against bone loss," he explains.

Norplant: A Five-Year Plan

What it is: Six flexible, matchstick-sized capsules inserted by a doctor just beneath the skin of the upper arm. They release progestin to suppress ovulation for five years.

Benefits: It's effective and convenient—you can't mess up. Norplant is also easily reversible; after removal, any remaining drugs leave the body in about three days. In addition, experts believe Norplant may be as good as the Pill at reducing the risk of endometrial and ovarian cancer.

Drawbacks: Norplant won't protect you from STD's, and it can cause irregular bleeding during the first year. There have also been a number of lawsuits filed by Norplant users, primarily because of problems such as pain or scarring upon removal. Despite the bad press, experts say such problems shouldn't arise if you use an experienced doctor. (For referrals, call your local Planned Parenthood clinic.)

What you may not know: Norplant is very expensive if used for fewer than three years.

When to consider it: If you're breastfeeding (unlike estrogen in the Pill, progestin doesn't reduce milk flow) and plan to wait several years before having another child or if you've completed your family. You also may want to try it if you absolutely don't want to worry about an accidental pregnancy.

Depo-Provera: Convenience Without Long-Term Commitment

What it is: This injection of synthetic progestin suppresses ovulation for 11 to 13 weeks.

Benefits: Depo-Provera provides many of the health perks of the Pill, and you don't have to take it every day. After about a year, periods may stop completely, which many women consider a welcome side effect.

Drawbacks: Doctor's visits are required four times a year to get the shots, and the effects are not immediately reversible (fertility may not return for an average of 10 months after the last dose). Side effects may include headaches, weight gain, depression and heavier, more frequent periods. Depo-Provera also provides no protection against STD's.

Six Reasons to Switch

If you've been using the same contraceptive since college, it's probably time to take a fresh look at your birth control options. Here are some compelling reasons to reconsider your method:

1. **You've settled down with one partner.** Provided neither one of you has a sexually transmissible disease, you can switch from condoms to a method you both like better and will use consistently.

2. **Your health has changed.** If you develop heart disease, high blood pressure or diabetes, you should re-evaluate your current method with your doctor.

3. **You're breast-feeding.** Consider a nonhormonal contraceptive, such as condoms, a diaphragm or a copper intrauterine device (IUD), or a progestin-only method, such as the minipill, Norplant or Depo-Provera.

4. **You've completed your family.** Sterilization is only one long-term option. Also consider Norplant, Depo-Provera, the IUD and the Pill.

5. **You're contemplating pregnancy.** If you're on the Pill, doctors recommend stopping two to three months before conceiving to re-establish your natural cycle. If you use Depo-Provera, it can take up to a year after your last shot to conceive.

6. **You dislike your current method.** If you hate inserting your diaphragm or can't remember to take the Pill every day, don't grin and bear it—switch.

What you may not know: Though many American women **Women who use triphasic birth control pills report experiencing a heightened sex drive.** think of this method, approved here in 1992, as new, Depo-Provera has been used by more than 30 million women in 100 other countries over the past 30 years.

When to consider it: If you're nursing or trying to space out the arrival of new children, or you can't remember to take the Pill every day.

The Reality Female Condom:

Women in the Driver's Seat

What it is: The Reality Condom is a floppy polyurethane tube with an inner ring at the closed end that fits over the cervix, like a diaphragm, and an outer ring at the open end that hangs outside the vagina.

Benefits: Protection against AIDS and other STD's; more spontaneity than with male con-

doms, since it can be inserted in advance.

Drawbacks: It has about as much sex appeal as a sandwich bag.

What you may not know: The device is reputed to squeak during use (adding a little extra lubricant can alleviate this distraction).

When to consider it: If you're not in a stable relationship or you have a partner who refuses to wear a condom.

Tubal Ligation: No More Hassles

What it is: This surgical procedure blocks the fallopian tubes so that sperm and egg never meet.

Benefits: No-worry, contraceptive-free sex for the rest of your life. And, after the cost of the surgery ($1,000-$2,500), you'll never spend another dime on birth control.

Drawbacks: This procedure isn't foolproof: Though only five in 1,000 users become pregnant in the first year, surprisingly, over 10 years the failure rate is one in 50 (2%). And, as with any surgery, the procedure carries risks. Finally, depending on how it's done it can't easily be undone.

What you may not know: Sterilization is the most popular method of birth control in the U.S., chosen by a whopping 42% of contraceptive users.

When to consider it: If you're *sure* you don't want any more children.

The Mini-Pill: Fewer Annoying Side Effects

What it is: This pill contains no estrogen and a very small dose of progestin—hence the name.

Benefits: Since it contains no estrogen, the mini-pill has fewer side effects than the Pill and is not associated with any increased risk of blood clots or breast cancer. It also causes lighter than normal periods, making it a good choice for women who are anemic or who tend to bleed heavily. And it does-

n't require a waiting period to get pregnant after you stop taking it.

Drawbacks: It can cause irregular bleeding, offers no protection against STD's and has a significantly higher failure rate than combined oral contraceptives, particularly if you have trouble remembering to take a pill every day.

What you may not know: This method has almost no margin for error. Missing even one day can result in a pregnancy.

When to consider it: If you're nursing (which naturally reduces—but doesn't rule out—fertility); it also seems to slightly increase the quantity and quality of breast milk.

Barrier Methods: STD Protection

What they are: This group includes condoms; diaphragms and cervical caps used with spermicidal jellies or foam; inserts and film. All prevent sperm from reaching eggs.

Benefits: They're safe, cheap and available without a prescrip-

tion; barrier methods also guard against STD's. Latex condoms provide the best protection against the AIDS virus.

Drawbacks: They interfere with spontaneity and can be messy, and your partner may complain of lessened sensation during sex with condoms. Also, caps can be tricky to insert and diaphragms may increase the risk of urinary tract infections in women.

What you may not know: Lubricated condoms and spermicides help counteract vaginal dryness, a common perimenopausal and postpartum problem.

When to consider them: If you're breast-feeding, planning to get pregnant relatively soon or having sex infrequently. Condoms are the best choice if you want iron-clad protection against AIDS and other STD's. Barrier methods are also handy backups when you forget to take a Pill.

 Article Review Form at end of book.

What are some of the repercussions of unplanned pregnancy?

It's Not Only Mammographies and Menopause

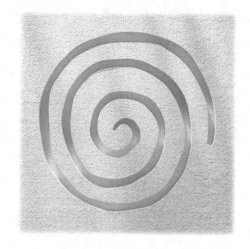

Margaret Comerford Freda

Margaret Comerford Freda, a member of the New York State Nurses Association, is an associate professor and director of patient education programs in the Department of Obstetrics and Gynecology and Women's Health, Albert Einstein College of Medicine, Montefiore Medical Center, Bronx, NY; director of education and community affairs for the Program to Reduce Obstetrical Problems and Prematurity at Albert Einstein; and an adjunct associate professor at Molloy College in Rockville Center, NY.

Everyone seems to be talking about mammographies and menopause these days. Finally, women's health has become a hot topic for policymakers. Issues ranging from hormone replacement therapy to the inclusion of women in clinical trials of drugs and other research have come to be recognized as vital areas of concern. Now it's time to add to this growing list another essential issue that must be addressed: unplanned pregnancy.

I venture to guess that for most people, the phrase "unplanned pregnancy" conjures up images of teenage pregnancy rates run amok. But did you know that 60% of *all* pregnancies

are unplanned? While the rates among teenagers are highest (82%), 50% of pregnancies among all women ages 20 to 34 and 40% of pregnancies among married women are unintended. These startling statistics speak volumes about how far we have yet to go in improving women's health in the United States.

The failure of the health system, and the country, to recognize and face this problem has far-reaching repercussions. Statistics show that women with unintended pregnancy have shorter interpregnancy intervals, are less likely to obtain early prenatal care, have more low-birthweight babies, and have babies with higher rates of infant mortality. In addition, although I am loath to mention the very politicized "A" word, it's obvious that unintended pregnancies lead directly to the 1.5 million abortions in the United States each year.

The consequences of unplanned pregnancies aren't limited to the realm of health. There are numerous economic effects,

> **The consequences of unplanned pregnancies aren't limited to the realm of health.**

including inability to continue at a job, cessation of schooling, and escalating day care costs. The appropriate planning and spacing of pregnancies remains a rarely discussed topic, but one with which nurses, as teachers of health, must become more familiar.

The Institute of Medicine's comprehensive 1995 report on this subject—a must-read for every nurse—led to the recommendation of a new social norm: All pregnancies should be intended—in other words, consciously and clearly planned. Other recommendations included:

- a major campaign to promote the benefits of planned pregnancy and to improve the public's knowledge about contraception and reproductive health;

- increased access to contraception;

- attention to the major roles that feelings, attitudes, and motivation play in avoiding unintended pregnancy;

- development and evaluation of a variety of local programs to reduce unintended pregnancy; and

- support for research on new methods of contraception for men and women and on the determinants and antecedents of unintended pregnancy.

This action plan is custom-made for nursing, since client education is an integral function of independent nursing practice. Every health assessment of every client of childbearing age could include family planning assessment and instruction, for both men and women. Our master's-prepared cadre of clinical nurse specialists and nurse practitioners can increase their knowledge base about the topic, educate their individual clients, and begin working in their practices and health care communities to develop and evaluate programs aimed at reducing unplanned pregnancies. Nurse researchers can attack the problem of reducing unintended pregnancy with the same vigor they've brought to other important issues.

In 1997, there is no reason for any woman to be pregnant if she doesn't desire it. As members of a profession peopled mostly by women, we nurses need to take up the call to address this problem. Education is the key. Research is an essential cause that the National Institute of Nursing Research should support by offering research funds to address the problem.

What can you do? Start by reading the Institute of Medicine report. Educate yourself. Become enraged that not enough is being done. Vow to do more for your clients. We need to stop thinking of family planning as a separate issue that's taught and discussed within the confines of an OB/GYN visit. Every woman and every man of childbearing age, at every health encounter with a nurse, should be assessed for family planning knowledge and practice, and then appropriately informed of their options. We owe this new commitment to the health care consumers of the 21st century.

 Article Review Form at end of book.

What does the term "safer sex" refer to according to Wenger, Kusseling, and Shapiro?

Misunderstanding of 'Safer Sex' by Heterosexually Active Adults

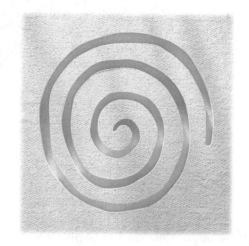

Neil S. Wenger, MD, MPH
Francoise S. Kusseling, MOB
Martin F. Shapiro, MD, PhD

The authors are with the Division of General Internal Medicine and Health Services Research at the University of California, Los Angeles.

To assess the understanding of safer sex among heterosexual adults, people enrolled in human immunodeficiency virus (HIV) education trials at a sexually transmitted disease (STD) clinic and a university student health service were surveyed concerning sexual behavior with their latest reported partner.

Of 646 sexually active persons enrolled in the trials, 233 (36 percent) reported having had safer sex with their latest partner; 124 of them (53 percent) also reported having vaginal or anal intercourse without a condom during that sexual encounter. Among the 124 who reported safer sex despite having intercourse without a condom, only 23 percent reported asking partners about their HIV status, 46 percent had asked about intravenous drug use, and 47 percent had asked about the number of prior sexual partners.

For 34 percent of those surveyed, the length of the sexual relationship with their latest partner was 1 month or less, and 18 percent estimated that this partner had had 11 or more prior sexual partners. STD clinic participants characterized intercourse without a condom as safer sex more often than student health service enrollees (76 percent versus 39 percent, P < 0.001).

The concept of safer sex is often misunderstood by persons engaging in behavior at risk for HIV transmission, and the level of misunderstanding differs among samples. Interventions to reduce transmission of HIV must confront misconceptions about the risk of sexual intercourse without condoms and include specific instructions understood by the targeted group.

An important part of public health efforts to stop the spread of the human immunodeficiency virus (HIV) is the reduction of behaviors that place people at risk of becoming infected. To reduce the chance of sexual transmission of HIV, public health interventions promote "safer" sexual behavior among persons who are sexually active. Consistent use of a condom and an accurate evaluation of a partner's risk of infection with HIV are important aspects of the public health strategy to reduce sexually transmitted disease transmission (1) and are the principal components of safer sex (2).

Interview and focus group evaluations of people's understanding of safer sex in a theoretical context suggest, however, that many persons do not understand the concept (3,4). This might seriously hamper the effectiveness of prevention efforts encouraging behavioral changes. We examined the understanding of safer sex in the context of their latest sexual encounter among persons enrolled in two trials of HIV education and testing.

Methods

There were 691 English speaking heterosexual adults enrolled in these trials—256 at an urban sexually transmitted disease (STD) clinic and 435 at a university student health service (SHS) clinic. Detailed descriptions of subject

Source: From Neil S. Wenter, et al., "Misunderstanding of 'Safer Sex' by Heterosexually Active Adults" in *Public Health Reports,* Volume 110, September/October, 1995 U.S. Public Health Service, Department of Health and Human Services.

enrollment and the trials are available elsewhere (5,6). Of the total, 646 (93 percent) responded to our questions about sexual behavior with their most recent sexual partner including whether they had safer sex with that partner. Our questionnaire contained questions about demographics, history of sexual behavior, and understanding of a most recent sexual partner's risk factors for HIV infection.

We compared responses about specific sexual activities during an encounter with the person's latest partner and about questions that they asked of that partner with their opinion on whether or not they had practiced safer sex. We defined safer sex to be any sexual activity other than vaginal or anal intercourse without a condom. Anyone who had vaginal or anal intercourse without a condom and reported safer sex was classified as inaccurate; all other safer sex assessments were considered to be accurate.

The proportion of those with inaccurate safer sex assessments was compared between the two study samples using a chi square test. For people with inaccurate safer sex assessments, we evaluated their understanding of their partner's risk factors for HIV infection to determine whether they might have believed the behavior was "safer" because of the partner's reported low risk profile. Partners' risk factors for HIV infection were compared between the two study samples with chi-square tests.

Results

The 646 sexually active persons who responded to the question about whether they had safer sex

Table I Demographic characteristics and sexual history of people in the two samples—STD and SHS—surveyed on safer sex

Characteristics	Total N=646	STD N=256	SHS N=390	P value for group comparison
Mean age (years) and standard deviation	25 ± 6	27 ± 8	23 ± 4	0.0001
Male (percent)	44	66	29	0.0001
Never married (percent)	83	67	94	0.0001
Race (percent)				
White	39	7	61	0.0001
Black	38	84	8	...
Hispanic	11	7	13	...
Asian	9	0	15	...
Other	3	1	4	...
Mean schooling (years) and standard deviation	14 ± 3	13 ± 2	15 ± 2	0.0001
Monthly income less than $1,000 (percent)	78	73	82	0.01
Lifetime number of STDs (median)	0	2	0	0.0001
Lifetime number of sexual partners (median)	8	12	4	0.0001
Mean age (years) at first sexual intercourse and standard deviation	17 ± 3	15 ± 3	18 ± 2	0.0001

during their latest sexual encounter had a mean age of 25 years; 44 percent were male, 83 percent had never married, 39 percent were white, 38 percent black, 11 percent hispanic, 9 percent Asian, and 3 percent of other ethnicity. The median number of sexual partners lifetime was 8. The demographics and sexual histories of the two study samples were different with those in the SHS sample more likely to be white and Asian, female, never married, and younger. Those in the STD sample had sex at an earlier age, were more likely to have had an STD, and had more lifetime sexual partners (table 1).

Of the total, 36 percent said they had safer sex with their latest sexual partner; 53 percent reported having vaginal or anal intercourse without a condom during that sexual encounter. Of the 413 who used a condom or had only oral sex, 91 percent reported having safer sex; the other 9 percent (who reported not having safer sex) all had oral sex without using a condom.

Among the 124 persons who said that they had safer sex but had intercourse without a condom, 23 percent reported that they had asked their sexual partner about his or her HIV status (10 percent indicated that their

Table 2 Characteristics of partners of survey sample members who were inaccurate about safer sex

Information about most recent sexual partner	Total N=124 (Percent)	STD N=66 (Percent)	SHS N=58 (Percent)
Questions asked most recent sexual partner:			
About HIV status	23	20	28
Partner was HIV-negative	10	11	10
About intravenous drug use	46	52	40
About past sexual experience[1]	47	27	69
Estimate of most recent partner's previous sexual experience:			
Never had sex before	8	3	14
1–3 partners	38	37	40
4–6 partners	18	23	12
7–10 partners	18	15	21
11 partners or more	18	22	14
Length of relationship with most recent sexual partner:			
First time	22	26	17
1 week to 1 month	12	14	9
1–6 months	20	14	26
More than 6 months	43	38	49

[1]P < 0.0001 for comparison between STD and SHS samples.

partner was HIV-negative), 46 percent asked their sexual partner about intravenous drug use, and 47 percent asked about their partner's number of prior partners. People estimated that their latest sexual partner had a median of 5 previous partners and that 18 percent of sexual partners had 11 or more prior partners. For 34 percent of these, the length of the sexual relationship with the latest partner was 1 month or less (table 2).

Those from the STD clinic were more likely to report that intercourse without a condom was safer sex than SHS subjects (76 percent versus 39 percent, P < 0.001), even though STD clinic subjects also were less likely to have asked sexual partners about their prior sexual partners (P < 0.0001), and there was a trend toward shorter relationships with these sexual partners for STD

clinic enrollees than for those from the SHS clinic (table 2).

Discussion

Although it is an important goal in preventing the spread of HIV, safer sex was often misunderstood among people in this study engaging in behavior at risk for HIV transmission. Despite the fact that this finding was suggested in previous studies asking about safer sex in a theoretical context, we believe that this is the first demonstration of misunderstanding safer sex concerning a recent sexual partner. Of all those who had vaginal or anal intercourse without a condom, 19 percent stated that they had safer sex. These persons either did not understand the risk involved in their latest sexual encounter or did not understand the meaning of safer sex. In either case, the misunderstanding likely places them at in-

creased risk of contracting a STD—including HIV—and makes it unlikely that public health messages promoting safer sex would succeed in achieving a desired change in behavior.

If both the people in this study and their partners had none or very low risk of infection with HIV, then sexual intercourse without a condom might be considered safer sex (2,7), but fewer than a quarter of them had ever asked about their sexual partner's HIV status, and only 10 percent stated that they knew their partner was not HIV-infected. Less than half of the total sample had asked their sexual partner about intravenous drug use and past sexual experience. For 22 percent of them, this sexual encounter was the first with this partner, and they estimated that 18 percent of these partners had had more than 10 prior sexual partners. On the other hand, public health recommendations would consider oral sex with a possibly HIV-infected partner as potentially unsafe (8). Thus, our estimates of misunderstanding may be conservative.

A more elaborate classification of HIV risk (9) is beyond the scope of these data. Furthermore, the study enrollees themselves may have been at risk of carrying HIV and of infecting their partner; more than half presented to a STD clinic with a presumed sexually transmitted disease. Thus, for the majority of them, the latest sexual encounter should not have been considered safer sex from a HIV prevention point of view. These people did not understand the concept of safer sex.

Interventions to decrease sexual behavior at risk of HIV transmission using the "safer sex" terminology would be unlikely to elicit the desired response among people who misunderstand the subject. More importantly, this finding might indicate that people consider factors other than the mutual chance of transmitting HIV in weighing the safety of a sexual encounter. Adequate pregnancy protection without condom use (10) or the belief that a partner's lack of risk factors made it very unlikely that the partner would transmit an infection (regardless of whether the person could infect the partner) might have been the basis on which people stated that intercourse without a condom was safer sex.

Although these hypotheses merit further exploration, including qualitative evaluation of people's perceptions of HIV risks and prevention strategies, the findings in this study suggest a number of caveats for HIV prevention interventions:

First, the term "safer sex" should not be used alone but always should be explained in terminology understood by the targeted sample. Second, the perceptions of risk associated with sexual intercourse should be explored so that the intervention can focus on correcting misunderstandings and sending messages to change behavior that are congruent with the sample's understanding of risky sexual behavior. Thirdly, these data show that samples differ in their understanding of the meaning of safer sex.

People from the STD clinic were much more likely to misunderstand safer sex than those from the SHS clinic. In addition, differences in sexual partner characteristics suggest that people at the SHS clinic may have believed that their latest sexual encounter was safer sex because their partner was extremely low-risk (14 percent had no prior sex, an additional 40 percent had an estimated three or fewer sexual partners, and 75 percent had had a sexual relationship with this partner for at least 6 months). STD clinic attenders may have misinterpreted safer sex for other reasons. Effective interventions to decrease HIV-risk behavior would need to be different for these two samples.

In conclusion, safer sex was commonly misinterpreted by persons engaging in behavior at risk for HIV transmission, and the degree of misunderstanding was different in two samples in need of HIV prevention interventions. Interventions to reduce transmission of HIV must include specific information targeted to the sample and should avoid such jargon as "safer sex."

References

1. 1993 Sexually transmitted diseases treatment guidelines. MMWR Morb Mortal Wkly Rep 42: 4–6, Sept. 24, 1993.
2. Goedert, J. J.: What is safe sex? Suggested standards linked to testing for human immunodeficiency virus. N Engl J Med 316: 1339–1341, May 21, 1987.
3. Macintyre, S., and West, P.: 'What does the phrase "safer sex" mean to you?' Understanding among Glaswegian 18-year-olds in 1990. AIDS 7: 121–125, January 1993.
4. Weiss, S. H., Weston, C. B., and Quirinale, J.: Safe sex? Misconceptions, gender differences and barriers among injection drug users: a focus group approach. AIDS Educ Prev 5: 279–293, winter 1993.
5. Wenger, N. S., Linn, L. S., Epstein, M., and Shapiro, M. F.: Reduction of high-risk sexual behavior among heterosexuals undergoing HIV antibody testing: a randomized clinical trial. Am J Public Health 81: 1580–1585, December 1991.
6. Wenger, N. S., et al.: Effect of HIV antibody testing and AIDS education on communication about HIV risk and sexual behavior. Ann Intern Med 117: 905–911, Dec. 1, 1992.
7. Davies, P. M.: Safer sex maintenance among gay men: are we moving in the right direction? AIDS 7: 279–280, June 1993.
8. Surgeon General's report to the American public on HIV infection and AIDS. Centers for Disease Control and Prevention, June 1993.
9. Campostrini, S., and McQueen, D. V.: Sexual behavior and exposure to HIV infection: estimates from a general-population risk index. Am J Public Health 83: 1139–1143 (1993).
10. Gold, R. S., Karmiloff-Smith, A., Skinner, M. J., and Morton, J.: Situational factors and thought processes associated with unprotected intercourse in heterosexual students. AIDS Care 4: 943–951 (1992).

Article Review Form at end of book.

This work was performed with the support of funds provided by the State of California (No. R88LA074) and allocated on the recommendation of the Universitywide Task Force on AIDS.

Which group of men is more likely to contract sexually transmitted diseases: circumcised or uncircumcised?

Circumcision in the United States

Prevalence, Prophylactic Effects, and Sexual Practice

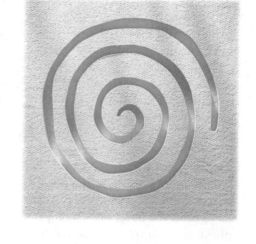

Edward O. Laumann, PhD;
Christopher M. Masi, MD;
Ezra W. Zuckerman, MA

From the Department of Sociology (Dr Laumann and Mr Zuckerman) and the School of Social Services Administration (Dr Masi), University of Chicago, Chicago, Ill.

Objective.—To assess the prevalence of circumcision across various social groups and examine the health and sexual outcomes of circumcision.

Design.—An analysis of data from the National Health and Social Life Survey.

Participants.—A national probability sample of 1410 American men aged 18 to 59 years at the time of the survey. In addition, an oversample of black and Hispanic minority groups is included in comparative analyses.

Main Outcome Measures.—The contraction of sexually transmitted diseases, the experience of sexual dysfunction, and experience with a series of sexual practices.

Results.—We find no significant differences between circumcised and uncircumcised men in their likelihood of contracting sexually transmitted diseases. However, uncircumcised men appear slightly more likely to experience sexual dysfunctions, especially later in life. Finally, we find that circumcised men engage in a more elaborated set of sexual practices. This pattern differs across ethnic groups, suggesting the influence of social factors.

Conclusions.—The National Health and Social Life Survey evidence indicates a slight benefit of circumcision but a negligible association with most outcomes. These findings inform existing debates on the utility of
circumcision. The considerable impact of circumcision status on sexual practice represents a new finding that should further enrich such discussion. Our results support the view that physicians and parents be informed of the potential benefits and risks before circumcising newborns.

Numerous recent studies have attempted to assess the value of neonatal circumcision. Several have determined that the procedure has positive effects. For example, an association has been found between circumcision and lower rates of urinary tract infections in infancy,[1,2] as well as lower rates of certain sexually transmitted diseases (STDs).[3,4] As a result of these and other findings, the 1989 American Academy of Pediatrics (AAP) Task Force on Circumcision shifted its previous position,[5] acknowledging that circumcision has potential medical benefits that must be weighed against its risks.[6]

Male satisfaction has also been debated. Some believe that circumcision reduces male sensitivity and coital enjoyment while others argue that circumcision may afford greater ejaculatory control.[7,8] Masters and Johnson reported no clinically significant difference in the tactile sensitivity of the glans.[9] More recent reports suggest the sensitivity of the circumcised glans may in fact be reduced.[10,11] Such claims of reduced sexual satisfaction for circumcised men have spurred a significant movement against the circumcision of infants and the reversing of circumcision in adult men. A technique of uncircumcising has even been introduced.[12] Nevertheless, little consensus exists regarding the role of the foreskin in sexual performance and satisfaction.

The present study attempts to shed light on the circumcision debate by exploiting the National Health and Social Life Survey (NHSLS), a unique data source on the sexual, attitudinal, and health-related experiences of circumcised and uncircumcised Americans. Our analysis of these data proceeds as follows. First, we describe the prevalence of circumcision in the NHSLS sample. Beyond limited records on historical circumcision rates, very little is known regarding how the practice is distributed across various groups and strata of Americans. Second, we illustrate how the NHSLS data speak to current debates regarding the effect of neonatal circumcision on outcomes such as STDs and sexual dysfunctions. Finally, we present results indicating significant differences between circumcised and uncircumcised men in terms of their sexual practices.

Methods

Survey

The NHSLS, conducted in 1992, is a nationally representative probability sample of 1511 men and 1921 women between the ages of 18 and 59 years living in households throughout the United States. It covers about 97% of the population in this age group—roughly 150 million Americans. It excludes people living in group quarters such as barracks, college dormitories, and prisons as well as those who do not know English well enough to be interviewed. There is an oversample of African Americans (n=458) and Hispanics (n=267). The sample completion rate was greater than 79%. Checks with other high-quality samples (eg, Census Bureau's Current Population Survey) suggest that the NHSLS succeeded in getting a truly representative sample of the population. Each person was surveyed in person by experienced interviewers, who matched respondents on various social attributes, for an interview averaging 90 minutes in duration. Extensive discussion of the sampling design and evaluation of sample and data quality can be found in Laumann et al.[13]

A respondent's circumcision status was ascertained by asking him whether he was circumcised. He was not asked, however, if the procedure was performed as a newborn or later in life. Experience with STDs was measured by asking respondents whether they had ever been told by a doctor that they had any of a specified list of such diseases, which were identified by medical names as well as by vernacular terms (eg, gonorrhea, clap, or drip). Experience of sexual dys-

function was ascertained with the following question:

Sometimes people go through periods in which they are not interested in sex or are having trouble achieving sexual gratification. I have just a few questions about whether you have experienced this in the past twelve months. During the past twelve months, has there been a period of several months or more when you. . . .

This question was asked regarding a series of sexual dysfunctions ranging from the inability to climax to lacking interest in sex. Respondents were also asked regarding their engagement in various sexual practices. Lifetime experience of a series of partnered behavior was ascertained by asking whether they had engaged in various sexual acts during their lifetimes. Respondents were also asked to describe the frequency with which they masturbated on a 10-point scale ranging from "never" to "every day."

We used a series of univariate and multivariable analyses to chart the distribution of circumcision and examine its effects. In assessing the prevalence of circumcision for various social groups, we performed multiple logistic regression of group membership on circumcision status and calculated adjusted odds ratios (ORs) that reflected the odds of being circumcised for group members relative to all others in the sample. In addition, we examined how such differences have changed over time by repeating the analyses within 3 broad age cohorts.

In assessing the impact of circumcision on the contraction of STDs and susceptibility to sexual dysfunction, we performed a series of 2-tailed *t* tests to uncover significant differences between circumcised and uncircumcised men across a wide array of related outcomes. Next, we estimated logistic equations for each of the STDs and dysfunctions on circumcision status and a series of control variables. These factors included the number of lifetime sexual partners; education; race/ethnicity; religion; nativity; residence in urban, suburban, or rural areas; a 7-point scale indicating how liberal or conservative were the respondent's sexual attitudes[13]; and the respondent's age. Net of these controls, we calculated adjusted ORs for the odds of having the various STDs and dysfunctions for circumcised relative to uncircumcised respondents. Finally, we repeated these comparisons within categories of a critical third variable—for STDs, the number of lifetime sexual partners reported by the respondent, and for sexual dysfunction, the respondent's age.

We conducted similar analyses to assess the association between circumcision status and various sexual practices. We performed logistic regression to assess this association with the respondent's lifetime experience with various practices. As it is an ordinal variable, we employed ordered logit to analyze the association between circumcision status and the respondent's masturbation experience. In addition, we repeated this analysis as a logistic regression with a critical cutoff point, masturbating at least once a month, as the dependent variable. As results from this analysis matched that from the ordered logit, we present the logistic regression results to afford comparability with the other analyses conducted. In all of the models of

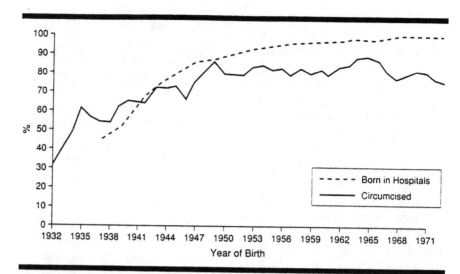

Circumcision rate and rate of hospitalization at delivery for US-born males. The rate for those born in hospitals is from the Vital Statistics of the United States. The rate for the 3-year moving average of circumcision is from the National Health and Social Life Survey.

sexual practices, we controlled for the same factors listed above. However, we excluded the number of lifetime sexual partners, a variable that is confounded with the tendency to engage in various practices. When this variable is included as a regressor, results for masturbation remain significant and findings regarding heterosexual oral sex weaken somewhat. In addition, we repeated the analyses for each of the 3 major ethnic groups featured in the survey, whites, blacks, and Hispanics. All analyses were performed using Stata version 4.0.[14]

Results

Prevalence of Circumcision

Since the age range of males participating in the NHSLS was 18 to 59 years, estimates of the prevalence of neonatal circumcision can be calculated for the years 1933 to 1974. As shown in the Figure, the steady increase in circumcision rates among respondents during much of this period reflects the increase identified by other investigators.[2] The proportion of

newborns that were circumcised reached 80% in the years after World War II and climaxed in the mid 1960s. This rise mirrors the increasing prevalence of hospital births. In addition, a slight decline in the proportion of newborns circumcised occurred in the last years covered by the survey, about the time when the medical establishment began to question the value of routine neonatal circumcision. Overall, 77% of the 1284 US-born men surveyed in the main NHSLS sample were circumcised, compared with 42% of the 115 non–US-born men.

Table 1 analyzes circumcision rates for religious, racial, and socioeconomic groupings of US-born respondents. We see that differences in circumcision rates across religious groups are not great. As may be expected, Jewish men report the largest proportion circumcised. However, given the small number of Jews surveyed in the NHSLS, this does not result in a significant adjusted OR. Mainline Protestants (including, eg, Methodists, Presbyterians, Lutherans, and Episcopalians) are somewhat more likely than conservative Protestants (including, eg, Baptists and Pentecostals) to be circumcised (see Laumann et al[13(pp146-147)] for rationale and details on coding of religious groups). However, as indicated by the insignificant adjusted OR, this difference disappears when race is controlled. Indeed, the predominant pattern is one of high circumcision rates for all major American religious groups.

Differences in circumcision levels across racial and ethnic groups are more revealing. In particular, whites are considerably more likely to be circumcised than are blacks or Hispanics (81% vs 65% or 54%). These differences remain significant when other variables are controlled. Net of these factors, the odds of a black being circumcised are roughly half (95% confidence interval [CI], 0.40-0.85) that of whites; the odds for Hispanics are about one third (95% CI, 0.26-0.44) that of whites. There has been some convergence in circumcision rates for the 3 groups across cohorts, though differences among groups have persisted (Table 1).

Circumcision rates vary significantly by the level of education attained by a respondent's mother. The critical break occurred between respondents whose mothers did and did not earn a high school diploma. While 62% of respondents whose mothers did not finish high school were circumcised, the rate for all other respondents varied from 84% to 87%. These differences remained significant when other factors were controlled. Net of such factors, the odds of being circumcised for respondents whose mothers earned at least a high school diploma was about 2.5 times (95% CI, 1.9-3.8) that of

those whose mothers were less educated. This discrepancy appeared to be narrowing in more recent cohorts. Among the youngest group of respondents, only those whose mothers had finished college displayed a significantly higher circumcision rate than those whose mothers had not earned a high school diploma.

Sexually Transmitted Diseases

Table 2 compares the incidence of various STDs reported by circumcised and uncircumcised respondents. Note that in this and subsequent tables, circumcision status serves as an independent variable rather than a dependent variable. Dependent variables are listed in the first column of these tables.

Several instructive features of the data presented in Table 2 deserve attention. First, circumcision status does not appear to lower the likelihood of contracting an STD. Rather, the opposite pattern holds. Circumcised men were slightly more likely to have had both a bacterial and a viral STD in their lifetime. While these differences are not statistically significant, they do not lend support to the thesis that circumcision helps prevent the contraction of STDs. Indeed, for chlamydia, the difference between circumcised and uncircumcised men is quite large. While 26 of 1033 circumcised men had contracted chlamydia in their lifetime, none of the 353 uncircumcised men reported having had it.

Table 2 shows a marked increase in the experience of STDs as the number of partners increases. The small, nonsignificant tendency for circumcised men to contract STDs at greater rates ap-

peared for each category of sexual experience. In addition, contraction of bacterial STDs occurred at a significantly greater rate for men who have had more than 20 sexual partners in their lifetimes. Among circumcised men with such a sexual background, the odds of contracting a bacterial STD are estimated at 2.88 that for uncircumcised men. While significant, the exact size of this difference is difficult to establish as indicated by the wide confidence interval (95% CI, 1.03-8.03). Note as well that this difference is driven largely by differential contraction of gonorrhea.

Sexual Dysfunction

While some difficulties, such as experiencing pain during sex, were rare, Table 3 demonstrates that sexual dysfunction is a relatively common event for American men. Approximately 45% of both circumcised and uncircumcised men experience at least one of these dysfunctions in the year prior to the survey. In addition, the data indicate a slight tendency for such dysfunctions to plague uncircumcised men. When all age groups are considered, almost every dysfunction is slightly more common among men who have not been circumcised. In particular, the likelihood of having difficulty achieving or maintaining an erection is significantly lower for circumcised men. When other factors are considered, the difference in the odds of experiencing this dysfunction for circumcised men is significantly less than that for uncircumcised men (OR, 0.66), but only at the 0.07 level (95% CI, 0.42-1.03).

Significant differences are more prominent when we examine the association between sexual dysfunction and circumcision status within age cohorts. While there appears to be little relationship between circumcision status and sexual dysfunction for the younger 2 cohorts, the association is quite strong for the older group of respondents (Table 3). Of the sexual dysfunctions considered, uncircumcised older men were more likely to experience every one of these difficulties than are their circumcised peers. The results of these differences are statistically significant even in the presence of contraceptives. The odds of a circumcised man of this type experiencing anxiety about his performance were approximately half that of his uncircumcised peers (95% CI, 0 0.95); the odds of a member of the former group having difficulty achieving or maintaining an erection are about 0.40 for the latter group. Overall, the odds that a circumcised man of the oldest cohort experienced sexual dysfunction was 0.48 that for uncircumcised man of the same age group (95% CI, 0.28-0.79). Thus, while circumcised men did not generally appear to experience different rates of sexual dysfunction, older circumcised men did display lower levels of dysfunction.

Sexual Practice

As shown in Table 4, NHSLS data indicate that circumcised men engaged somewhat more elaborated set of sexual practices than do men who are not circumcised. For each of the practices examined, lifetime experience of various forms of oral and anal sex and masturbation frequency in the past year, circumcised men engaged in these behaviors at greater rates. The difference between circumcised and uncircumcised men was greatest for masturbation—ironically, a prac-

tice that circumcision was once thought to limit. A total of 47% of circumcised men reported masturbating at least once a month vs 34% for their uncircumcised peers. This difference remains significant even when various attitudinal and demographic factors are controlled. The odds of a circumcised man masturbating at least once a month are estimated at 1.4 (95% CI, 1.04-1.89) that for uncircumcised men. In terms of lifetime sexual experience, the greatest differences occurred for heterosexual oral sex. In models with controls, circumcision status was associated with active heterosexual oral sex with a probability of insignificance of 0.07 (OR, 1.37; 95% CI, 0.97-1.92) and with passive heterosexual oral sex with a probability of insignificance of 0.08 (OR, 1.36; 95% CI, 0.96-1.93).

The association between circumcision status and the various sexual practices exhibited differences across ethnic groups (Table 4). While circumcised men of all 3 ethnic groups tended to engage in a more elaborated set of sexual practices, this was less true of blacks and Hispanics. For white men, the difference between circumcised and uncircumcised men was quite stark. Circumcised white men exhibited a greater likelihood of experiencing each of the various practices. In particular, the estimated ratio of the odds of masturbating at least once a month for circumcised men was 1.76 that for uncircumcised men (95% CI, 1.24-2.51). The adjusted ORs for both forms of heterosexual oral sex were significant as well. These associations were less consistent for blacks and Hispanics. While circumcised Hispanic men did masturbate at a slightly higher rate than their uncircumcised peers, no such difference appeared for blacks.

Similarly, while circumcised black men exhibited a greater tendency to engage in passive oral sex than did uncircumcised black men (this difference was insignificant when other factors are controlled), the reverse was true among Hispanic men. Thus, while circumcision status appeared to be significantly linked with a higher likelihood to engage in various sexual practices, this applied mostly to whites and considerably less for blacks and Hispanics.

Comment

The United States stands apart from the rest of the Western world for its high rates of neonatal circumcision. Nevertheless, medical research on the topic has generated an ambiguous set of results regarding the impact of circumcision status on the lives of men. As a result, rhetoric has reached a fever pitch as each side of the debate appeals to divergent criteria to make its case. Recognizing the merit of each position, the AAP has counseled that parents be fully informed of the risks and benefits of the procedure before deciding to have their sons circumcised.

Our analysis of the NHSLS furnishes information that should be useful in such decision-making processes. We examined the prevalence of circumcision among American men as well as its impact on sexually transmitted diseases, sexual functioning, and sexual practice and preferences. Each of these areas generated noteworthy findings.

Prevalence

With respect to prevalence, we demonstrated that circumcision rates are greatest among whites and better-educated respondents and that Americans of various religions do not display significantly different rates. The latter fact illustrates the unique cultural status maintained by circumcision in the United States. While circumcision has been employed as a religious marker in other Western societies, it has clearly lost such an association in America. American religious organizations have never strongly objected to the circumcision of its members, as they have instead deferred to medical authority on the subject.

Several factors may account for differential rates across ethnic groups. First, as race is associated with socioeconomic differences between Americans, these differences may reflect the greater tendency for middle-class parents to desire circumcision for their sons. Similarly, blacks and Hispanics are concentrated in such regions as the South or Southwest where circumcision is less prevalent. However, the fact that differences in circumcision rates remain significant when region and class are controlled suggests that the various racial groups may have different preferences for circumcision. Members of groups for whom circumcision is less common may avoid circumcision for their sons so that a sense of shared physical appearance is retained. Indeed, a recent study revealed that such social considerations typically outweigh various medical issues in determining parents' circumcision decisions.[15]

As with race, differences among socioeconomic groupings may result from a differential likelihood of being born in a hospital. However, this difference remained salient even in later periods where hospital births were virtually universal. Thus, it again appears likely that significant social variation exists in the prefer-

ence for and acceptance for circumcision. Better-educated parents, who are more likely to be exposed to the prevailing scientific wisdom favoring circumcision and to be exposed to significant social pressure to conform to this wisdom, circumcised their sons at greater levels than less educated parents.

In sum, we see that just as significant social institutions have played critical roles in the propagation of neonatal circumcision in the United States, the practice spread and persisted differentially across social groups. In contrast to societies where circumcision has indicated religious or cultic difference, the popularity of circumcision in 20th century United States clearly reflects social distinctions that are salient in contemporary society. Those social groups that had the education and cultural affinity for following the recommendations of medical and state authorities adopted circumcision while those groups who maintain a more distant relationship to such institutions did not embrace the practice to a comparable degree.

Note that these results should be treated with some caution when applied to rates of neonatal circumcision. The NHSLS respondents were asked whether they were circumcised, but not if the procedure was performed as a newborn or later in life. Given the rarity of circumcision on nonnewborns[16] and the match of our data with existing records on neonatal circumcision, we feel that it is reasonable to assume that different rates across social groups reflect differential experience at the time of birth. Note that this assumption is not necessary for examining the association between circumcision status and various outcomes. In such cases, the procedure must only

have been performed before the outcome in question. A second source of ambiguity concerns the accuracy of respondents' reports of their circumcision status. Research from the 1950s[17] and on adolescents in the 1980s[18] suggests that up to a third of men may not know their circumcision status. While we have no means of independently verifying respondents reports, we control for education in all of our models, a variable that should significantly impact knowledge of circumcision status.

Sexually Transmitted Diseases

With respect to STDs, we found no evidence of a prophylactic role for circumcision and a slight tendency in the opposite direction. Indeed, the absence of a foreskin was significantly associated with contraction of bacterial STDs among men who have had many sexual partners in their lifetimes. These results suggest reexamination of the prevailing wisdom regarding the prophylactic effect of circumcision. While circumcision may have an impact that was not picked up in the NHSLS data, it seems unlikely that this effect is great enough to justify the claim made by those who base their support for widespread circumcision on it.

Several cautions apply to these findings, however. The NHSLS self-reports of STD contraction were almost certainly underreports, because respondents may have lacked knowledge that they had the STD, if it was asymptomatic or never diagnosed, or if they did not understand the diagnosis. Moreover, given the social stigma associated with having STDs, some respondents may have been reluctant to report that they had such a condition.

Considerable effort was expended in minimizing underreporting by devising an interview protocol that gave a maximum sense of privacy and confidentiality, that persuaded the respondent of full disclosure for public health reasons, and provided memory aids to facilitate respondent recall. Even if these procedures were especially effective, and we think they were, we must still acknowledge that the self-reports understate the incidence of STDs to a substantial but unknown extent. In addition, there may have been systematic biases in underreporting related to particular attributes of respondents. In particular, we might expect better-educated people to be more knowledgeable about disease labels than less well-educated people. By contrast, however, better-educated persons may be more sensitive to the social stigma associated with having an STD. Controlling for education in the various models helped but probably did not fully redress these issues.

Results may also have been affected by the possibility that some respondents did not know whether they had been circumcised. If one assumes that respondents were more likely to say that they were circumcised (ie, the default answer is to give an affirmative response to any question) and that the same people report higher levels of STDs, this may account for any association found. While we feel that such distortions are small, it is worth reiterating that the principal result of the presented analysis is that no discernible differences in STD experience can be found to distinguish circumcised and uncircumcised men.

Sexual Dysfunctions

The NHSLS data suggest a benefit of circumcision with respect to sexual dysfunction. Circumcised men were slightly less likely than those who had not been circumcised to experience various sexual difficulties. This difference was significant among the oldest age group. Interestingly, this age group presents the best test for establishing differences between circumcised and uncircumcised men as it contains comparable numbers of both. It would seem then that NHSLS data supply some support for those who see circumcision as performing a positive role in promoting healthy sexual behavior. This appears most true for older men. While there may be many sources for this relationship, it is possible that the association between masturbation frequency and circumcision status (discussed below) provides a clue. If older men require more direct stimulation to function sexually, men for whom masturbation is part of their sexual script[13] may be better able to adapt sexually as they age. Clearly, such reasoning must remain speculative until further research is performed.

Sexual Practice

Our findings regarding sexual practice pose the greatest challenge for future research. NHSLS results reveal a clear pattern in that circumcised men report a more highly elaborated set of sexual practices. In particular, the association between circumcision status and masturbation frequency was quite strong. Similar results, at a somewhat weaker level, occurred for heterosexual oral sex. These results escape easy interpretation. Certainly, they cast doubt on the Victorian-era notion that circumcision reduces the urge to masturbate.

While we do not wish to push speculation too far, differences in the association between circumcision status and sexual practice across ethnic groups suggest that cultural, rather than physiological, forces may be responsible. In particular, the presented results may reflect attitudes regarding the cultural acceptability of the uncircumcised penis. Note that the association of circumcision with experience of sexual practices is weakest among ethnic minorities for whom circumcision is less prevalent. Among whites by contrast, uncircumcised men are relatively uncommon. A consequence of this may be that a certain stigma is attached to the uncircumcised penis in the white population. If the uncircumcised penis assumes somewhat negative cultural associations among whites, this may lead uncircumcised white men to engage in a somewhat less-elaborated set of sexual practices.

Conclusion

While NHSLS results do not lend clear support to either side of the circumcision debate, they make a significant contribution to our knowledge regarding the potential risks and benefits of circumcision. In addition to documenting the prevalence of circumcision across various social groups, we have discovered that circumcision provides no discernible prophylactic benefit and may in fact increase the likelihood of STD contraction; that circumcised men have a slightly lessened risk of experiencing sexual dysfunction, especially among older men; and that circumcised men displayed

Table 1 Circumcision Rates Across Social Groups by Cohort: US-Born Men*

Predictor Variable	All Men (N=1369) Circumcised, No. (%)	Adjusted OR (95% CI)†	Born 1933-1947 (n=358) Circumcised, No. (%)	Adjusted OR (95% CI)†	Born 1947-1962 (n=653) Circumcised, No. (%)	Adjusted OR (95% CI)†	Born 1963-1973 (n=488) Circumcised, No. (%)	Adjusted OR (95% CI)†
Religion								
No religion	179 (80)	Referent	28 (71)	Referent	77 (82)	Referent	73 (82)	Referent
Mainline Protestant	301 (82)	1.24 (0.78-1.98)	85 (64)	0.88 (0.37-2.09)	143 (87)	1.83 (0.88-3.79)	73 (93)	1.73 (0.69-4.34)
Conservative Protestant	394 (71)	0.81 (0.65-1.00)	101 (53)	0.78 (0.51-1.20)	164 (76)	1.14 (0.58-2.21)	129 (81)	0.86 (0.42-1.76)
Catholic	324 (79)	1.16 (0.91-1.47)	80 (68)	1.19 (0.50-2.83)	150 (84)	1.53 (0.74-3.17)	94 (80)	1.03 (0.48-2.21)
Jewish	25 (96)	...(...)	...(...)	...(...)	...(...)	...(...)	...(...)	...(...)
Ethnicity‡								
White	1067 (81)	Referent	251 (65)	Referent	478 (86)	Referent	332 (86)	Referent
Black	189 (65)	0.58 (0.40-0.85)	46 (49)	0.63 (0.31-1.29)	89 (64)	0.37 (0.21-0.65)	58 (76)	0.62 (0.30-1.27)
Hispanic	90 (54)	0.34 (0.26-0.44)	23 (35)	0.38 (0.17-0.86)	31 (61)	0.15 (0.10-0.22)	36 (56)	0.21 (0.10-0.46)
Mother's education								
Less than high school	372 (62)	Referent	142 (52)	Referent	153 (68)	Referent	76 (66)	Referent
High school graduate	538 (84)	2.56 (1.90-3.46)	107 (69)	2.17 (1.30-3.62)	264 (89)	2.78 (1.66-4.64)	167 (84)	1.48 (0.68-3.21)
Some college	167 (84)	2.72 (2.15-3.47)	21 (57)	1.12 (0.48-2.60)	72 (93)	4.62 (1.90-11.71)	74 (84)	1.86 (0.87-3.96)
College graduate	148 (87)	2.93 (2.25-3.81)	22 (82)	3.06 (1.13-8.32)	58 (81)	1.74 (1.14-2.39)	68 (94)	4.07 (1.54-10.72)

*Source: National Health and Social Life Survey.
†Estimated ratio of odds of being circumcised for members of the specified group to odds for reference group. Derived from logistic regression model performed on all US-born respondents. The model includes all predictor variables as well as controls for residence in rural, suburban, or urban areas. OR indicates odds ratio; and CI, confidence interval. Ellipses indicate 20 cases or fewer.
‡Asians and American Indians were also included in the full model but are excluded here because they represent too few cases for reliable results.

Table 2 Lifetime Experience of Sexually Transmitted Diseases by Circumcision Status and Number of Sexual Partners*

Criterion Variable	All Men Rate per 1000 C	UC	Adjusted OR (95% CI)†	1-4 Lifetime Partners Rate per 1000 C	UC	Adjusted OR (95% CI)†	5-20 Lifetime Partners Rate per 1000 C	UC	Adjusted OR (95% CI)†	21+ Lifetime Partners Rate per 1000 C	UC	Adjusted OR (95% CI)†
Gonorrhea	94.7	104.8	1.42 (0.79-2.56)	22.1	20.4	2.22 (0.25-19.77)	108.4	143.9	0.79 (0.38-1.62)	237.3	196.4	3.26 (0.96-11.11)
Syphilis	9.3	10.8	2.14 (0.41-11.30)	2.5	6.8	...(...)	9.9	7.6	0.77 (0.07-8.87)	28.2	0.0	...(...)
Chlamydia	25.1‡	0.0	...(...)	7.4	0.0	...(...)	32.2	0.0	...(...)	56.5	0.0	...(...)
Nongonococcal urethritis	24.4	19.1	1.33 (0.43-4.09)	2.5	6.8	...(...)	27.2	23.1	1.17 (0.20-6.93)	74.3	56.6	1.53 (0.27-8.76)
All bacterial	129.9	112.9	1.61 (0.94-2.78)	29.5	20.4	2.46 (0.35-17.13)	157.6	151.5	0.99 (0.50-1.94)	316.4	232.1	2.88 (1.03-8.03)
Herpes	14.9	8.1	1.18 (0.23-5.94)	2.5	0.0	...(...)	9.9	15.5	...(...)	62.1	17.9	1.27 (0.12-12.95)
Hepatitis	24.2	24.4	1.22 (0.43-3.46)	14.6	13.7	1.53 (0.19-12.36)	32.1	15.3	1.50 (0.30-7.42)	28.2	72.7	0.04 (0.00-2.59)
Human immunodeficiency virus	1.9	5.4	...(...)	0.0	6.8	...(...)	2.5	7.8	...(...)	5.7	0.0	...(...)
All viral	35.3	32.3	1.30 (0.52-3.22)	17.2	13.7	1.35 (0.19-9.57)	32.0	30.3	1.84 (0.36-9.51)	90.4	89.3	0.70 (0.15-3.24)
No. of respondents	1449	1118		554	449		538	444		233	190	

*Source: National Health and Social Life Survey. C indicates circumcised; and UC, uncircumcised.
†Estimated ratio of odds of circumcised men having experienced the specified sexually transmitted disease relative to odds for uncircumcised men. Derived from logistic regression model performed in which experience of the sexually transmitted disease is the dependent variable and independent variables, in addition to circumcision status, include ethnicity, religion, residence in rural, suburban, or urban areas, education and, in models for "all men," the number of sexual partners. OR indicates odds ratio: and CI, confidence interval. Ellipses indicate unstable estimates.
‡Indicates $P \leq .05$ t test for difference between circumcised and uncircumcised men.

Table 3 Sexual Dysfunction in Past Year by Circumcision Status and Age*

Criterion Variable	All Men Comparison, %		Adjusted OR (95% CI) †	Age, 18-29 y Comparison, %		Adjusted OR (95% CI)†	Age, 30-44 y Comparison, %		Adjusted OR (95% CI)†	Age, 45-59 y Comparison, %		Adjusted OR (95% CI)†
	C	UC		C	UC		C	UC		C	UC	
Lacked interest in sex	15	17	1.04 (0.71-1.53)	14	15	1.39 (0.62-3.13)	16	12	1.59 (0.79-3.20)	14	23	0.52 (0.27-1.02)
Unable to ejaculate	8	10	1.05 (0.64-1.72)	6	9	0.58 (0.25-1.82)	9	5	1.86 (0.76-4.54)	9	16	0.70 (0.30-1.22)
Ejaculated prematurely	28	31	0.87 (0.64-1.18)	29	27	1.00 (0.54-1.84)	29	28	1.17 (0.68-2.00)	25§	37	0.59 (0.34-1.03)
Experienced pain during sex	3	3	1.14 (0.49-2.68)	4	4	0.93 (0.22-3.94)	3	1	...(...)	2	5	1.49 (0.25-9.04)
Did not enjoy sex	8	9	0.76 (0.46-1.26)	10	7	1.04 (0.39-2.77)	8	8	1.09 (0.44-2.69)	5	10	0.33 (0.11-0.97)
Was anxious about performance	17	18	0.87 (0.60-1.27)	20	15	1.35 (0.62-2.94)	18	17	1.05 (0.55-2.00)	13§	22	0.50 (0.22-0.95)
Had trouble achieving/ maintaining erection	10§	17	0.66 (0.42-1.03)	7	9	0.85 (0.30-2.44)	10	7	1.28 (0.53-3.11)	13‡	29	0.38 (0.16-0.77)
Had any dysfunction	43	48	0.85 (0.64-1.13)	47	46	0.99 (0.57-1.72)	44	39	1.33 (0.81-2.18)	40‡	58	0.47 (0.28-0.79)
No. of respondents	1221		1203	378		399	586		519	340		285

*Source: National Health and Social Life Survey. C indicates circumcised; and UC, uncircumcised.

†Estimated ratio of odds of circumcised men having experienced the specified dysfunction relative to odds for uncircumcised men. Derived from logistic regression model performed in which experience of the dysfunction is the dependent variable and independent variables, in addition to circumcision status, include number of sexual partners, religion, residence in rural, suburban, or urban areas, education and, in models for "all men," ethnicity. OR indicates odds ratio; and CI, confidence interval. Ellipses indicate unstable estimates.

‡Indicates $P \leq .05$ t test for difference between circumcised and uncircumcised men.

§Indicates $P \leq .10$ t test for difference between circumcised and uncircumcised men.

greater rates of experience of various sexual practices. While evidence regarding STD experience contributes to ongoing debates, our results concerning sexual dysfunction and practice represent largely unprecedented effects.

We benefited greatly from the support of National Institutes of Health grant 5 R01 HD28356, the Ford Foundation grant 940-1417, and the Program in Medicine, Arts, and the Social Sciences at the University of Chicago.

We wish to acknowledge the following people for their helpful comments and suggestions: Anne E. Laumann, MD, William Parish, PhD, Nancy Roizen, MD, and Robert L. Rosenfield, MD.

These findings suggest the need for continued research that should further aid parents in weighing the benefits and risks of circumcising their sons.

References

1. Wiswell T, Smith FR, Bass JW. Decreased incidence of urinary tract infections in circumcised male infants. *Pediatrics.* 1985;75:901-903.
2. Herzog L. Urinary tract infections and circumcision: a case control study. *Am J Dis Child.* 1989;143:348-350.
3. Parker S, Stewart AJ, Wren MN, et al. Circumcision and sexually transmissible disease. *Med J Aust.* 1983;2:288-290.
4. Task Force on Circumcision. Report of the task force on circumcision. *Pediatrics.* 1989;84:388-391.
5. Committee on Fetus and Newborn. Report of the ad hoc task force on circumcision. *Pediatrics.* 1975;56:610-611.
6. Masi CM. *Circumcision: The Medical Issues.* Chicago, Ill: University of Chicago School of Social Services Administration; 1995. Working paper.
7. Morgan W. Penile plunder. *Med J Aust.* 1967;1:1102-1103.
8. Burger R, Guthrie T. Why circumcision? *Pediatrics.* 1974;54:362.
9. Masters W, Johnson V. *Human Sexual Response.* Boston, Mass: Little Brown & Co; 1966.
10. Preston EN. Whither the foreskin? a consideration of routine neonatal circumcision. *JAMA.* 1970;213:1853-1858.

Table 4 Sexual Practice by Circumcision Status, Ethnicity, and Control Factors*

Criterion Variable	All Men Comparison, % — C	UC	Adjusted OR (95% CI) †	Whites Comparison, % — C	UC	Adjusted OR (95% CI)†	Blacks Comparison, % — C	UC	Adjusted OR (95% CI)†	Hispanics Comparison, % — C	UC	Adjusted OR (95% CI)†
Lifetime experience												
Active heterosexual oral sex	80‡	65	1.37 (0.97-1.92)	84‡	73	1.57 (1.04-2.37)	52	47	0.96 (0.40-2.28)	75	67	0.96 (0.70-1.32)
Passive heterosexual oral sex	81‡	61	1.36 (0.96-1.93)	84‡	73	1.57 (1.04-2.38)	71‡	57	1.38 (0.56-3.37)	71	75	0.26 (0.05-1.26)
Active homosexual oral sex	5	2	2.15 (0.85-5.42)	6	3	2.22 (0.73-6.74)	3	3	...(...)	10‡	2	...(...)
Passive homosexual oral sex	8	6	1.59 (0.85-2.96)	9	6	1.88 (0.73-6.74)	6	8	...(...)	10	5	...(...)
Heterosexual anal intercourse	27	23	0.80 (0.56-1.14)	27	22	0.69 (0.45-1.06)	24	22	1.16 (0.40-3.38)	35	36	1.10 (0.35-3.48)
Masturbation ≥ 1/mo in past year	47‡	34	1.40 (1.04-1.89)	50‡	34	1.76 (1.24-2.51)	27	28	0.92 (0.35-2.39)	44	38	0.55 (0.22-1.96)
No. of respondents	1404		1143	1046		903	190		126	119		74

*Source: National Health and Social Life Survey. C indicates circumcised; and UC, uncircumcised.

†Estimated ratio of odds of circumcised men having experienced the specified sexual practice relative to odds for uncircumcised men. Derived from logistic regression model performed in which experience of the sexual practice is the dependent variable and independent variables, in addition to circumcision status, include number of sexual partners, religion, residence in rural, suburban, or urban areas, education and, in models for "all men," ethnicity. OR indicates odds ratio; and CI, confidence interval. Ellipses indicate unstable estimate.

‡Indicates P≤.05 t test for difference between circumcised and uncircumcised men.

11. Cleary T, Kohl S. Overwhelming infection with group B beta-hemolytic streptococcus associated with circumcision. *Pediatrics.* 1979;64:301-303.
12. Goodwin W. Uncircumcision: a technique for plastic reconstruction of a prepuce after circumcision. *J Urol.* 1990;144:1203-1205.
13. Laumann EO, Michael RT, Gagnon JH, et al. *The Social Organization of Sexuality: Sexual Practices in the United States.* Chicago, Ill: University of Chicago Press; 1994:chapt 2, appendixes A, B.
14. Stata Corporation. *STATA Version 4.0.* College Station, Tex: Stata Corp; 1994.
15. Brown MS, Brown CA. Circumcision decision: prominence of social concerns. *Pediatrics.* 1987;80:215-219.
16. Graves EJ. Detailed diagnoses and procedures: National Hospital Discharge Survey, 1993, from the National Center for Health Statistics. *Vital Health Stat 13.* 1995;122:128.
17. Lilienfeld AM, Graham S. Validity of determining circumcision status by questionnaire as related to epidemiological studies of cancer of the cervix. *J Natl Cancer Inst.* 1958;21:713-720.
18. Schlossberger NM, Turner RA, Irwin CE Jr. Early adolescent knowledge and attitudes about circumcision: methods and implications for research. *J Adolesc Health.* 1991;12:293-297.

Article Review Form at end of book.

How can the use of over-the-counter feminine products potentially harm women?

Feminine Needs

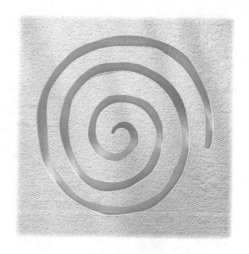

Karyn Snyder

Last year, American women spent $250 million on over-the-counter antifungals, $120 million on douche products, and $50 million on vaginal deodorants, according to Sharon Hillier, Ph.D., director of reproductive infectious disease research at Magee-Women's Hospital at the University of Pittsburgh. While these products may offer convenient relief from vaginal discomfort, they are often misused by consumers who unwittingly purchase remedies that are improper or ineffective treatments for their symptoms. This news was presented by a panel of doctors speaking at a recent conference sponsored by the National Vaginitis Association (NVA), Barrington, Ill.

According to these health-care specialists, women often buy OTC products that do little more than mask unpleasant symptoms rather than provide a cure to the underlying problem. More important, improper self-medication can delay the medical intervention necessary to prevent potentially serious reproductive problems. These health-care professionals were especially concerned that women who believe their vaginal discharge is either normal or the result of a yeast infection may actually be suffering from bacterial vaginosis (BV) or a sexually transmitted disease (STD), both of which can lead to problems as serious as infertility.

Experts believe some women are misusing vaginal OTCs

Though BV is much more common and much more serious than a yeast infection, many women know little about the condition. It is also very easy for women to mistake more serious infections for a yeast infection, because the symptoms can be very similar. The NVA reported that a recent survey of 390 gynecologists found an estimated 44% of patients diagnosed with BV had initially treated themselves with OTC products for what they thought were yeast infections. Hillier claimed that only one in three women visiting her clinic in Pittsburgh with complaints of vaginal itching was actually suffering from a yeast infection. The rest were, instead, suffering from afflictions such as BV, STDs, or urinary tract infections.

Many women use douches or vaginal deodorants to mask odor, believing it is simply the result of a hygiene problem. Others use OTC remedies that are effective against yeast infections but not other types of vaginitis. Still others use creams that have not been proven effective against any type of vaginitis.

Can misuse, or even use, of OTC products harm women? Yes, according to the panelists. In addition to delaying proper treatment, these products can turn a normally healthy balance of protective bacteria in the vagina into what the NVA calls "an ecological disaster." For this reason, the doctors were critical of the practice of douching. "It completely changes a woman's balance between the good guys and the bad guys . . . and strips her of her natural defense system," said Anita Nelson, associate professor of obstetrics and gynecology at Harbor-UCLA Medical Center. Hillier agreed, saying that douching had "no medical benefit" and that many studies have found that douching may be a risk factor "in pelvic in-

Reprinted with permission of *Drug Topics*, Medical Economics Co., January 6, 1997.

flammatory disease, ectopic pregnancy, and future infertility." Most douche products do warn about these risks on their packages.

Some manufacturers of douche products were contacted for a response, but did not return calls to *Drug Topics* by press time.

Misuse of OTC antifungals may also cause problems for women. Edward Hook, professor of medicine and epidemiology for the department of infectious diseases at the University of Alabama, suggested that the use of OTC antifungals in the absence of a yeast infection could similarly disrupt the vaginal flora or mask a more severe infection. He and his colleagues stressed that only women with symptoms identical or similar to those previously diagnosed by a doctor as a yeast infection are candidates for OTC treatment. The packaging of these products reinforces that message, advising women to see a doctor if this is their first experience with a yeast infection and also to seek medical help if their symptoms don't improve after three days of OTC antifungal use.

"I am particularly concerned about younger women and adolescents who have not had a documented yeast infection confirmed by a provider and who may be covering up the signs and symptoms of an STD because they think the cause of their discharge and vulvar itching is actually vaginitis as opposed to an STD," said David Soper, professor and director of the department of obstetrics and gynecology at the Medical University of South Carolina.

The doctors also expressed concern about overuse of OTC products in lieu of proper medical treatment. Hillier said that many women who have treated themselves over and over with multiple products "have so assaulted their vaginal ecosystems that they get almost an allergic reaction in their vagina, and they have symptoms that are not related to any infection but rather are an allergic reaction to overuse of too many products." Alabama's Hook echoed her concerns, saying that women should not be using two and three courses of OTC therapy before seeking professional help. He said that one failed OTC treatment is enough cause for a woman to make a visit to her doctor's office.

Given the potential problems associated with improper use of these products, is there any way pharmacists can assist women?

"Pharmacists actually are becoming increasingly interested in educating their patients and are counseling them, but I guess I see it as a difficult role for a pharmacist to play," said Soper, referring to the fact that only clinical tests performed by a doctor can really determine what kind of infection a woman might have. But he did say that R.Ph.s can play an important role in product selection. "Where [the pharmacist] might play a major role would be that if [a patient] picked up an unstudied and less effective brand of topical medication, that he might be able to direct [her] to what probably will be a more expensive but truly efficacious medication."

Nelson, too, hoped that R.Ph.s might help women differentiate between vaginal medications and what Hillier called "vaginal cosmetics." Unfortunately, she said, pharmacists are often "out of the loop" because women simply come into the drugstore, select a product from the shelf, and pay the cashier for it, but she said it "ought to be in big letters" who is a proper candidate for which remedy.

Pharmacists might also benefit from learning more about the myths associated with vaginal health and the traditions handed down from mother to daughter. Hook stressed that patient education is very important, "It's a very pervasive problem that cuts across and is not limited to individuals fitting any race, ethnicity, cultural, or geographic distinction."

The doctors also stressed that, contrary to popular belief, women are not embarrassed to talk about vaginal health. A recent Gallup poll found that 52% of women were very comfortable talking about it, and another 26% were somewhat comfortable.

 Article Review Form at end of book.

What is homophobia?
How is homophobia harmful to the health of gays and lesbians?

Homophobia Is a Health Hazard

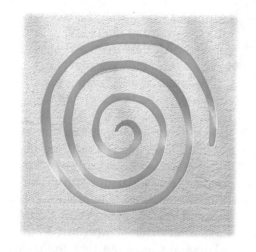

Katherine A. O'Hanlan, M.D.;
Patricia Robertson, M.D.;
Robert Paul Cabaj, M.D.;
Benjamin Schatz;
and Paul Nemrow, M.D.

Dr. O'Hanlan, assistant professor, Department of Obstetrics and Gynecology, Stanford University School of Medicine, Palo Alto, Calif., is president emerita, Gay and Lesbian Medical Association, Palo Alto. Dr. Robertson is associate professor, Department of Obstetrics, Gynecology, and Reproductive Sciences, University of California, San Francisco. Dr. Cabaj, associate clinical professor of psychiatry, University of California, San Francisco, is president, Gay and Lesbian Medical Association. Mr. Schatz is executive director, Gay and Lesbian Medical Association. Dr. Nemrow is an attending physician in physical medicine, St. Mary's Hospital, San Francisco.

Physicians can not avoid the fact that as many as six percent of the patients they currently see are gay, lesbian, or bisexual with medical problems that often are radically different from the heterosexual population.

To a large extent, American society has made gay men and lesbians the brunt of multiple levels of prejudice, with negative assumptions about their morality, trustworthiness, employability, and integrity. (Similar accusations have been made against African-Americans, Jews, and other ethnic groups.) As a result, gay men and lesbians developed a hidden subculture among themselves that only recently has become much more open, and now weaves throughout all segments of society. Surveys of the homosexual community suggest that medical practitioners may lack knowledge of the issues salient in the lives of gay men and lesbians and inadvertently and sometimes purposely have alienated their patients. The gay and lesbian community is much more visible today and is asking for health care that recognizes its unique medical demographic profile and is provided with the same degree of knowledge, sensitivity, and respect afforded other segments of America's large and diverse society.

Homophobia is defined as the "unreasoning fear of or antipathy toward homosexuals and homosexuality." It operates on two levels: internally and externally. Internal homophobia represents prejudices that individuals incorporate into their belief systems as they grow up in societies biased against gays and lesbians. External homophobia is the overt expression of those biases, ranging from social avoidance to legal and religious proscription to violence.

There is no scientific basis for homophobic prejudice. The initial classification of homosexuality as a mental disorder in the *Diagnostic and Statistical Manual* (DSM-III) has been reviewed extensively and found to be reflective only of the social mores at the time it was inserted. The extensive psychiatric literature reveals no major differences in levels of maturity, neuroticism, psychological adjustment, goal orientation, or self-actualization between heterosexuals and homosexuals. A few studies, though, have revealed slightly higher lifetime rates of depression, attempted suicide, psychological help seeking, and substance abuse among the latter. These rates are attributed to the chronic stress from the endurance of societal hatred or the ascription of inferior status. This stress may have worse mental health implications than other stressors because of the frequent loss of familial support systems and the concealment and suppression of feelings and thoughts.

The developmental steps gay men and lesbians must negotiate helps explain the psychological injury to which they are vulnerable. These include recognizing and accepting their homosexual orientation despite pervasive familial and societal condemnation; developing a new identity as a gay/lesbian person, a process labeled "coming out"; and confronting ubiquitous homophobia.

Children, sometimes as young as two to eight years old, who experience homosexual feelings often are isolated and alienated from family members who perceive that heterosexuality is the only acceptable "norm." In American society, some religious organizations promote homophobia by depicting homosexuality as an immoral proclivity that must be resisted, often telling gay and lesbian children they are wicked and condemned to hell. Educational institutions do not teach children about diversity of orientation, particularly at the ages when most youths begin to discern their orientation. The paucity of gay and lesbian role models in society, combined with negative stereotypes in the media, further diminishes the ability of gay and lesbian youth to develop a positive self-identity and gain respect and understanding from their peers.

The Committee on Adolescence of the American Academy of Pediatrics acknowledged in 1993 that gay and lesbian youth, while attempting to reconcile their feelings with negative societal stereotypes, confront a "lack of accurate knowledge, [a] scarcity of positive role models, and an absence of opportunity for open discussion. Such rejection may lead to isolation, run-away behavior, homelessness, domestic violence, depression, suicide, substance abuse, and school or job failure."

Children often attempt to conceal their orientation from friends and relatives for fear of reprisals and discrimination, allowing a presumption of their heterosexuality to prevail. In one study, awareness of sexual orientation typically occurred at age 10, but disclosure to another person did not take place until six years later. Homosexual youth find it difficult to maintain a positive self-image, having created a double-life that is not satisfactory in either realm.

Though survey data suggests that the majority of lesbians and gay men are in long-term relationships, misconceptions persist about their ability to form committed and stable involvements, even though researchers have found that 90% of surveyed homosexual couples shared income, lived together, were mutually dependent, and said they were committed for life. Relationship instability in homosexual pairings can occur because of the same common conflicts of all couples, and it can be compounded by effects of cultural homophobia. Internalized homophobia, with its self-doubt and shame, may make some feel they can not develop any relationship at all.

Complications of isolation from the family of origin by gay and lesbian individuals can be manifested in medical crisis. The definition of "family," for gays and lesbians, necessarily involves creation of a network of close and accepting friends as a family of choice, especially if their family-of-origin has rejected them. Yet, hospitals may restrict visitation privileges of "non-relatives." Sometimes, when domestic partners have visited their loved ones in the intensive care unit, displays of affection have been met with open disdain by the hospital staff. During a hospitalization, conflict can arise if the couple has not signed contracts for mutual medical conservatorship. Without them, a blood relative, automatically vested with medico-legal authority as next of kin, can override the role and input of the domestic partner, even though the domestic partner may be the primary caretaker and more knowledgeable of his or her partner's religious and ethical beliefs.

Many studies demonstrate that Americans who had close friends and relatives had a lower mortality rate than people lacking such connections. A 1992 report from the International Conference on AIDS found a positive correlation between the number of social supports for HIV patients and how well their immune systems fight the disease. Other studies demonstrate that participation in psychologically supportive networks and frequent social interactions are associated with reduced morbidity or mortality from cancer, HIV, and stroke.

Stress in the gay community derives from anxiety, depression, and guilt from being viewed as immoral and deviant, and has been compounded by the effects of the HIV epidemic. Individuals who carry multiple socially marginalized statuses—*e.g.,* race, ethnicity, sexual orientation—are at higher risk of depressive stress.

Substance use can serve as an easy relief, as well as provide acceptance. It numbs painful feelings, tempering the sting of homophobia, and serves as a social lubricant, facilitating the expression of forbidden sexual behavior. For some individuals, alcohol or other substance use and coming out become interconnected. Legal prohibitions and societal disdain effectively have restricted gay and lesbian social outlets to bars and private homes or clubs that typically promote alcohol use. Although there are increasing alternatives to bars and parties, these sites remain the usual initial social outlet for many gay or lesbian individuals, who, in reality, are seeking a wider network of friends.

Homophobia reduces the success of treatment and recovery for gay and lesbian substance abusers. Failure to acknowledge a gay or lesbian identity makes recovery more difficult and increases likelihood of relapse. While gay and lesbian clients are more willing to attend a treatment program which addresses gay issues and provides gay or lesbian counselors, most detoxification and rehabilitation programs show little sensitivity to issues of sexual orientation and generally do not encourage its disclosure. Although research supports the genetic, biological, and biochemical components of both drug use and homosexuality, there are no correlations between the two traits, and there is no suggestion of any linkage.

Domestic violence. Although there is growing awareness in the medical community concerning domestic violence among heterosexuals, there is little awareness that it also occurs in gay and lesbian relationships. Victims and perpetrators may need medical care, but rarely feel able to talk openly about their problems, thus perpetuating a cycle of denial and continuing violence. The National Lesbian Health Care Survey reported that 11% of lesbians had been victims of domestic violence by their partner, while the incidence of domestic violence in gay male couples is estimated at 15-25%.

Public violence. The Hate Crime Statistics Act requires the Federal government to collect data obtained by police agencies. However, only 12 states include homophobic violence in their definition of hate crimes; 17 have hate crime laws that do not count violence based on sexual orientation; and 21 do not count hate crimes.

The 1994 National Gay and Lesbian Task Force Report on Violence described 1,813 instances of harassment, threats, assault, vandalism, arson, kidnapping, extortion, and murder over 12 months in the six cities they monitor—New York, Minneapolis/St. Paul, Chicago, Denver, Boston, and San Francisco. Homicides against gay men and lesbians appear to be more grizzly and more likely to involve mutilation and torture, and are more likely to go unsolved, according to a two-year national study, reflecting the intensity of anti-gay hatred.

While physical harm caused by anti-gay violence is immediately obvious, psychological and emotional injury also can occur. These include post-traumatic stress and chronic pain syndromes, phobias, eating disorders, and, most commonly, depression.

Effects on earnings and medical insurability. In an analysis of the 1990 census data, in which gay and lesbian couples could identify themselves as such, it was found that, while 38% of lesbian respondents were college graduates, compared to 34% of male homosexuals and 18% of married heterosexuals, lesbian couples had the lowest income of the three groups. A reduced earning potential may result from experienced or anticipated discrimination, thus inhibiting gays and lesbians from seeking higher-profile, higher-paying jobs.

Barriers to insurance for both lesbians and gay men may keep them from obtaining yearly screening tests and seeking care early in the course of a disease. In one study, 58% of lesbians reported not seeking medical care when they felt they needed it because they lacked insurance or the financial resources. Recently, some health insurers have begun to deny insurance to men *perceived* to be gay (*e.g.,* over 30 years of age and unmarried), regardless of their HIV status.

Effects on the Doctor-Patient Relationship

Homophobia can lead to misrepresentation of facts by patients and misinterpretation of facts by physicians. Numerous studies have revealed a significant prevalence of homophobic attitudes among all types of health care practitioners in the U.S.

In the 1994 survey of the 1,311 members of the American Association of Physicians for Human Rights, now called The Gay and Lesbian Medical Association, more than half of the respondents specifically had observed the denial of care or provision of reduced or sub-optimal care to gay or lesbian patients, and 88% have heard their physician colleagues make disparaging remarks about gay or lesbian patients relating to their orientation. While 98% of respondents felt that it was medically important for patients to inform their physicians of their orientation, 64% believed that, in so doing, they risked receiving substandard care. Additionally, 17% of practicing physicians reported being refused medical privileges, employment, educational opportunities, and referrals from other doctors because of their orientation. Social ostracism and verbal harassment or insults by their medical colleagues because of their orientation were reported by one-third of physicians and one-half of medical student respondents. Summarizing the survey results, just 12% of respondents felt that "gay, lesbian or bisexual physicians are accepted as equals in the medical profession."

Medical students have reported frequently hearing overtly hostile comments made about lesbians and gay people by attending physicians during clinical teaching rounds. They express frustration with the limited information about homosexuality in their curricula, and have requested that medical educators present lectures that are updated, inclusive, and deal directly and honestly with gay and lesbian-related health issues.

Homophobic attitudes of nurses, medical students, and physicians are perceived by patients and negatively affect their experience of and the quality of their medical care. In one study, 72% of lesbians surveyed reported experiencing ostracism, rough treatment, and derogatory comments, as well as disrespect for their partners by their medical practitioners. Several studies document extremely negative reactions from health care practitioners commencing after gay or

lesbian patients revealed their orientation. More than two-thirds of lesbians report having withheld information about their sexual behavior, fearing sanctions or repercussions if they did. As a result, 84% were hesitant to return to their physicians' offices for new ailments and were less likely to come back for indicated medical screening tests—e.g., Pap smears, blood pressure, cholesterol, stool blood assays, etc. One respondent indicated: "It's like putting your health in the hands of someone who really hates you."

Many physicians have informed their lesbian patients that they do not require Pap smears because they are assumed to be in a low-risk category, having no sex with males. However, most studies reveal that 77-91% of lesbians have had at least one prior sexual experience with men. The interval between Pap smears for lesbians was reported to be more than twice that for heterosexual women. As many as five-10% of respondents in two large surveys never have had a Pap smear or had one more than 10 years ago. Moreover, one-fourth of lesbians over age 40 in a Michigan study never have had a mammogram.

Lesbians, in one study, weighed more and had less concern for appearance and thinness than heterosexual women. High body mass increases risk for breast and endometrial cancer, diabetes, heart and gall bladder disease, and hypertension. Some studies suggest that single women have higher rates of cigarette abuse. Considering all of these factors, lesbians may experience greater morbidity or mortality from multiple cancers and heart disease, especially if they defer seeing a physician until symptoms or signs become extreme or acute.

Outside the context of HIV, representative data on health and psychology issues have not been obtained from the gay and lesbian community because researchers have not considered sexual orientation an important question in national probability health surveys. In a review of journal articles reporting research on lesbian and gay men, it was observed that authors rarely involved research participants beyond the role of generating data, frequently failed to report conditions of consent, hardly ever cited feedback to participants, and virtually never indicated using the data to promote social action. This is critical because, if reliable demographic information about gay and lesbian health showed a higher incidence, morbidity, or mortality from cancers or heart disease, screening or health education programs could be instituted and targeted to the population at risk. The psychological needs of the gay and lesbian population also could be addressed more effectively, as well as the issues of ethnic minority gays and lesbians.

Once AIDS was detected among gay men in 1981, scientists at the U.S. Centers for Disease Control (CDC) quickly recognized its potential for rapid spread and lobbied their superiors for funds to research and prevent the epidemic. Given the perception of AIDS as a gay disease, though, such funding was nearly impossible to obtain from an administration that owed much of its election victory to political conservatives. It was not until two years later, after more than 1,000 Americans already had been diagnosed with AIDS, that the Reagan Administration finally requested funds from Congress to address the epidemic.

While AIDS research funding has increased dramatically in recent years, persistent antipathy towards homosexuals has made it difficult to obtain Federal funds for prevention of HIV infection among gay and bisexual men. In 1987, an amendment was passed by the Senate prohibiting the CDC from funding any materials that would "promote or encourage . . . homosexual activities," which precluded creation of any prevention informational material specific to the gay community. While this law eventually expired, other obstacles took its place. Regulations subsequently required any CDC-supported prevention materials aimed at gay or bisexual men to be reviewed by a panel representing a "reasonable cross-section of the general population" to ensure that the materials were not "offensive to a majority of adults beyond the target audience." A Federal court struck down these regulations, finding that they hampered AIDS prevention efforts.

After a *Reader's Digest* article criticized the CDC for "promoting homosexuality" by funding an AIDS prevention agency targeting gay and bisexual men of color, CDC funding to that agency was cut. A similar difficulty was encountered in obtaining information from the medical professions about lesbian and gay health in general. Numerous requests by members of the American College of Obstetricians and Gynecologists to its Patient Education Committee to include information about sexual orientation in brochures dealing with teenage sexuality, teaching children about sexuality, sexual dysfunction, and sexually transmitted diseases have been ignored.

Upon inquiry regarding the absence of HIV prevention materials directed towards individuals and communities at highest risk, U.S. Assistant Secretary for Health James O. Mason responded: "There are certain areas which, when the goals of science collide with moral and ethical judgment, science has to take a time out." Health and Human Services spokesman William Grigg explained that, "when you're fighting a fire, you control it from the outside and let the center burn. The same holds true for medicine."

Creating and Implementing Solutions

It is important to recognize that being gay or lesbian is not inherently—genetically or biologically—hazardous, but that risk factors are conferred through "homophobic fallout." Therefore, homophobia—the socialization of heterosexuals against homosexuals and concomitant conditioning of gays and lesbians against themselves—must be recognized by physicians as a legitimate health hazard.

Progress already has been made in multiple precedent-setting examples. The American Medical Association (AMA), at its 1993 annual meeting, voted to include the words "sexual orientation" in its non-discrimination statement, after having rejected this motion for four consecutive years. The American Medical Women's Association (AMWA), the 12,000-member association of female physicians, passed, without opposition, a policy statement urging an end to discrimination by sexual orientation. Moreover, AMWA encouraged: "national, state, and local legislation to end discrimination based on sexual orientation in housing, employment, marriage and tax laws, child custody and adoption laws; to redefine family to encompass the full diversity of all family structures; and to ratify marriage for lesbian, gay and bisexual people . . . creation and implementation of educational programs . . . in the schools, religious institutions, medical community, and the wider community to teach respect for all humans."

Recognizing the importance of knowledge about diversity of sexual orientation in clinical practice is an important part of the solution. Physicians must be aware that as much as six percent of the patients they see—about 15,000,000 Americans—are gay, lesbian, or bisexual, and that these individuals express part of the normal range of human sexuality. Their unique health issues need to be heard, respected, and addressed. A prerequisite is the learned genuine appreciation of the diversity that exists in America today. Such information must come from organized curricula in medical school and/or residency training programs. The Temple University School of Medicine provides its medical community with a resource guide that addresses many of the issues described above. The American Psychiatric Association has sponsored "A Curriculum for Learning About Homosexuality and Gay Men and Lesbians in Psychiatric Residencies," which describes educational objectives, learning experiences, and implementation strategies for sound clinical practice.

Health care providers can do much to reduce homophobia within their practices. The need for a trusting, supportive, and open doctor-patient relationship is critical in compiling a thorough and accurate medical history of each patient. There are numerous ways physicians can make their practices more welcoming of gay and lesbian patients.

- Physicians routinely should ask, when discussing sexual behavior, whether the patient is sexual with men, women, both, or neither. Doctors clearly should dispel any assumption of heterosexuality by using inclusive language with all patients, inquiring about behavior, not labeling the orientation, and accepting the information with neutrality. Simply having a non-judgmental, non-homophobic attitude is not enough. A responsible practitioner must convey that attitude to all patients.

- Using generic terms such as "partner" or "spouse" rather than "boyfriend" or "girlfriend" will encourage trust in the physician by removing assumptions. It would be useful for health care providers to become familiar with language commonly utilized in naming sexual behaviors. Comfortable use of these terms will facilitate taking the health history by enhancing clarity of communication.

- Registration forms and questionnaires that require patients to identify themselves in heterosexual terms such as single or divorced should be revised to include "significantly involved" or "domestic partner," in order to avoid excluding gay or lesbian patients.

- Informational brochures for patients—especially those dealing with aspects of human sexuality—need to include facts about homosexuality. Educational pamphlets in the offices of gynecologists,

pediatricians, and family practitioners could provide life-affirming information to youngsters and become an educational source for parents, possibly impacting rates of youth suicide as well as public violence and discrimination.

- If the lesbian or gay patient is partnered, the health care provider should welcome the patient's significant other and routinely encourage the couple to consider obtaining a medical power of attorney document, especially prior to any elective surgery or obstetrical delivery. Just as for married individuals, the physician should provide support for the stability of the patient's relationship. The doctor should have the skills to counsel for gay-related anxieties and safeguard against referrals to homophobic colleagues.

In order to provide general information as well as specific education for all adolescents, physicians should not reserve their questions about orientation for the gender-atypical individuals, the "sissy" boys and "tomboy" girls. It is impossible to predict which youth are struggling with issues of orientation, and all youngsters can benefit from the non-biased demonstration of the health care provider's positive attitude toward issues of orientation. While gender-atypical youth ultimately may develop a homosexual orientation, negative parental attitudes serve only to alienate the parent and isolate the child. It is irrational to classify such behavior in youth as abnormal when homosexuality in adults is not considered in that manner. The American Academy of Pediatrics (AAP), recognizing homosexuality as a natural sexual expression, recommends psychotherapy for gay and lesbian

youth who are uncertain about their orientation or need help addressing personal, family, and environmental difficulties that are concomitant with coming out. The AAP also recognizes that families may experience some stress and need information while supporting an individual's newly expressed orientation and recommends that families contact organizations such as Parents, Family, and Friends of Lesbians and Gays or obtain therapy.

The AAP further states: "Therapy directed at changing sexual orientation is contraindicated, since it can provoke guilt and anxiety while having little or no potential for achieving changes in orientation." Conversion therapy is ineffective, unethical, and harmful to the individual. In 1994, the American Medical Association issued its concurrence in an updated policy statement regarding the medical treatment of gay men and lesbians. One of the conclusions of the report was that therapy to change sexual orientation no longer is recommended, but psychotherapy may be necessary to help gays or lesbians become more comfortable with their sexuality and deal with society's prejudicial response to them. The AMA report agreed on the importance of obtaining an accurate, unbiased sexual history from all patients with a focus on behavior, recognizing the alienation of many gay men and lesbians from the medical system, the ubiquity of prejudice against homosexuals, and the psychological effects of the prejudice.

Physicians can encourage their practice group and medical centers to make available benefit packages that insure all committed couples. Regardless of their orientation and political or religious affiliation, doctors must provide the highest standard of care to all patients by discarding those views which science does not validate. They have a responsibility to examine their attitudes about homosexuality and recognize the views they hold which are not consistent with facts. Health care providers have a unique opportunity to influence others in American society to align their attitudes with objective information. Public education of both adults and children about the diversity of orientation will reduce the pervasive, unfounded disdain for homosexuals and maintain lesbian and gay individuals' self-respect. Civil rights legislation proscribing discrimination and providing legal recognition for the unions of lesbian and gay families will restore legal, societal, and financial equity to the marginalized population. Improved access to health care, increased integration into family and society, and heightened life satisfaction and productivity will result when homophobia is recognized as the major health hazard it poses to gays and lesbians.

 Article Review Form at end of book.

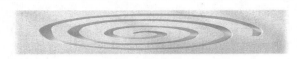

WiseGuide Wrap-Up

- Various health conditions and emotional circumstances, your choice of contraceptive method, and

family planning practices can have serious sexual and reproductive health consequences.

- Common health aspects of sexuality, such as safer sex practices, circumcision, and homosexuality, are not always well understood by those who are sexually active.

R.E.A.L. Sites

This list provides a print preview of typical **coursewise** R.E.A.L. Sites. (There are over 100 such sites at the **courselinks**™ site.) The danger in printing URLs is that Web sites can change overnight. As we went to press, these sites were functional using the URLs provided. If you come across one that isn't, please let us know via email at webmaster@coursewise.com. Use your Passport to access the most current list of R.E.A.L. sites at the **courselinks**™ site.

Site name: Atlanta Reproductive Health Centre

URL: http://www.ivf.com/index.html

Why is it R.E.A.L.? Thorough, reliable, current, and searchable information about a wide variety of women's health topics including infertility and reproductive health.

Key topics: reproductive health, women's health

Activity: Use this site as a starting point for researching term papers on women's health topics. After viewing this site, you should be able to narrow down your topic to manageable size.

Site name: Planned Parenthood

URL: http://ppfa.org/ppfa/

Why is it R.E.A.L.? Searchable information about sexual and reproductive health for women, men, parents, and teenagers. Social advocacy and job opportunities listed.

Key topics: women's health, reproductive health, health statistics

Activity: Consider applying for a job with Planned Parenthood. See if your personal philosophy matches with the Planned Parenthood mission. Find out what qualifications you would need. Decide if it's a place you'd like to work.

Site name: SIECUS (Sexuality Information and Education Council)

URL: http://www.siecus.org

Why is it R.E.A.L.? SIECUS is a professional organization dedicated to providing sexuality education information to the public. Information provided is very current, objective, thoroughly researched, and accurate.

Key topics: sexual health, reproductive health, health statistics

Site name: American Social Health Association

URL: http://sunsite.unc.edu/ASHA/faq/faq.html

Why is it R.E.A.L.? Objective answers to frequently asked questions about safer sex in a non-threatening format for personal discovery.

Key topics: sexual health and sexually transmitted disease, reproductive health

Activity: The Legislative Advocacy option will "Let Your Voice Be heard." Participate as an active citizen by sending a message to Congress about the need for greater efforts to prevent sexually transmitted disease.

Site name: Men's Health Issues

URL: http://medic.med.uth.tmc.edu/ptnt/00000391.htm

Why is it R.E.A.L.? Provides basic information about men's health issues.

Key topics: men's health

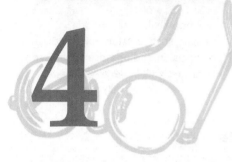

section

4

Key Points

- People with chronic disabilities can be healthy, given an appropriate definition of health.

- Care must be taken to avoid becoming a victim of health fraud when living with illness, disease, or disability.

- Critical thinking skills, good preparation, and assertiveness can help you make the most of your healthcare interactions and health information sources.

- Some medical conditions with common and vague symptoms are particularly difficult to diagnose.

- Specific measures can be taken to reduce your risk of developing cancer and increase your chances of being cured from cancer.

Living Well with Illness, Disease, and Challenge

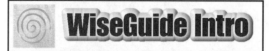 **WiseGuide Intro**

In some ways, engaging in a healthy lifestyle can give us a false sense of security. Despite all our best efforts to get and stay healthy, we can still get sick from influences beyond our control. Under these circumstances, becoming a critical consumer of healthcare and health information and learning as much as possible about a condition are far more effective strategies than ignoring symptoms and doggedly pursuing positive health habits. Symptoms are often viewed as problematic, yet identification of symptoms is necessary for diagnosis, treatment, and management. Begin to view symptoms as tools to gaining control over illness, disease, and disability rather than as barriers to good health.

Two alternative notions of health are presented in the first two articles ("Redefining Health for People with Chronic Disabilities" and "An FDA Guide to Choosing Medical Treatments"). The next articles ("Let's Get a Physical" and "To Get Top Health Care, Be Sure to Consult a Trusted Advisor—Yourself") provide advice to health consumers about how to make the best of their healthcare opportunities. The remaining articles describe the risks, diagnosis, and management of immune disorders, heart disease, and cancer. Audre Lorde ("A Burst of Light") poignantly describes her struggle with cancer and the healthcare system from her perspective as an African-American woman.

? Questions ?

R19. Why are existing medical and holistic concepts of health meaningless for people with chronic disabilities?

R20. What makes older adults especially vulnerable to health fraud?

R21. What tests might men expect when they get a physical examination?

R22. What are three ways that you can screen medical advice from health information resources?

R23. What are some conditions that are particularly difficult to diagnose?

R24. What are two symptoms of heart disease in women that often go unrecognized?

R25. What is the single most important and preventable cause of cancer death? What are some other measures you can take to reduce your risk of cancer?

R26. Who was Audre Lorde? What did living fully mean to Audre Lorde?

Why are existing medical and holistic concepts of health meaningless for people with chronic disabilities?

Redefining Health for People with Chronic Disabilities

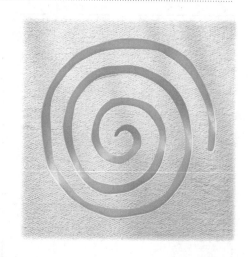

Youngkhill Lee
Thomas K. Skalko

The term health appears to be one of the recent recurring themes in allied health professions, including therapeutic recreation (TR). Although health is an important concept, little discussion has been made to examine the relevance of health in the lives of people with disabilities. Most health care agencies, and thus, TR service within health care systems, follow a medical view and/or World Health Organization's (WHO) holistic concept. These concepts may not respond well in the context to the lives of people with disabilities. The medical concept excludes individuals with chronic disabilities who persevere and succeed in spite of their disabilities. The holistic concept sets unrealistic criteria for people with chronic disabilities who adapt to their circumstances. Accordingly, there is no definitive health state for individuals with these characteristics, and therefore, their health status thus remains undefined. In order to conceptualize health for people with chronic disabilities, one important conceptual premise—life story—should be woven into existing concepts of health.

Life Story

Life story combines the life plans in the past with the life plans of the future (see Brody, 1987; Kleiber, Brock, Lee, Dattilo, & Caldwell, 1995). For most people, current life story is a reflection of the recollected past and the desired future. Life story is defined as "a person's story of his or her life, or of what he or she thinks is a significant part of that life" (Tilton, 1980, p. 276). The state of "illness" occurs when people with chronic disabilities experience a threat to their story. As they change, and as the physical and social world around them changes, they rewrite their stories accordingly. People with chronic disabilities constantly attempt to discover an alternative story to help them make sense of a life that involves adjustment and acceptance of limitations. One im-

portant conceptual suggestion focuses on the particular role individuals find for health in the new stories they write for themselves after illness/disability. In rewriting one's life stories, Goffman (1961) offered two contrasting life stories that people with disabilities might write:

If the person can manage to present a view of his current situation which shows the operation of favorable personal qualities in the past and a favorable destiny awaiting for him, it may be called a *success story*. If the facts of a person's past and present are extremely dismal, then about the best he can do is to show that he is not responsible for what has become of him, and the term *sad tale* is appropriate (pp. 150-151).

The possible stories that people with chronic illness might write are either *success stories* or *sad tales*. When rewriting one's life stories, it is a *success story* if one indicates successful adjustment to illness/disability, while *sad tales* would reflect unsuccessful adjustment to the changed circumstances. Identification of what

From Youngkhill Lee and Thomas K. Skalko. This article is reprinted with permission from the *Journal of Physical Education, Recreation & Dance*, November/December, 1996, pp. 64-65. JOPERD is a publication of the American Alliance for Health, Physical Education, Recreation and Dance, 1900 Association Drive, Reston, VA 20191.

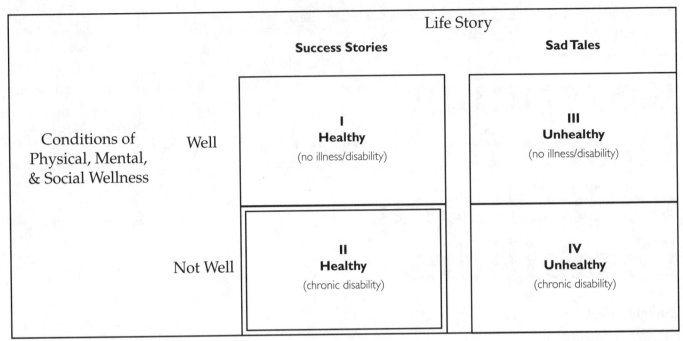

Figure 1

stories one writes can be an important consideration for determining the health status of these individuals.

Reconceptualized Model of Health

Using the life story component in the concept of health, we developed a model of health that contextualizes the lives of people with chronic disabilities. Figure 1 represents our model, in which two dimensions are important: conditions in physical, mental and social wellness (CPMS) and life story. The CPMS dimension (vertical) reflects existing concepts of health. In this dimension, one end signifies "well" and the other end "not well." In the life story dimension (horizontal), one end indicates "success stories" and the other end "sad tales" (Goffman, 1963).

In cell I of figure 1, "success stories" in the life story dimension merges with "well" in the CPMS dimension. People who meet these two conditions can without doubt be considered healthy. This cell may include individuals without disabilities who are satisfied with their lives.

In cell II, "success stories" merges with "not well." This cell represents those people who are able to write success stories in spite of their physical disabilities. These people feel healthy even though they do not meet traditional criteria for health. Therefore, they can be classified as healthy.

In cell III, "sad tales" merges with "well." This cell represents people without disabilities who may be considered well under existing concepts but whose life stories place them in a questionable state of health. In our model, they are classified as unhealthy.

Cell IV represents people with sad tales who are not well. These people may not have accepted their disabilities, and their life stories suffer accordingly.

This model reflects the reality of the lives of people with chronic disabilities and supplies a revised definition of health. Our definition of health does not negate existing concepts, but rather weaves them together with the concept of life story.

References

Brody, H. (1987). *Stories of sickness*. New Haven, CT: Yale University Press.

Goffman, E. (1963). *Stigma: Notes on the management of spoiled identity*. Englewood Cliffs, NJ: Prentice-Hall.

Kleiber, D. A., Brock, S., Lee, Y., Dattilo, J., & Caldwell, L. (1995). The relevance of leisure in an illness experience: The realities of spinal cord injury. *Journal of Leisure Research, 27*(3), 283-299.

Tilton, J. T. (1980). The life story. *Journal of American Folklore, 93*, 276-292.

Youngkhill Lee is an assistant professor of School of Recreation and Sport Sciences at Ohio University, Athens, OH 45701; Thomas Skalko is a professor and chair of Department of Health, Physical Education, and Recreation at East Carolina University, Greenville, NC 27858-4353.

 Article Review Form at end of book.

Editor's Note: Because of space limitations, this article has been condensed. An in-depth article on the subject is planned for future publication. Contact the author for more information.

What makes older adults especially vulnerable to health fraud?

An FDA Guide to Choosing Medical Treatments

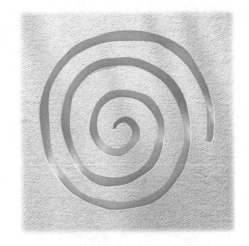

Isadora B. Stehlin

Medical treatments come in many shapes and sizes. There are "home remedies" shared among families and friends. There are prescription medicines, available only from a pharmacist, and only when ordered by a physician. There are over-the-counter drugs that you can buy—almost anywhere—without a doctor's order. Of growing interest and attention in recent years are so-called alternative treatments, not yet approved for sale because they are still undergoing scientific research to see if they really are safe and effective. And, of course, there are those "miracle" products sold through "back-of-the-magazine" ads and TV infomercials.

How can you tell which of these may really help treat your medical condition, and which will only make you worse off—financially, physically, or both?

Many advocates of unproven treatments and cures contend that people have the right to try whatever may offer them hope, even if others believe the remedy is worthless. This argument is especially compelling for people with AIDS or other life-threatening diseases with no known cure.

Clinical Trials

Before gaining Food and Drug Administration marketing approval, new drugs, biologics, and medical devices must be proven safe and effective by controlled clinical trials.

In a clinical trial, results observed in patients getting the treatment are compared with the results in similar patients receiving a different treatment or placebo (inactive) treatment. Preferably, neither patients nor researchers know who is receiving the therapy under study.

To FDA, it doesn't matter whether the product or treatment is labeled alternative or falls under the auspices of mainstream American medical practice. (Mainstream American medicine essentially includes the practices and products the majority of medical doctors in this country follow and use.) It must meet the agency's safety and effectiveness criteria before being allowed on the market.

In addition, just because something is undergoing a clinical trial doesn't mean it works or FDA considers it to be a proven therapy, says Donald Pohl, of

FDA's Office of AIDS and Special Health Issues. "You can't jump to that conclusion," he says. A trial can fail to prove that the product is effective, he explains. And that's not just true for alternative products. Even when the major drug companies sponsor clinical trials for mainstream products, only a small fraction are proven safe and effective.

Many people with serious illnesses are unable to find a cure, or even temporary relief, from the available mainstream treatments that have been rigorously studied and proven safe and effective. For many conditions, such as arthritis or even cancer, what's effective for one patient may not help another.

Real Alternatives

"It is best not to abandon conventional therapy when there is a known response [in the effectiveness of that therapy]" says Joseph Jacobs, M.D., former director of the National Institutes of Health's Office of Alternative Medicine, which was established in October 1992. As an example he cites childhood leukemia, which has an 80 percent cure rate with conventional therapy.

Source: From Isadora B. Stehlin, "An FDA Guide to Choosing Medical Treatments" in *FDA Consumer*, June 1995, U.S. Food and Drug Administration Office.

But what if conventional therapy holds little promise?

Many physicians believe it is not unreasonable for someone in the last stages of an incurable cancer to try something unproven. But, for example, if a woman with an early stage of breast cancer wanted to try shark cartilage (an unproven treatment that may inhibit the growth of cancer tumors, currently undergoing clinical trials), those same doctors would probably say, "Don't do it," because there are so many effective conventional treatments.

Jacobs warns that, "If an alternative practitioner does not want to work with a regular doctor, then he's suspect."

Alternative medicine is often described as any medical practice or intervention that:

- lacks sufficient documentation of its safety and effectiveness against specific diseases and conditions

- is not generally taught in U.S. medical schools

- is not generally reimbursable by health insurance providers.

According to a study in the Jan. 28, 1993, *New England Journal of Medicine,* 1 in 3 patients used alternative therapy in 1990. More than 80 percent of those who use alternative therapies used conventional medicine at the same time, but did not tell their doctors about the alternative treatments. The study's authors concluded this lack of communication between doctors and patients "is not in the best interest of the patients, since the use of unconventional therapy, especially if it is totally unsupervised, may be harmful." The study concluded that medical doctors should ask their patients about any use of unconventional treatment as part of a medical history.

Many doctors are interested in learning more about alternative therapies, according to Brian Berman, M.D., a family practitioner with the University of Maryland School of Medicine in Baltimore. Berman says his own interest began when "I found that I wasn't getting all the results that I would have liked with conventional medicine, especially in patients with chronic diseases.

"What I've found at the University of Maryland is a healthy skepticism among my colleagues, but a real willingness to collaborate. We have a lot of people from different departments who are saying, let's see how we can develop scientifically rigorous studies that are also sensitive to the particular therapies that we're working with."

Anyone who wants to be treated with an alternative therapy should try to do so through participation in a clinical trial. Clinical trials are regulated by FDA and provide safeguards to protect patients, such as monitoring of adverse reactions. In fact, FDA is interested in assisting investigators who want to study alternative therapies under carefully controlled clinical trials.

Some of the alternative therapies currently under study with grants from NIH include:

- acupuncture to treat depression, attention-deficit hyperactivity disorder, osteoarthritis, and postoperative dental pain

> **Anyone who wants to be treated with an alternative therapy should try to do so through participation in a clinical trial.**

- hypnosis for chronic low back pain and accelerated fracture healing

- Ayurvedic herbals for Parkinson's disease. (Ayurvedic medicine is a holistic system based on the belief that herbals, massage, and other stress relievers help the body make its own natural drugs.)

- biofeedback for diabetes, low back pain, and face and mouth pain caused by jaw disorders. (Biofeedback is the conscious control of biological functions, such as those of the heart and blood vessels, normally controlled involuntarily.)

- electric currents to treat tumors

- imagery for asthma and breast cancer. (With imagery, patients are guided to see themselves in a different physical, emotional or spiritual state. For example, patients might be guided to imagine themselves in a state of vibrant health and the disease organisms as weak and destructible.)

While these alternative therapies are the subject of scientifically valid research, it's important to remember that at this time their safety and effectiveness are still unproven.

Avoiding Fraud

FDA defines health fraud as the promotion, advertisement, distribution, or sale of articles, intended for human or animal use, that are represented as being effective to diagnose, prevent, cure, treat, or mitigate disease (or other conditions), or provide a beneficial effect on health, but which have not been scientifically proven safe and effective for such purposes. Such practices may be deliberately deceptive, or done without adequate knowledge or understanding of the article.

Health fraud costs Americans an estimated $30 billion a year. However, the costs are not just economic, according to John Renner, M.D., a Kansas City-based champion of quality health care for the elderly. "The hidden costs—death, disability—are unbelievable," he says.

To combat health fraud, FDA established its National Health Fraud Unit in 1988. The unit works with the National Association of Attorneys General and the Association of Food and Drug Officials to coordinate federal, state and local regulatory actions against specific health frauds.

Regulatory actions may be necessary in many cases because products that have not been shown to be safe and effective pose potential hazards for consumers both directly and indirectly. The agency's priorities for regulatory action depend on the situation; direct risks to health come first.

Unproven products cause direct health hazards when their use results in injuries or adverse reactions. For example, a medical device called the InnerQuest Brain Wave Synchronizer was promoted to alter brain waves and relieve stress. It consisted of an audio cassette and eyeglasses that emitted sounds and flashing lights. It caused epileptic seizures in some users. As a result of a court order requested by FDA, 78 cartons of the devices, valued at $200,000, were seized by U.S. marshals and destroyed in June 1993.

Indirectly harmful products are those that do not themselves cause injury, but may lead people to delay or reject proven remedies, possibly worsening their condition. For example, if cancer patients reject proven drug therapies in favor of unproved ones and the unproven ones turn out not to work, their disease may advance beyond the point where proven therapies can help.

"What you see out there is the promotion of products claiming to cure or prevent AIDS, multiple sclerosis, cancer, and a list of other diseases that goes on and on," says Joel Aronson, director of FDA's Health Fraud Staff, in the agency's Center for Drug Evaluation and Research. For example, he says, several skin cream products promise to prevent transmission of HIV (the virus that causes AIDS) and herpes viruses. They are promoted especially to health-care workers. Many of the creams contain antibacterial ingredients but, "there is no substantiation at all on whether or not [the skin creams] work" against HIV, says Aronson. FDA has warned the manufacturers of these creams to stop the misleading promotions.

People at Risk

Teenagers and the elderly are two prime targets for health fraud promoters.

The NIH Office of Alternative Medicine recommends the following before getting involved in any alternative therapy:

- Obtain objective information about the therapy. Besides talking with the person promoting the approach, speak with people who have gone through the treatment— preferably both those who were treated recently and those treated in the past. Ask about the advantages and disadvantages, risks, side effects, costs, results, and over what time span results can be expected.

- Inquire about the training and expertise of the person administering the treatment (for example, certification).

- Consider the costs. Alternative treatments may not be reimbursable by health insurance.

- Discuss all treatments with your primary care provider, who needs this information in order to have a complete picture of your treatment plan.

For everyone—consumers, physicians and other health-care providers, and government regulators—FDA has the same advice when it comes to weeding out the hopeless from the hopeful: Be open-minded, but don't fall into the abyss of accepting anything at all. For there are—as there have been for centuries—countless products that are nothing more than fraud. ■

Teenagers concerned about their appearance and susceptible to peer pressure may fall for such products as fraudulent diet pills, breast developers, and muscle-building pills.

Older Americans may be especially vulnerable to health fraud because approximately 80 percent of them have at least one chronic health problem, according to Renner. Many of these problems, such as arthritis, have no cure and, for some people, no effective treatment. He says their pain and disability lead to despair, making them excellent targets for deception.

Arthritis

Although there is no cure for arthritis, the symptoms may come and go with no explanation. According to the Arthritis Foundation, "You may think a new remedy worked because you took it when your symptoms were going away."

Some commonly touted unproven treatments for arthritis are harmful, according to the foundation, including snake venom and DMSO (dimethyl sulfoxide), an industrial solvent similar to turpentine. FDA has approved a sterile form of DMSO called Rimso-50, which is administered directly into the bladder for treatment of a rare bladder condition called interstitial cystitis. However, the DMSO sold to arthritis sufferers may contain bacterial toxins. DMSO is readily absorbed through the skin into the bloodstream, and these toxins enter the bloodstream along with it. It can be especially dangerous if used as an enema, as some of its promoters recommend.

Treatments the foundation considers harmless but ineffective include copper bracelets, mineral springs, and spas.

Cancer and AIDS

Cancer treatment is complicated because in some types of cancer there are no symptoms, and in other types symptoms may disappear by themselves, at least temporarily. Use of an unconventional treatment coinciding with remission (lessening of symptoms) could be simply coincidental. There's no way of knowing, without a controlled clinical trial, what effect the treatment had on the outcome. The danger comes when this false security causes patients to forgo approved treatment that has shown real benefit.

Some unapproved cancer treatments not only have no proven benefits, they have actually been proven dangerous. These include Laetrile, which may cause cyanide poisoning and has been found ineffective in clinical trials, and coffee enemas, which, when used excessively, have killed patients. (See "Hope or Hoax? Unproven Cancer Treatments" in the March 1992 *FDA Consumer.*)

Ozone generators, which produce a toxic form of oxygen gas, have been touted as being able to cure AIDS. To date this is still unproven, and FDA considers ozone to be an unapproved drug and these generators to be unapproved medical devices. At least three deaths have been connected to the use of these generators. Four British citizens were indicted in 1991 for selling fraudulent ozone generators in the United States. Two of the defendants fled

Medical Guides

Whether looking for an alternative therapy or checking the legitimacy of something you've heard about, some of the best sources are advocacy groups, including local patient support groups. Those groups include:

American Cancer Society
1599 Clifton Road, N.E.
Atlanta, GA 30329
(404) 320-3333, (1-800) ACS-2345

Arthritis Foundation
P.O. Box 19000
Atlanta, GA 30326
(1-800) 283-7800

National Multiple Sclerosis Society
733 Third Ave.
New York, NY 10017-3288
(212) 986-3240, (1-800) 344-4867

HIV/AIDS Treatment Information Service
P.O. Box 6303
Rockville, MD 20849-6303
(1-800) 448-0440, TDD/Deaf Access:
(1-800) 243-7012

Federal government resources on health fraud and alternative medicine are:

FDA (HFE-88)
Rockville, MD 20857
(301) 443-3170

Office of Alternative Medicine/
NIH Information Center
6120 Executive Blvd., EPS
Suite 450
Rockville, MD 20852
(301) 402-2466

U.S. Postal Inspection Service
(monitors products purchased by mail)
Office of Criminal Investigation
Washington, DC 20260-2166
(202) 268-4272

Federal Trade Commission
(regarding false advertising)
Room 421
6th St. and Pennsylvania Ave., N.W.
Washington, DC 20580
(202) 326-2222

Other agencies that may have information and offer assistance include local Better Business Bureaus, state and municipal consumer affairs offices, and state attorneys general offices.■

to Great Britain, but the other two pleaded guilty and served time in U.S. federal prisons.

The bottom line in deciding whether a certain treatment you've read or heard about might be right for you: Talk to your doctor. And keep in mind the old adage: If it sounds too good to be true, it probably is.■

Isadora B. Stehlin is a staff writer for FDA Cosumer.

 Article Review Form at end of book.

What tests might men expect when they get a physical examination?

Let's Get a Physical

When it comes to managing your health, you're the boss, right? So here's everything you need to do to keep tabs on your personal bottom line

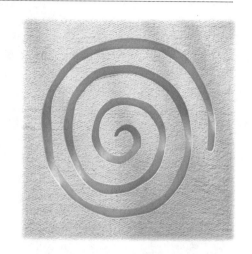

Dan Rutz

Being a television reporter is a glamorous job, filled with excitement, intrigue and danger. I try to remind myself of these facts as I lie here, on my side, a CNN camera rolling while physician Larry Gibbons, M.D., uses a flexible sigmoidoscope to inspect the state of my lower bowel—and describe it to a potential audience of millions.

As senior medical correspondent for CNN, I've asked more than a thousand people to let us in on the most private details of their medical past and present. Sometimes I'm amazed by their willingness. "Hell," I've thought, "*I* wouldn't do it." But in honor of National Men's Health Week, I sold myself on my own pitch. "Maybe it'll help someone else. It might even help me."

So let's take this physical together. Why now? If you're older than 40 and it's been more than two years since your last head-to-toe, like me, you're overdue. For younger men, if it's been more than five years since your last date with the doctor, your appointment is waiting to be made. We don't have to *like* getting a physical. We just have to *do* it. Stick with me to find out why.

The Private Parts

A good physical is like school in reverse. First your get the test, then the lesson. And a checkup at the world-renowned Cooper Clinic is thorough. Thousands are drawn to Dallas on the reputation of the clinic's founder, Kenneth Cooper, M.D., the father of aerobic exercise. While growing older is inevitable, Dr. Cooper believes that many of the maladies of old age are optional.

They say guys are gutless when it comes to doctors. I am, too, especially when it comes to somebody poking around in private places. But I can honestly tell you that none of the below-the-belt stuff is as bad as it sounds. Here's what it entails:

• **Colon exam.** Because the risk of colon cancer jumps sharply when men hit their mid-40s, a complete mid-life exam includes the lower tract. I've already completed the first part of this test before arriving at the office. All it takes is a minuscule stool sample, smeared on a sensitized card. A lab technician determines whether there's any blood hidden in the specimen. Cancer (or the growths that precede it) often causes bleeding, so a "positive" test is reason for further investigation.

The second part of the test utilizes the amazing power of modern optics to spot suspicious growths inside the bowel. About half of all colorectal cancers or polyps are within range of the flexible sigmoidoscope. Trust me: The exam is finished in minutes with no pain. For me the news is good—nothing out of the ordinary. This year, about 70,000 men won't be as lucky. But still only 5 to 10 percent of those who should be screened for colorectal cancer have the test.

• **Digital rectal exam (DRE).** As a man, you have a one-in-five chance of developing prostate cancer at some point in your life. My risk is even higher: I take after my grandfather, who died of the disease before his time. There's a good chance that, besides looking like him, I may have inherited his tendency to develop prostate cancer at an early age. He couldn't do much to protect himself, but I can, by detecting it early. Thirty seconds in awkward contemplation is a fair trade for ruling out a potential killer. The doctor's gloved finger does the walking through the rectum, where it is possible to feel the back side of the gland for increased size or hard bumps. Starting at age 40, you should have this exam once a year. It's a bit uncomfortable, but surprisingly painless and quick.

- **PSA.** The letters stand for *prostate-specific antigen.* It can be a reassuring acronym if, like me, your risk of prostate cancer is higher than average. Where prostate cancer runs in the family, and for all African-American men, it's a good idea to combine the digital rectal exam with the PSA blood test, starting at age 40. A high level may mean cancer is present. The doctor can conduct further tests if necessary. A sigh of relief: My PSA is well within normal limits.

The Heart Parts

The leading killer of men is still heart disease, which explains why so much of a physical exam is dedicated to your ticker.

- **Blood-pressure test.** Pressures are reported in two numbers—as the heart is actually pumping blood, and during its "resting" phase between beats. Consistent

readings above 140/90 indicate an increased risk of stroke or heart disease. Mine is in this range, but my doctor is not concerned: He and I both suspect the presence of the TV camera has something to do with it. In fact, so many guys show signs of "white-coat hypertension" that doctors usually don't sound the alarm unless the readings run consistently high. I'm advised to have my pressure rechecked in a more relaxed setting, and sure enough, it has been in the normal range (130/80) subsequent times.

- **Stethoscope exam.** The familiar stethoscope amplifies sounds of the heart and lungs. Yeah, it's cold, but it's necessary. Trained ears can pick up many irregularities. Be sure your doctor also listens to the arteries in your neck. "Noisy" carotids may be an early warning sign of stroke.

- **Stress test.** My Cooper Clinic physical includes a trip on the gerbil trail—the treadmill from hell. "Nothing to it, sir. Just hop up here and walk until your legs give out." The longer you go, the steeper the hill. At 26 minutes I give. "Hey, Dr. Gibbons says, "you're in better shape than I thought."

"Damn right," I mutter to myself. This makes up for all the sleep I've missed with those 4-mile runs at the crack of dawn. But there's more to this exercise than affirming male pride. It shows the doctor how well the heart performs during heavy labor. The exercise stress test is 90 percent accurate in ruling out

heart disease, and 75 percent reliable for finding it. It provides an excellent measure of overall fitness, and how we compare with other men our age.

- **Chest x-ray.** I don't smoke, and I'm guessing you're smart enough not to, either. But even for those of us who have never smoked, the chest x-ray provides a good way to find the 10 percent of lung cancers in men that aren't caused by tobacco. The test also reveals how big a heart you have. And we're not talking about your generosity. Medically speaking, your heart should be about the size of your clenched fist. An enlarged heart is a sign that the vital organ is overworked and headed for early failure, unless steps are taken to lessen the stress on it.

The Obscure Parts

Besides the obvious tests you'd expect from a physical, there is a battery of additional examinations you can undergo. Each of them gives you more information about the state of your health. And the more information you have, the better decisions you can make.

- **Body-fat percentage test.** It is possible to be both fit and fat. That, the experts say, describes me the day of my exam. Crouched naked on a submersible scale, I exhale fully and duck underwater. A computer takes measurements, figures the relative buoyancy of lean tissue versus fat and determines that nearly 21 percent of me is blubber. I'm informed that 19 percent fat would be better—and that I'd need even less to qualify for an "athletic" build. This translates into a 7- to 12-pound loss, which I decide on the spot is both doable and desirable.

- **Melanoma exam.** If you're fair skinned, as I am, the sun is your enemy. Dr. Gibbons spends an extra few minutes thoroughly looking over my skin. Malignant melanoma can start out looking like a common mole, but instead of being uniform and round, it often develops an irregular shape and varying color tones. Unless it is caught early, melanoma can kill by spreading to organs throughout the body. Less-dangerous skin cancers are far more common than melanoma, often appearing as red, scaly patches or small, pesky sores that don't heal.

- **Neurological exam.** If a cop ever suspects you've had one drink too many when he pulls you over, he may ask you to perform a few simple tasks, such as standing on one foot or touching your nose with your eyes closed. When the doctor asks you to do the same, it's to find out something about the condition of the part of the brain that controls movement. A rubber hammer in the right spot should produce a knee-jerk reaction. This is a sign your nerves are healthy. And muscle strength should be approximately the same on both sides of the body. Such symmetry gives a reassuring sign that both sides of the brain are healthy and are receiving enough blood and nourishment.

The Pointed Parts

Needles? Don't like them. But you have to have them. A drop of blood is an open book on some of the accidents of our inheritance as well as the most health-threatening excesses in our lives. My blood work includes close to four dozen specific measurements for signs of disease. At minimum, you should be tested for at least these typical male health risks:

- **Diabetes.** Half of us who have diabetes don't know it, so a positive lab test provides a chance for correcting the body's sugar/insulin imbalance—often through diet and exercise—before serious complications arise.

- **Cholesterol.** At 149, my cholesterol level is well within the normal range. Consistent readings of more than 200 are cause for concern because high cholesterol may add to the risk of heart disease. The HDL portion of my total cholesterol, the "good cholesterol" that helps protect against heart attacks, is 49. A reading above 35 is considered normal. Exercise has been shown to boost HDL.

- **Complete blood count.** Low levels of red blood cells may be a sign of a polyp or an unknown cancer, or it might just mean you're not eating right. Fatigue may be a sign of anemia.

- **Uric acid and liver function (AST) tests.** Too much of the former could increase your risk of gout or kidney stones. High levels of the enzyme AST suggest liver disorders.

- **HIV.** The test for the AIDS virus depends on your sexual lifestyle. If yours is a mutually faithful, long-standing commitment to a one-and-only, this test can safely be skipped. But, if you are an active player in the sexual arena, consider including the HIV test as protection for you and your partners.

- **Urinalysis.** This one requires a paper cup instead of a needle. The small urine sample tells how well your kidneys function, whether you take in enough water and whether you may have kidney stones, prostate or urinary infections, or even some cancers.

Most components of the Cooper Clinic physical can be arranged at any doctor's office or clinic. Underwater weighing is less common, but a manual fat-measurement test is generally available and almost as accurate. It may be up to you to ask for certain tests, such as the PSA blood test for prostate cancer or an HIV test for the virus linked to AIDS. It's important to review your family's medical history and your lifestyle to determine which blood tests to include. Every physical should include the basics: examinations of your ears, eyes and mouth, any of which may turn up signs of disease or help determine overall health. Insist that your skin, including the scalp, be checked for suspicious growths that could spell trouble. The doctors should press deliberately around the neck, underarms and groin for swollen lymph glands, which may signal the presence of an infection or tumor. He should check your resting pulse rate—in general, the lower it is, the fitter your heart—and perform the classic "turn your head and cough" test for hernias.

Perhaps just as important as any of these tests is how you and your doctor converse. He should ask you about your past and present health, your diet and exercise program, your drinking and smoking habits and your family history. And you should ask him for specific advice about managing any element of your health that turns up troubling test results. After all, he's only the mechanic. You're the guy driving into the future in this valuable vehicle called your body.

 Article Review Form at end of book.

What are three ways that you can screen medical advice from health information resources?

To Get Top Health Care, Be Sure to Consult a Trusted Adviser—Yourself

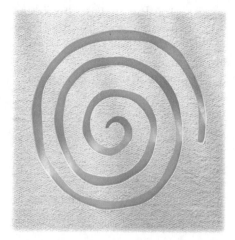

Lani Luciano

Now that some health insurance companies limit how much time your doctor spends with you and even which tests and treatments you get, who can you count on to make sure you're receiving the right care? For a growing number of patients, the answer is—themselves. These days, there's an abundance of self-help health material—books, newsletters, videos, CD-ROMs and Internet sites—offering information on topics ranging from the mundane to the technical. But which type of resource is best depends on what you're trying to find out. Here's how to match your needs to the best self-help sources:

- **For advice on treating minor symptoms.** A clear, comprehensive book or CD-ROM featuring video animation—such as the *Mayo Clinic Ultimate Medical Guide* (IVI Publishing, $40)—is best for quick, reliable advice on how to handle minor maladies and for recommendations on when it's time to see an expert. For instance, a quick scan of *Self-Care* (People's Medical Society, $29.95) will tell you that itchy, red eyes could be conjunctivitis but that it's okay to wait a day to see if the problem gets better while you try home remedies. Meanwhile, though, don't wear your contact lenses, or you may irritate the eyes further. People over 50 might browse through *Healthwise for Life* (Healthwise Inc., $9.95), which has large print and includes techniques for managing chronic conditions such as arthritis.

- **For help deciding among alternative tests and treatments.** When there are several ways to handle your condition, you probably hope your physician will make a recommendation. But if not, you may want to turn to one of the 10 treatment videos produced by the Foundation for Informed Medical Decision-Making, a nonprofit patient-education group formed by researchers at Dartmouth Medical School and Massachusetts General Hospital ($56 each; 603-650-1180). The 20- to 60-minute videos describe research backing your therapy choices, the advantages and drawbacks of each and testimony from patients who've chosen a particular alternative. Topics include benign prostate disease, prostate cancer, breast cancer surgery, follow-up treatment for breast cancer, lower-back pain, ischemic heart disease, mild hypertension, hormone-replacement therapy, benign uterine conditions and the prostate-specific antigen (PSA) test.

A computer online chat group devoted to your medical problem is another useful way to learn from others who have your condition or have had it. Of course, you can't take the opinions of strangers as gospel. But many patients find terrific advice and support this way, says Tom Ferguson, a leading expert in on-line self-help who is a physician and senior associate at the Center for Clinical Computing, a Boston think tank. Ferguson's new paperback, *Health Online* (Addison-Wesley, $17), can steer you through the many Internet newsgroups, mailing lists and other person-to-person medical services available via computer.

- **For advice about the quality of your care.** Worried that you're not getting the best treatment? Topnotch experts—as well as crackpots—produce newsletters, books, magazines and Websites. Jennifer Wayne-Doppke, editor of *Healthcare Guide to the Internet* (COR Healthcare Resources, $68), suggests screening advice in the following three ways:

First, consider the bias of the organization or individual providing the tips. Look for the names behind the names. If there's no way to trace the information to a sponsor, be skeptical.

Second, verify all health statistics and data with the original source. If no source is cited, view the information with caution.

And third, don't assume any medical material you read is true unless you have three or more independent sources for it.

You can likely find information about common medical conditions in periodicals at your library. For unusual or complex problems, however, you may need to turn to esoteric journals or other erudite repositories. The easiest way to find them is via computer. One way to streamline such a trek is by tapping into a patient-oriented Website such as the WellnessWeb (http://www.wellweb.com), which has links or referrals to hundreds of medical sources. Another is to hire a professional medical information service, such as the Health Resource (800-949-0090, or e-mail the group at more-info@thehealthresource.com). For $250 ($350 for cancer questions), the well-respected team of researchers will crawl through medical databases for the latest research on your problem. Within five business days, you'll get a bound report covering both mainstream and alternative therapies.

 Article Review Form at end of book.

What are some conditions that are particularly difficult to diagnose?

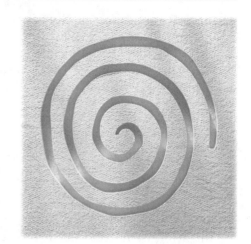

Mysterious Maladies

Separating real from imagined disorders presents frustrating challenges

Sasha Nemecek

As a physician in Tanzania in 1988, Robert Aronowitz struggled to isolate the cause of the arthritis-like joint aches and pains he saw in dozens of his patients. Local doctors had also been stumped by the condition—they name it *hapa-hapa*, or "here and there," because the symptoms were so difficult to pin down. Aronowitz, now a clinician and medical historian at the Robert Wood Johnson Medical School in New Jersey, never could determine what was behind his patients' complaints.

Such confusion is not unusual: most of us have on occasion left the doctor's office wondering if something important has been missed. Explaining sickness can become especially complicated when the medical community disagrees over whether a particular disease even exists. Consider the condition known as chronic fatigue syn-drome (CFS), characterized by fatigue, pain and cognitive disorders, which has been riding a roller coaster of medical opinion since it was first described in the mid-1980s. A recent book—*Osler's Web: Inside the Labyrinth of the Chronic Fatigue Syndrome Epidemic*—recounts the history of this controversial ailment.

The author, Hillary Johnson, a journalist and CFS patient, traces the syndrome from its early connection with the Epstein-Barr virus to the current search for a novel retrovirus that some claim may cause CFS. Along the way, she criticizes health officials for dismissing the syndrome as psychological and notes that CFS is not the first condition to be overlooked—in the early part of this century, for instance, multiple sclerosis was known as "the faker's disease."

People complaining of CFS and similarly disputed maladies, such as Gulf War syndrome, multiple chemical sensitivity and the complications supposedly connected to silicone breast implants, generally blame stress on the immune system for their problems. According to advocates of these syndromes, an overload of toxins—nerve gas, insecticides, silicone gel or a virus—somehow overwork the body's natural defenses, leaving its immune system in disarray.

Charles Rosenberg, a historian and sociologist of science at the University of Pennsylvania, notes that immune disorders have traditionally been difficult to identify. "Even well-established diseases such as lupus are elusive and complicated to diagnose," he says. (On average, patients with lupus, a disease in which the immune system attacks healthy tissue and damages the skin, joints, blood and kidneys, go undiagnosed or misdiagnosed for about four years.) Aronowitz suggests that because of science's incomplete understanding of the immune system, physicians and patients—no doubt influenced by the specter of AIDS—often implicate immune disorders in mysterious illnesses. "They point to things like environmental exposure and the battle of the immune system" to explain why some people get sick and others do not, Aronowitz says.

Of course, not every ache and pain heralds a bona fide disease. So how do doctors distinguish between hypochondria and hidden illness? An organic agent, such as a bacterium, virus or mutated gene, certainly establishes a disease as real. But many diseases—multiple sclerosis, for example—lack a well-understood biochemical cause yet are still considered legitimate. What makes these disorders easier to accept? Edward Shorter, a medical historian at the University of Toronto, observes that although doctors may not always understand the cause of a disease, they are good at finding organic changes triggered by the ailment, such as the damage to nerve fibers seen in multiple sclerosis.

Shorter goes on to argue that "these mystery diseases share many of the same symptoms—chronic pain, chronic fatigue, slight cognitive changes, maybe some dizziness," adding that "these symptoms are as common as grass." He notes that some patients simply need the "gift of time"

from family doctors who will listen to these recurring complaints.

Regardless of how the debates on CFS and other disputed syndromes are resolved, physicians will no doubt continue to face mysterious ailments as medical research and the health care system both attempt to keep up. When pressed further to explain the "here and there" problems of his Tanzanian patients, Aronowitz turns philosophical, suggesting that an undercurrent of as yet unexplained suffering may be at work in many ailments—a frustrating diagnosis, to be sure.

 Article Review Form at end of book.

What are two symptoms of heart disease in women that often go unrecognized?

Women and Their PCPs Lack Understanding of Heart Disease Symptoms and Risks

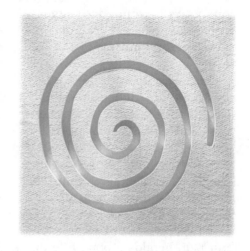

Not only are women and their primary care physicians unaware of the risks of heart disease that women face, they also have a poor understanding of the symptoms that are prevalent among women, a study has found.

Cardiovascular disease kills more the 479,000 women in the United States each year, making it the leading cause of death among women, according to the Washington Hospital Center in Washington, D.C., which commissioned the study. (By comparison, breast cancer kills about 44,000 women annually; all forms of cancer kill about 242,000 women each year.)

However, when asked what they believe is the greatest health risk facing women under age 50, 34% of physicians surveyed in *Women and Heart Health: A Study of Primary Care Physicians*, said breast cancer is the greatest risk. Only 15% named heart disease.

The nationwide survey of 256 internists and family practitioners, which was conducted by the Gallup Organization, also found that 56% of PCPs believe the risk factors for heart disease are different for women and men and that 64% feel that the symptoms of heart disease are the same in women as in men.

Similarly, women don't recognize the risks and symptoms. The hospital surveyed 1,000 women and found that women place heart disease behind breast cancer and stress. Another Gallup survey found that 70% of women believe the symptoms of heart disease are the same for women and men.

While chest pain is a major indicator of heart disease in both women and men, symptoms such as shortness of breath and chronic fatigue should not be ignored in women.

"Women's heart disease develops differently than men's, often progressing over a longer period of time," said Elizabeth Ross, M.D., a Washington Hospital Center cardiologist and author of *Healing the Female Heart*. "Their symptoms can also be more subtle. While women do experience chest pain, they often describe it as a tightness in the chest that moves to the left arm or jaw, rather than the crushing or severe chest pain that men often experience. And it is very important to recognize that two major symptoms in women are shortness of breath, sometimes occurring in the middle of the night, and chronic, unexplained fatigue."

A lack of training could be part of the problem in diagnosing and treating heart disease among women. Only 39% of the doctors surveyed reported that they had extensive training in diagnosing heart disease in women. Meanwhile, 69% reported extensive training in reporting the same disease in men. Also, even though postmenopausal women are at higher risk for heart disease because of the loss of estrogen hormones, only 45% of the physicians surveyed said they've had extensive training in the use of hormone replacement therapy.

The survey is the first part of a program called "Listen to your Heart," a three-year campaign to raise awareness and understanding of the heart disease risks that women face. The hospital is developing a physician education and awareness program to address issues identified in the survey. The Washington Hospital Center and Parke-Davis also have developed a risk assessment quiz for women.

 Article Review Form at end of book.

For more information and a free copy of the quiz, call the Washington Hospital Center at 202/877-DOCS.

What is the single most important and preventable cause of cancer death?

What are some other measures you can take to reduce your risk of cancer?

Winning the War on Cancer

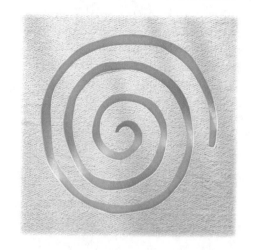

R. Grant Steen

R. Grant Steen is on the faculty of St. Jude Children's Research Hospital, where he studies brain tumor biology, and has conducted cancer research at Johns Hopkins Medical School.

Cancer is one of today's most-feared diseases, but you can do a lot to lower your risk.

Cancer is probably the most dreaded of all diseases; nearly everyone has close friends or relatives who have fallen victim to it. Cancer is now the leading cause of death for women and the second leading cause of death overall, after heart disease. Cancer has been projected to become the leading overall killer in the United States by the year 2000.

Cancer will probably never be completely preventable. Yet it has been calculated that about two-thirds of all human cancers could be prevented.

In this article, I will compile and rank the major *preventable* cancer risk factors—i.e., those that are not inherited. While hereditary cancers carry a high risk if they run in your family, they are *very* rare otherwise. By focusing on preventable cancer risk factors,

we can direct our personal choices and public policies toward achieving the maximum possible reduction in cancer mortality.

The top 25 preventable cancer risks in the United States are listed in the table at right.

Preventable Causes of Cancers

Of the top 25 completely preventable causes of cancer in the United States, about 84% are lifestyle-related. Those few that are not clearly lifestyle-related (such as hepatitis B virus infection, DDT exposure, and secondhand smoke) nevertheless can have a significant component of lifestyle choice involved. For example, hepatitis B virus (HBV) infection is more prevalent among homosexual men who engage in anal sex, high-level DDT exposure is usually occupational and can be minimized through careful application of the pesticide, and secondhand smoke is often avoidable.

At least 48% of the top 25 preventable causes of cancer are related to diet. This shows that the current emphasis on dietary pre-

vention of cancer is not a misplaced effort, since diet is more easily changed than certain other lifestyle risk factors, such as tobacco use or obesity.

At least 28% of the top 25 preventable causes of cancer are specifically related to an inadequate intake of fruits and vegetables. This would seem to be a relatively easy dietary change to make, since modern farming and shipping practices make fresh fruits and vegetables available year-round to virtually everyone in the United States. Many cookbooks provide recipes that make vegetables more palatable, so all that may be required is the impetus to try these recipes. It is hoped that our analysis of cancer risk factors will provide such impetus.

One-fifth of the top 25 preventable causes of cancer are arguably stress-related, since stress can cause an increased intake of tobacco, alcohol, and total calories, and since many people respond to stress by becoming obese. Dealing productively with stress can therefore play a critical role in maintaining a healthy lifestyle and minimizing the risk of cancer. Perhaps the most effective way to

Originally appeared in the March/April 1997 issue of *The Futurist*. Used with permission from the World Future Society, 7910 Woodmont Avenue, Suite 450, Bethesda, Maryland 20814. 301/656-8274; fax 301/951-0394; http://www.wfs.org/wfs.

deal with stress is to establish a regular routine of exercise.

Other preventable risks are exposure to carcinogenic chemicals, such as tobacco smoke, hair dye, and DDT; HBV, for which a vaccine exists; and of course tobacco, which is known to cause at least 85% of all lung cancers and up to 30% of all other cancers.

Actual Causes of Death

A recent study examined the actual causes of death in the United States, with the specific goal of identifying the major nongenetic factors that contribute to death. Of the 2.1 million people who died in 1990, death certificates show that more than half a million people died of cancer, and that cancer was the second leading cause of death overall, after heart disease.

But medical terms (e.g., cancer), used to describe the physical condition at death, do not reveal the actual root causes of death. In order to get at the root causes of death in the United States, a large number of separate studies were analyzed in a sort of meta-analysis. The actual (nongenetic) causes of death identified in this meta-analysis were, in descending order of importance:

1. Tobacco.

2. Diet and activity patterns.

3. Alcohol.

4. Microbial agents.

5. Toxic agents.

6. Firearms.

7. Sexual behavior.

8. Motor vehicles.

9. Illicit use of drugs.

The Top 25 Risk Factors for Preventable Cancer

Rank	Risk Factor	Related Cancer
1.	Hepatitis B virus infection	Liver
2.	Tobacco smoking (two packs or more per day, 10 years)	Lung
3.	Human papilloma virus (HPV-16 or -18)	Cervical
4.	High dietary intake of saturated fat	Lung
5.	Low dietary intake of folate	Cervical
6.	Heavy drinking (any alcohol)	Oropharyngeal
7.	DDT in pesticides	Breast
8.	Frequent red meat consumption	Colon
9.	*Hellcobacter* infection	Stomach
10.	Highly stressful life events (more than two in last year)	All cancers
11.	Low dietary intake of Vitamin E	Colon
12.	Low dietary intake of Vitamin C	Cervical
13.	Oral contraceptive use (at 40-44 years of age)	Breast
14.	Long-term use of black hair dye	Lymphoma
15.	Low dietary intake of raw fruits and vegetables	Lung
16.	Chronic obesity	Colon
17.	Low carbohydrate intake	Colorectal
18.	Secondhand smoke (more than 22 years)	Lung
19.	High total caloric intake	Prostate
20.	Low activity (less than 1,000 kilocalories per week)	Colorectal
21.	Low dietary intake of selenium	Lung
22.	Low dietary intake of fiber	Colorectal
23.	Never bearing children	Breast
24.	Low dietary intake of peas and beans	Lung
25.	More than 30 years old at first childbirth	Breast

Source: *Changing the Odds* by R. Grant Steen

Together, these causes accounted for about half of all deaths in the United States in 1990.

Tobacco was the major root cause of death identified in the United States, taking 400,000 lives in 1990. Tobacco is responsible for about 19% of all deaths, 30% of all cancer deaths, 30% of all chronic lung disease deaths, 24% of all pneumonia and influenza deaths, 21% of all cardiovascular deaths, and a substantial fraction of deaths from cerebrovascular disease and diabetes. Without doubt, smoking is the most damaging carcinogen to which humans are regularly exposed.

Diet and activity patterns were the next most important root cause of death identified, taking 300,000 American lives in 1990. Dietary factors are responsible for deaths from cardiovascular disease, cancer, and diabetes, while physical inactivity is responsible for deaths from heart disease and cancer. Together, these factors account for at least 20% of all

Genetic Screening for Cancer

Cancer screening is the use of medical tests to examine people with no symptoms of cancer in order to determine if these people are in the early stages of developing disease. Current screening tests include the Pap smear, mammography, prostate-specific antigen test, fecal occult blood test, and colonoscopy. These tests are an important weapon in the war on cancer. According to the American Cancer Society, 100,00 people could have been saved in 1992 if there had been full implementation of current tests.

The ideal cancer screening test is reliable, inexpensive, easy to use, accurate, and gives adequate warning, so that the cancer can be successfully treated. It is fair to say that such a test does not yet exist. However, in the future, it may become possible to develop new tests based on an understanding of the genetic basis of cancer.

Genetic screening would be analogous to taking a genetic "fingerprint" of individuals to determine if they have mutations of tumor suppresser genes. Genetic screening might be able to determine which cancer each person is most likely to get, to identify a cancer-prone person years before developing the disease, and to help a person avoid specific risk factors for cancer.

—*R. Grant Steen*

---

cancer deaths, 30% of all diabetes deaths, and 22% of all cardiovascular deaths.

Alcohol was the third most important root cause of death identified, taking 100,000 lives. An estimated 18 million people in the United States suffer from alcohol dependence, and 76 million are affected by alcohol abuse at some time during their lives. Alcohol abuse is responsible for at least 3% of all cancer deaths, 60% of all cirrhosis deaths, 40% of all motor vehicle fatalities, and 16% of all other injuries.

More than 20 times as many people died from cancer in 1990 as died from AIDS. Despite the public attention given to HIV/AIDS, various other viruses were far more important as a cause of death in the United States in 1990. Viruses caused about six times as many deaths from cancer as from AIDS in 1990, and the death toll from virally induced cancer is rising at a rate comparable to the death toll from AIDS in the United States. Thus, cancer must remain a major focus of the medical research enterprise.

Summary: Ten Things You Can Do To Lessen Your Risk of Cancer

1. Stop smoking. No rationale is possible for this devastating habit. Stop those you love from smoking or hound them senseless. Don't allow anyone to smoke in your house or your office, and make it as difficult as possible for smokers to abuse themselves. Smokeless tobacco is really no better than smoked tobacco—it just causes cancers that are somewhat less uniformly fatal than lung cancer.

2. Learn your familial risk factors and be especially vigilant about those cancers that seem to run in your family. Ask your older relatives for as full a description as possible of the cause of death of your deceased relatives, then specifically avoid the risk factors for these cancers.

3. Increase your consumption of fresh fruits and vegetables. A broad variety of each is best, with special emphasis on whatever is freshest in your produce department or store.

4. Decrease your consumption of red meat. This does not mean become a vegetarian, but rather place greater dietary emphasis on white meats, such as chicken and fish. An appropriate dietary modification might be as simple as having red meat fewer than four times per week, or having chicken or fish at least three times per week. Vegetarian dishes or dishes rich in complex carbohydrates (e.g., pasta) can also be substituted for red meat.

5. Exercise at least three times per week, for at least 20 minutes each time. This will help to maintain your weight at an appropriate level as well as conferring other benefits.

6. Get vaccinated against hepatitis B virus if at all possible and avoid other viral exposures. This may mean using a condom, minimizing the number of different sexual partners, or avoiding intercourse with someone you suspect to be infected with human papilloma virus.

7. Practice moderation in all things. Overuse or abuse of alcohol, prescription drugs, and fast foods takes a very high toll in the modern world, as does overexposure to sunlight.

8. Make a yearly visit to a physician if you are over 40 years old, and make biannual visits if you are over 30. This will certainly help to diagnose and treat current problems, but may also alert you to newly discovered cancer risk factors. In addition, there are several widely available cancer screening tests that should be used on the advice of your physician, including mammography, Pap test, fecal occult blood test, and prostate-specific antigen screening.

9. Avoid unnecessary exposure to the hormones used in estrogen-replacement therapy (ERT). Long-term ERT use by perimenopausal women is associated with an increased risk of breast cancer, especially if estrogen is combined with progestin. However, the benefits of ERT may outweigh the risks, since breast cancer risk may drop rapidly after discontinuation of the therapy.

10. Learn the 10 warning signs of cancer: (1) Swelling, thickening, or lump in any soft tissue, but especially the breasts. (2) Persistent or unexplained coughing or hoarseness. (3) A sore that does not heal or a mole that abruptly changes in size or color. (4) Unexplained fatigue. (5) Abrupt weight loss or loss of appetite. (6) Changes in bowel habits, including pain or bleeding on defecation, narrow stools, or constipation. (7) Changes in urinary function, particularly bleeding or difficulty in discharge. (8) Changes in menstrual function, especially unexpected or excessive bleeding. (9) Difficulty in swallowing or a feeling of bloat or fullness. (10) Pallor or abnormal bleeding.

Conclusion

Much of what we know about cancer prevention is common sense. Everyone should eat a balanced diet and practice moderation in all things. It is fair to say that cancer is a disease of abuse or disuse, and moderation may be key to avoiding both extremes.

Whenever possible, people should learn more about their personal risk factors. If there is a family history of cancer, especially if cancer has affected a particular organ in a large number of family members, special care should be taken to avoid known risk factors for that cancer. It would also be wise to be screened for that cancer whenever possible. In the absence of specific screening tests for a particular cancer, regular visits to a family physician can substantially reduce cancer risk. However, there is no substitute for common sense, moderation, and personal knowledge of cancer risk factors.

 Article Review Form at end of book.

Who was Audre Lorde?
What did living fully mean to Audre Lorde?

A Burst of Light

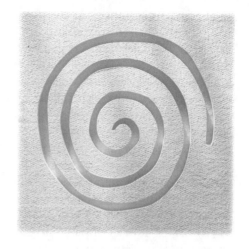

Audre Lorde

On February 1, 1984, two weeks before her fiftieth birthday, Audre Lorde—an extraordinary poet, essayist and social activist—was diagnosed with liver cancer. She chose homeopathic medicine and spiritual will instead of surgery and chemotherapy to wage her battle against that cancer. Earlier, in her book The Cancer Journals, *Lorde had given a breathtaking account of her initial experience with breast cancer and mastectomy in 1978. In June 1987 she underwent surgery again, this time for ovarian cancer, metastasized from the breast cancer. She chose surgery in this instance because the danger of spread was acute and because allopathic medicine (traditionally practiced in the West) has a better success record with ovarian than with liver cancer. After recuperation in Saint Croix, Virgin Islands, Lorde is living, writing and lecturing in Berlin. She treats the cancer homeopathically with an advanced formulation of a medicine that proved effective in containing the liver cancer. The following*

'Caring for myself is not self-indulgent; it is self-preservation, and that is an act of political warfare. . . . I train myself for triumph by knowing it is mine no matter what.' So writes an extraordinary woman whose battle against cancer is an inspiration for us all

excerpts are from A Burst of Light, *Lorde's journal from 1984 to 1987 (to be published this spring by Firebrand Books, Ithaca, New York).* —Ed.

If I am to put this all down in a way that is useful, I should start at the beginning. "Sizable tumor in the right lobe of the liver," the doctors said. "Lots of blood vessels in it means it's most likely malignant. Let's cut you open right now and see what we can do about it." "Wait a minute," I said. "I need to feel this thing out and see what's going on inside myself first." Not one of them said, "I can respect that, but don't take too long about it."

Instead, that simple claim to my body's own processes elicited such an attack from a reputable Specialist in Liver Tumors that my deepest—if not necessarily most useful—suspicions were totally aroused.

What that doctor could have said to me that I would have heard was, "You have a serious condition going on in your body,

and whatever you do about it you must not ignore it or delay deciding how you are going to deal with it, because it will not go away, no matter what you think it is." Acknowledging my responsibility for my own body. Instead, what he said to me was, "If you do not do exactly what I tell you to do right now without questions, you are going to die a horrible death." In exactly those words.

I felt the battle lines being drawn up within my own body.

I saw this Specialist in Liver Tumors in a leading cancer hospital in New York City, where I had been referred as an outpatient by my own doctor. The first people who interviewed me in white coats from behind a computer were interested only in my health-care benefits and proposed method of payment. Those crucial facts determined what kind of plastic ID card I would be given, and without a plastic ID card no one at all was allowed upstairs to see any doctor, as I was told by the uniformed, pistoled guards at all the stairwells.

From the moment I was ushered into the doctor's office and he saw my X-rays, he proceeded to infantilize me with an obviously well-practiced technique. When I told him I was having second thoughts about a liver biopsy, he glanced at my chart. Racism and Sexism joined hands across his table as he saw I taught at a university. "Well, you look like an *intelligent girl*," he said, staring at my one breast all the time he was speaking. "Not to have this biopsy immediately is like sticking your head in the sand." Then he went on to say that he would not be responsible when one day I wound up shrieking in agony in the corner of his office.

I asked this Specialist in Liver Tumors about the dangers of a liver biopsy spreading an existing malignancy or even encouraging it in a borderline tumor. He dismissed my concerns with a wave of his hand, saying, instead of an answer, that I really did not have any other sensible choice.

I would like to think that this doctor was motivated by his desire for me to seek what he truly believed to be the only remedy for my sickening body, but my faith in that scenario is considerably diminished by his two-hundred-and-fifty-dollar consultation fee and his subsequent medical report to my doctor containing numerous supposedly clinical observations such as *obese abdomen* and *remaining pendulous breast*.

In any event, I can thank him for the fierce shard lancing through my terror that shrieked, *There must be some other way: this doesn't feel right to me.* If this is cancer and they cut me open to find out, what is stopping that intrusive action from spreading the cancer, or turning a questionable mass into an active malignancy? All I was asking for was the reassurance of a realistic answer to my questions, and that was not forthcoming. I made up my mind that if I was going to die in agony

on somebody's office floor, it certainly wasn't going to be his! I needed information, and I pored for hours over books on the liver in a Barnes and Noble bookstore's medical-textbook section. I learned, among other things, that the liver is the largest, most complex and most generous organ in the human body. But that did not help me very much.

In this period of physical weakness and psychic turmoil, I found myself going through an intricate inventory of rage. First of all at my breast surgeon—had he perhaps done something wrong? How could such a small breast tumor have metastasized? Hadn't he assured me he'd gotten it all, and what was this now anyway about micrometasteses? Could this tumor in my liver have been seeded at the same time as my breast cancer? There was too much that I just did not understand.

But my worst rage was the rage at myself. For a brief time I felt like a total failure. What had I been busting my ass doing these past six years if it wasn't living and loving and working to my utmost potential? And wasn't that all a guarantee supposed to keep exactly this kind of thing from ever happening again? So what had I done wrong, and what was I going to have to pay for it, and *why me?*

But finally a little voice inside me said sharply, *Now really, is there any other way that you would have preferred living the past six years? And should or shouldn't isn't even the question; how do you want to live the rest of your life and what are you going to do about it? Time's a-wasting!*

Gradually, I felt myself shifting into another gear. My resolve strengthened as my panic lessened. Deep breathing, regularly. I'm not going to let them cut into my body again until I'm con-

vinced there is no alternative. And this time, the burden of proof rests with the doctors, because their record of success with liver cancer is not so good that it would make me jump at a surgical solution. And scare tactics are not going to work. I have been scared for six years, and that hasn't stopped me. I *hoped* scare tactics were not going to work. At any rate, thank the goddess, they were not working yet. One step at a time.

Medical textbooks on the liver were fine, but there were appointments to be kept, and bills to pay, and decisions about my upcoming trip to Europe to be made. And what do I say to my children?

I visited my breast surgeon, with whom I have always been able to talk frankly, and from him I got my first trustworthy, objective sense of timing. I learned that conventional forms of treating liver metastases made little more than a year's difference in the survival rate. My old friend Clem's voice came back to me through the dimness of 30 years: "I see you coming here trying to make sense where there is no sense. Try just living in it. Respond, alter, see what happens." I thought of the African way of perceiving life: as an experience to be lived rather than as a problem to be solved.

Homeopathic medicine calls cancer the cold disease. I understand that down to my bones that quake sometimes in their need for heat, for the sun, even for just a hot bath. Part of the way in which I am saving my own life is to refuse to submit my body to cold whenever possible.

In general, I fight to keep my treatment scene together in some coherent and serviceable way, integrated into my daily living, and absolute. Forgetting is no excuse. It's as simple as this: One missed shot [Lorde regularly injects herself with a homeopathic preparation] could make the difference between a quiescent malignancy and one that is growing again. This keeps me in an intimate relationship with my own health in a positive way and it also underlines the fact that I have the responsibility for attending my own health and cannot simply hand over that responsibility to anybody else. Which does not mean that I give in to the belief, arrogant or naive, that I know everything I need to know in order to make informed decisions about my body. But attending my own health and gaining enough information to help me participate in the decisions made about my body by people who know more medicine than I do are both crucial strategies in my battle for living. They also provide me with important prototypes for battle in all my other arenas of life.

Battling racism and battling heterosexism and battling apartheid share the same urgency inside me as battling cancer. None of these struggles is ever easy, and even the smallest victory is never to be taken for granted. And even the smallest victory must be applauded, because it is so easy not to battle at all, to just accept, and to call that acceptance inevitable. (11/8/86)

*   *   *   *

I have a privileged life or else I would be dead by now. It is two and a half years since the first tumor in my liver was discovered.

It was an accident of circumstance that brought me to Germany at a critical moment in my health, and another that introduced me to one holistic—homeopathic approach to the treatment of certain cancers. Not all homeopathic alternatives work for every patient. Time is a crucial element in the treatment of cancer, and I had to decide which chances I would take.

I think about what all this means to other Black women who are living with cancer, and to women in general. I think of how important it is for us to share with one another the powers released by the breaking of silence about our bodies and our health, even though we have been schooled to be secret and stoical about pain and disease. But stoicism and silence do not serve us or our communities, only the forces of things as they are. (11/11/86)

*   *   *   *

I have found something interesting in a book . . . on active meditation as a form of self-control. There are six steps:

1. **Control of thought.** Think of a small object (for instance, a paper clip) for five minutes exclusively; practice for a month.

2. **Control of action.** Perform a small act every day at the same time.

3. **Control of feeling (equanimity).** Become aware of feelings and introduce equanimity into experiencing them; that is, be afraid, not panic-stricken. . . .

4. **Positivity (tolerance).** Refrain from critical downgrading thoughts that sap energy from good work.

5. **Openness (receptivity).** Perceive even what is unpleasant in an unfettered, nonprejudiced way.

6. **Harmony (perseverance).** Work toward balancing the other five.

As a living creature I am part of two kinds of forces—growth and decay, living and dying—and at any given moment each one of us is actively located somewhere along a continuum between these forces.

(12/15/85, Arlesheim, Switzerland, the Lukas Klinik)

*   *   *   *

For Black women, learning to consciously extend ourselves to one another and call on one another's strengths is a lifesaving strategy. In the best of circumstances, we require an enormous amount of mutually consistent support to be emotionally able to look straight into the face of the powers aligned against us and still do our work with joy. It takes determination and practice.

Black women who survive have a head start in learning how to be open and self-protective at the same time. One secret is to ask as many people as possible for help, depending on all of them and on none of them at the same time. Some will help, others cannot. For the time being.

Another secret is to find something your soul craves for nourishment—a religion, a quiet spot, a dance class—and satisfy it. That satisfaction does not have to be costly or difficult. The need only has to be recognized, articulated and answered.

There is an important difference between openness and naïveté. Not everyone has good intentions, or means me well. I remind myself I do not need to change these people, only recognize them. (11/16/86)

*   *   *   *

Evil never appears in its own face to bargain, nor does impotence, nor does despair. After all, who believes anymore in the devil buying up souls? But I warn myself, don't even pretend no to say no, loudly and often, no matter how symbolically. Because the choices in our lives are never simple or fable-clear. Survival never comes as "Do this particular thing precisely as directed, and you will go on living; don't do that and, no question about it, you will surely die." Despite what the doctor said, it just doesn't happen that way.

Probably in some ideal world we would be offered clear choices, where we make our decisions from a clearly typed and annotated menu. But no life for any Black woman I know is that simple or that banal. There are as many crucial, untimed decisions to be made as there are dots in a newspaper photo of great contrast, and as we get close enough to examine them within their own terrain, the whole picture becomes distorted and obscure.

I do not think about my death as being imminent, but I live my days against a background noise of mortality and constant uncertainty. Learning not to crumple before these uncertainties fuels my resolve to print myself upon the texture of each day fully rather than forever.

(11/19/86)

* * * *

I'm glad I don't have to turn away anymore from movies about people dying of cancer. I no longer have to deny cancer as a reality in my life. As I wept over *Terms of Endearment* last night, I also laughed. It's hard to believe I avoided this movie for over two years.

Yet while I was watching it, involved in the situation of a young mother dying of breast cancer, I was also very aware of that standard of living, taken for granted in the film, that made the expression of her tragedy possible. Her mother's maid and the manicured garden, the unremarked but very tangible money so evident through its effects. Daughter's philandering husband is an unsuccessful English professor, but they still live in a white-shingled house with trees, not in some rack-ass tenement on the Lower East Side or in Harlem for which they pay too much rent.

Her private room in Lincoln Memorial Hospital has her mama's Renoir on the wall. No Black people are visible in that hospital in Lincoln, Nebraska, not even in the background. This may not make the death scenes any less touching, but it did strengthen my resolve to talk as a Black woman about my experiences with cancer.

(12/7/86, New York City)

* * * *

To acknowledge privilege is the first step in making it available for wider use. I have been very blessed in my life. I have been blessed to believe passionately, to love deeply and to be able to work out of those loves and beliefs. Accidents of privilege allowed me to gain information about holistic and biological medicine and their approach to cancers, and that information has helped keep me alive, along with that original gut feeling that said, "Stay out of my body." For me, living and the use of that living are inseparable, and I have a responsibility to put that privilege and that life to use.

For me, living fully means living with direct access to my experience and power, loving and doing work in which I believe. It means writing my poems, telling my stories and speaking out of my most urgent concerns and against the many forms of antilife surrounding us. Whatever life I have I wish to live as fully and as sweetly as possible, rather than refocus that life upon extending it for some unspecified time. I consider this a political decision, and a lifesaving one, one that I am fortunate to be able to make.

If one Black woman I do not know gains hope and strength from my story, then it will have been worth the difficulty of telling.

(1987, Carriacou, Grenada, Anguilla, British West Indies and Saint Croix, Virgin Islands)

 Article Review Form at end of book.

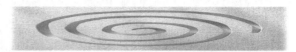

- You can live well with illness, disease, or disability with skills in gathering accurate medical information, being assertive, thinking critically, solving problems, and making decisions.

R.E.A.L. Sites

The adjacent list provides a print preview of typical **coursewise** R.E.A.L. sites. (There are over 100 such sites at the **courselinks**™ site.) The danger in printing URLs is that web sites can change overnight. As we went to press, these sites were functional using the URLs provided. If you come across one that isn't, please let us know via email at webmaster@coursewise.com. Use your Passport to access the most current list of R.E.A.L. sites at the **courselinks**™ site.

Site name: Go Ask Alice
URL: http://www.columbia.edu/cu/healthwise/alice.html
Why is it R.E.A.L.? Provides answers to health and medical questions posed by site visitors.
Key topics: self-help, general health and wellness
Activity: Submit a health question of interest to you then see what answer you get.

Site name: Medical Matrix
URL: http://www.medmatrix.org
Why is it R.E.A.L.? Searchable database for medical information on diseases, medical specialities, clinical practice, literature, education, healthcare professionals, medical technology, and the marketplace.
Key topics: disease, general health and wellness

Site Name: American Self-Help Clearinghouse
URL: http://www.cmhc.com/selfhelp/
Why is it R.E.A.L.? Homepage for organization dedicated to addressing self-help issues. Provides information about self-help resources and materials.
Key topics: self-help, community agency
Activity: Figure out how to go about setting up a new mutual self-help support group on some health issue of importance to you. Write up a detailed plan. How would you start?

Site name: American Cancer Society
URL: http://www.cancer.org/
Why is it R.E.A.L.? Homepage for nonprofit voluntary health organization dedicated to addressing cancer. Provides information about cancer resources and materials.
Activity: Go to "Statistics" then "Cancer Facts and Figures" to estimate the number of new cancer cases in 1997 in your own community. Find out where your local American Cancer Society is located. See if it's a place you'd like to volunteer.

Site name: American Lung Association
URL: http://www.lungusa.org/
Why is it R.E.A.L.? Homepage for nonprofit voluntary health organization dedicated to addressing lung disease. Provides information about lung disease resources and materials.
Key topics: community agency, disease

Site name: NOAH
URL: http://www.noah.cuny.edu/qksearch.html
Why is it R.E.A.L.? Consumer health resource on a variety of general health topics.
Key topics: general health, disease, consumer health

Site name: ACHOO

URL: http://www.achoo.com/index.htm

Why is it R.E.A.L.? Searchable and comprehensive database on health care along with health news, health care newsgroup discussions, and site of the week.

Key topics: general health, consumer health

Activity: Find out the latest health news. Did you already know any of it?

....

Site name: Centers for Disease Control and Prevention

URL: http://www.cdc.gov/diseases/diseases.html

Why is it R.E.A.L.? The CDC is a federal government agency charged with protecting the public's health. Provides searchable access to the latest information about specific diseases. Current information about specific diseases also available.

Key topics: governmental agency, disease

....

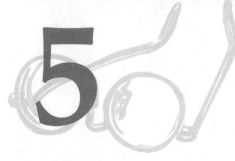

section 5

Key Points

- Poverty, unemployment, and health are interrelated.

- Along with greater access to self-care opportunities comes responsibility for one's own safety.

- Healthcare and healthcare coverage are not equal for all groups.

- Ageism negatively impacts the health of older adults.

- To gain greater access, healthcare consumers need to be active in their own healthcare.

Health for All: Access to Healthcare

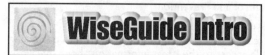
WiseGuide Intro

U.S. morbidity and mortality statistics indicate that minorities and women suffer disproportionately from certain illnesses, diseases, and disabilities. Except for a few genetic predispositions to specific diseases, differential access to healthcare, whether due to inadequate healthcare coverage or discrimination factors, seems to be the primary explanation.

The articles selected for Section 5 all address access to healthcare. In "Good Health for Sale," Barbara Ehrenreich humorously describes one way to improve access to healthcare by empowering health consumers with medication self-care opportunities. The next three articles ("Women's Health as a Human Rights Issue," "Equity in Biomedical Research," and "How Women Pay More Than Men for Less Health Coverage") detail the discrimination against women in terms of healthcare, health research, and healthcare coverage. After documenting the ways in which ageism impacts the health of older adults, Grant ("Effects of Ageism on Individual and Health Care Providers' Responses to Healthy Aging") offers specific solutions. Minority health issues are similarly addressed in the next article ("Concern About AIDS in Minority Communities"). Hagland describes a proactive approach to negotiating the healthcare system in the last article ("Power to the Patient").

Questions

R27. What are the advantages and disadvantages of increased availability of medication without a prescription?

R28. How are human rights violated in the area of women's health, according to Joel?

R29. What are two forms of gender bias in clinical research? What are some differences between females and males in terms of longevity, acute symptoms, chronic conditions, and disabilities?

R30. In what ways are men on Medicare at a greater advantage than women on Medicare? What three steps can women take to improve their health insurance coverage?

R31. How does ageism impact health? What is one way to combat ageism and its impact on health?

R32. What are barriers to prevention and treatment of AIDS among minorities?

R33. How have HIV/AIDS education and activism impacted healthcare?

What are the advantages and disadvantages of increased availability of medication without a prescription?

Good Health for Sale

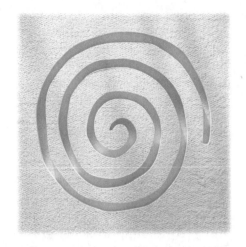

Barbara Ehrenreich

The writer Barbara Ehrenreich is a Dollars & Sense Fellow. Her latest book is The Snarling Citizen: A Collection of Essays.

You're feeling a little peckish perhaps, some indefinable malaise of the intestinal tract or maybe it's the thyroid gland. So you're surfing around for distraction and, suddenly there it is—Claritin! The commercial doesn't say what it does, but you sense, somehow, that whatever it does is going to work for you. The transcendent calm of those clear blue skies! The cool triumph of that goddess-like face! Rush out to the nearest physician, is the message, and get yourself a little of this!

Time was when the pharmaceutical companies were content to market to the physicians themselves—hosting them, for example, at free weekend-long "seminars" at important margarita-producing sites. But doctors are a rushed and harried bunch these days, struggling to survive in their HMOs. Only the consumers—still known in the medical business by the archaic term "patients"—have

the time to savor a well-crafted commercial and decide whether it suits their needs.

Hence the sudden expansion of "direct-to-consumer" prescription drug advertising, which began, innocently enough, with Rogaine, and extends now to remedies for everything from high blood pressure and prostate problems to fungus and migraines. Pharmaceutical companies spent $35 million on it in 1987 and almost ten times more—$308 million—in '94. And whatever the pills do, at least the advertising works: In 1989, 45% of doctors said they had patients who were able to specify, by brand name, exactly what they wanted prescribed. By 1995, 93% of doctors were encountering such medically gifted patients.

But why go to a doctor if you already know what you need? When an ad works, when it touches you in that deep subconscious layer of the brain where the ad-receptors are located, you don't want to diddle around with appointments and insurance

forms and long waits on cold plastic seats. It gets irritating, in fact, that you have to go through this odd ritual—undressing in front of strangers, answering personal questions—just to get hold of some product that a nice voice on TV has already told you that you need.

Then there's the cost. Drug prices, already giddily high, are rising at more than twice the rate of inflation. This makes sense when you realize that pharmaceutical companies, just like presidential candidates and breakfast cereals, have to spend hundreds of millions a year on high-concept prime-time commercials. But when you're already facing $90 or more for a little vial of chemical comfort, that $50 surcharge for a doctor's prescription begins to look like an inexcusable shakedown.

So the pressure will inevitably grow to cut the doctors out of the loop. We're already being groomed by the medical companies in the skills of kitchen-table diagnosis. Take that indefinable malaise you were feeling:

Why pay doctors $50 just for their bedside manner?

Dollars & Sense is a progressive economics magazine published six times a year. First-year subscriptions cost $18.95 and may be ordered by writing to *Dollars and Sense*, One Summer St., Somerville, MA 02143.

Now you can go to a drug store and, without any prescription at all, pick up a testing kit that will allow you to determine whether the problem is pregnancy or diabetes or possibly AIDS. So what are you paying the doctor for—$50 worth of bedside manner?

Think of it as the ultimate market-based health reform: A system in which consumers will decide what they need and then go out and get it, unimpeded by the need to support some gray-templed fellow with a serious golf habit. Americans currently spend billions a year on visits to physicians, and, despite the nice neighborly locution, most of these "visits" are purely bureaucratic formalities required to renew our antihistamine prescriptions. Why not go the way of Mexico and so much of the Third World and let consumers fill their shopping carts with beta-blockers and serotonin-uptake inhibitors as impulse demands? We don't, after all, require anyone to have a note from a fashion consultant before going home with a salmon-colored leisure ensemble.

There is of course the issue of safety. The drug with the most appealing packaging or cunning commercial could conceivably put an end to one's entire medical shopping career. But the truth is we're not doing so well on the safety front now, even with doctors manning the medical checkpoints. About 2 million people are hospitalized each year, and 140,000 actually die, as a result of dire reactions to drugs that were duly prescribed. Besides, if prescriptions are such an indispensable safeguard, why are the drug companies rushing to make their antacids and analgesics available over the counter, where we can O.D. on them to our hearts content?

Sadly, in a health system dominated by mega-corporations, the physician is fast becoming an evolutionary throwback. Today, the insurance companies that manage "managed care" don't even trust a doctor to monitor a routine blood pressure problem without some low-level bureaucrat looking over his or her shoulder for deviations from "cost effectiveness." And any loyalty the medical profession may have had from the long-suffering public evaporated last year when the AMA made a deal to let the Republicans cut Medicare without cutting doctors' fees. As for threatening us with serious trouble if we don't stop smoking and take off 15 pounds—well, what are spouses for?

So, Physician, heal thyself—is the message from Madison Avenue—and patients, heal thyselves too. Health reformers used to fantasize about networks of neighborhood clinics filled with nurturing, culturally sensitive, holistic providers. But in a health system ruled increasingly from Wall Street, where the only vital signs of interest are profits and market-share, doctor-free drug shopping may be the best we can hope for.

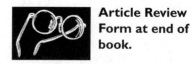 **Article Review Form at end of book.**

How are human rights violated in the area of women's health, according to Joel?

Women's Health as a Human Rights Issue

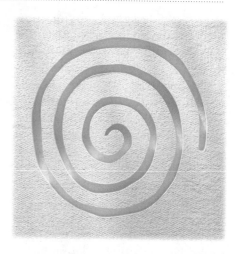

Lucille A. Joel, EdD, RN, FAAN

Lucille A. Joel, AJN Editor-at Large, is a professor in the College of Nursing, Rutgers, The State University of New Jersey, and past president at the American Nurses Association. She represents North America on the Board of the International Council of Nurses.

United Nations documents clearly define human rights as the entitlement of a healthy and productive life. They specify that the human rights of women and girls are an inalienable, integral, and indivisible part of universal rights. These guarantees have been reaffirmed at the World Conferences on Women and generations of conferences on population, social development, and human rights. To many, however, international human rights protections include torture, forced detention, and not much more. In reality, more often than not compromised health status is the link to human rights violations that are deeply ingrained in a culture.

Widespread poverty inhibits the enjoyment of human rights by its association with limited access to social and health services, illiteracy, environmental risk, high fertility, and low economic productivity. This is not just a Third World story; it can be observed in many areas of this country. Environmental risks in the home and workplace disproportionately affect women's health because of their unique susceptibility to some toxins. American business and industry are fully aware of these relationships and often require guarantees to avoid pregnancy or disclaimers of responsibility from the worker. Due to the persistence of women's rights advocates in this country, we have come to know that women have many different responses to illness and requirements for health.

Many women's health violations are associated with reproduction and sexuality. Freedom of choice about childbearing and protection from harmful practices such as female genital mutilation, virginal testing, child marriage, female infanticide, and unsafe sex are often at issue.

In less developed countries, discrimination against women is

In less developed countries, discrimination against women is demonstrated in serious sex-related discrepancies in nutrition, health, and education.

demonstrated in serious sex-related discrepancies in nutrition, health, and education. In the industrialized world these distinctions are played out in different but equally dangerous ways. A woman's cardiac disease may remain untreated until the damage is permanent. Health insurers may be slow to accept the newest diagnostic and treatment options for common women's diseases—for example, bone density testing and marrow transplant for breast cancer.

Neither do women always receive full information about options available to them. Their symptoms may be treated in a cavalier fashion, with subsequent unnecessary surgical intervention or inappropriate medication. The high incidence of the use of psychotropic drugs by women is cultural and associated with more sophisticated countries.

There should be a natural linkage between human rights and professional ethics. Among health care providers, the ethical responsibility to report violations and not participate in suspect practices or procedures seems indisputable.

Ethics were directly challenged several years ago when the

government gagged provider professionals, forbidding them to give full information about family planning, including the availability of abortion as an option, to clients funded through certain federal entitlement programs. The lobbying strength of professional associations forced the reversal of this policy.

Today we see a new twist in the involvement of health care professionals in human rights violations, and women are most frequently the victims. Claiming that their participation would make harmful procedures safer, health professionals are performing procedures such as female genital mutilation and virginity testing.

This medicalization of human rights violations represents the ultimate indignity to humankind.

An international consultancy focusing on the sexual and reproductive health of women was held recently in New York City. The meeting, sponsored by the Commonwealth Medical Association, brought together a select group of women's health, human rights, and social justice advocates. The nursing and physician communities were the only provider groups included. You were ably represented by the International Council of Nurses and the International Federation of Midwives, who were seen by all the participants as major allies

in this cause. A declaration drafted and approved during the meeting spoke boldly about some very controversial topics, such as the responsibility for professionals to stand up and be counted, the personal danger that sometimes ensues, and the protection that professional associations can provide.

Simply put, there is no safe haven around these issues, only the challenge to build a firm foundation for our ethical decision-making and to realize that human rights are violated in many subtle ways.

 **Article Review Form at end of book.**

What are two forms of gender bias in clinical research?
What are some differences between females and males in terms of
longevity, acute symptoms, chronic conditions, and disabilities?

Equity in Biomedical Research

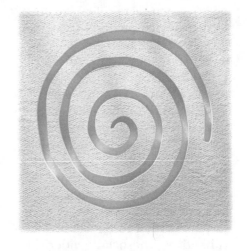

Vivian W. Pinn

V. Pinn is the Associate Director for Research on Women's Health at the National Institutes of Health.

Research on the health of women is expanding fundamental biological and clinical knowledge that will have a positive effect on global morbidity and mortality patterns of women. This research seeks to better understand conditions that are unique to women, as well as those that affect both sexes. Learning if and when differences exist between genders and their potential consequences for health should influence policies to improve the health status of both women and men.

In many cultures, women's health has been viewed traditionally in terms of the reproductive system. This view is yielding to a more comprehensive definition of women's health, so research must encompass other conditions and transcend scientific disciplines and the conventional fragmentation of women's health care.

Although women constitute a greater proportion of the elderly population in developing and developed countries, their longer life expectancy does not guarantee better health or quality of life than men. Women, in general, suffer more acute symptoms, chronic conditions, and short- and long-term disabilities. By virtue of their longer lives, women are more susceptible to emerging conditions that affect the aged. Research to elucidate genetic, hormonal, and other mechanisms that differentiate aging and longevity in men and women could lead to reductions in the economic burdens of illness and frailty.

Information is evolving from ongoing research, but further studies are needed to discover optimal preventive measures and interventions to reduce risk factors and improve health outcomes for women when there are gender differences in disease presentation, progression, or response to therapies. The debate over the merits of gender analyses and the inclusion of women in clinical studies has led to changes in traditional assumptions that tolerated gender bias and a narrow definition of women's health. Gender is now recognized as a parameter that must be appraised if results are to be generalized to whole populations.

In a 1994 report, "Women and Health Research," the Institute of Medicine in the United States identified two forms of gender bias in clinical research: male bias in designing and conducting studies, and the tendency to use males as the norm or standard. The report concluded that these biases impede research and produce findings that are not valid for large segments of the population. Increasing the number of women researchers who are involved in the formulation of scientific policies can alleviate male bias, but the inclusion of female participants in clinical studies is necessary to augment health care standards originally formulated on the male model with standards appropriate for women.

Although data on the actual numbers of female participants in past clinical studies have not always been available, ample evidence exists that many large clinical trials did not include women in numbers adequate to allow for analysis of the results by gender. Data are particularly lacking for pregnant women. For a variety of reasons, including purported protection for women who are pregnant or of childbearing

From Vivian W. Pinn, "Equity In Biomedical Research" in *Science*, Vol. 269, August 11, 1995. Dr. Vivian Pinn is the Associate Director for Research on Women's Health at the National Institutes of Health.

age, women were often excluded from research on conditions that affect both genders. Women, however, have not routinely been excluded from the clinical applications of such research. Thus, studies of the effects of sex hormones and comparisons of gender variations in the pharmacokinetics and pharmacodynamics of drug metabolism are needed. Standards of medical care and public health policies must be developed that recognize biological and psychosocial gender differences.

Policies and programs have been developed to ensure that research fills gaps in our knowledge of women's health. As an example, the Office of Research on Women's Health at the U.S. National Institutes of Health (NIH) has contributed to the formulation of comprehensive, multidisciplinary approaches to expand basic, clinical, and applied research and ensure that women are appropriately represented in biomedical and behavioral studies.

The challenge now inherent in women's health research is to establish a scientific knowledge base that will permit reliable diagnoses and effective prevention and treatment strategies for all women, including those of diverse cultural and ethnic origins, geographic locations, and economic status. The ultimate objective is good science to enhance biological wisdom and inform the development of policies and medical standards from which women and men can benefit equally.

 Article Review Form at end of book.

In what ways are men on Medicare at a greater advantage than women on Medicare?

What three steps can women take to improve their health insurance coverage?

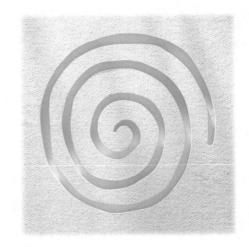

How Women Pay More than Men for Less Health Coverage

Karen Cheney

Two pieces of bad news for working women: You're less likely to have health insurance than your male counterparts are. And if you are insured, your coverage probably has serious holes. Those findings appear in a new study by Dr. Steven Miles and researcher Kara Parker of the Center for Biomedical Ethics at the University of Minnesota in St. Paul. In their *Gender and Health Insurance* report, the authors add that biases against women occur even under Medicare, the government's health insurance program for people 65 and older.

After analyzing more than 35 reports done by the Health Care Financing Administration and academics in the past 10 years, Parker and Miles found that 68% of men working full time are insured, compared with 61% of women. Further, only 17% of women working part time have health coverage, vs. 26% of men. The primary reason for the differences: Women tend to fill lower-paying jobs that lack health insurance benefits, says Parker. The study also discovered that health policies rarely pay benefits for some common preventive treatments for women. For example, only 25% of typical company-sponsored health plans cover Pap smears that detect cervical cancer.

Medicare is more generous to men too. The study found that Medicare pays 12% more a year, on average, to men than women. "Medicare has higher reimbursement levels for illnesses that are common among men," explains Parker. In reviewing the 10 most common illnesses with generally accepted treatments, Parker and Miles found that three of the four with the highest out-of-pocket costs (depression, arthritis and high blood pressure) were more prevalent among women than men. On the other hand, four of the five with the lowest out-of-pocket costs (enlarged prostate, heart attack, lung cancer and pneumonia) occur more often in men.

"Policies rarely pay benefits for some common preventive treatments for women."

Experts say women should take these three steps to improve their coverage:

- **Pressure your boss to provide better health benefits.** "If certain treatments in your plan aren't covered, the culprit is not always the insurer but the employer," says Dr. Timothy McCall, author of *Examining Your Doctor: A Patient's Guide to Avoiding Harmful Medical Care* (Citadel, $16.96). He suggests that women employees band together to demand better coverage. "If the boss wants to offer a benefit, he will make sure that the insurer provides the coverage," he says.

- **Make plans for long-term care.** Because women live an average of 6.3 years longer than men, they are more likely to need long-term-care insurance. Typical cost: $360 to $840 a year, depending on your age. Review your family's medical history and determine how much coverage you may need. Start looking into coverage by your fifties, earlier if your family has a history of Alzheimer's or Parkinson's disease, says Nancy Morith, a Princeton, N.J. specialist in financing long-term health care. The younger and healthier you are, the less your premium will cost you.

- **If you're on Medicare, buy supplemental coverage or join an HMO.** According to Parker, since men are more likely than women to have vested benefits, they are more apt to get retirement health benefits from their former employer that help fill Medicare's gaps. If you can't afford the $1,000 or so annual premium of a basic Medigap policy, consider joining a Medicare managed-care plan. For details, see "What You Need to Know About Medicare HMOs" in the March issue of MONEY. You can get help selecting the right plan for you by writing to the United Seniors Health Cooperative and requesting its 12-page report *Medicare, Medigap and Managed Care: 1997 Consumer Update* ($3.50; USHC, 1331 H St. N.W., Suite 500, Washington, D.C. 20005).

Article Review Form at end of book.

How does ageism impact health?
What is one way to combat ageism and its impact on health?

Effects of Ageism on Individual and Health Care Providers' Responses To Healthy Aging

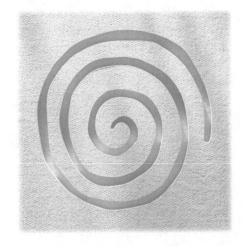

Lynda D. Grant

Lynda D. Grant, MA, is a doctoral student, Department of Counseling Psychology, University of British Columbia, 2125 Main Hall, Vancouver, British Columbia V6T 1L2.

Although misconceptions about the aging process have lessened over recent years, ageism is still having a detrimental effect on healthy aging. This article reviews the literature to support this contention and to demonstrate how stereotyping can affect the shape and nature of programs for elderly people. It is argued that for long-lasting change to occur, service providers need to directly target these negative attitudes in themselves, their professional institutions, their clients, and their communities. Suggestions are made for professional development, research, and program planning.

Key words

ageism

elderly people

health

stereotypes

Ageism has been described as "thinking or believing in a negative manner about the process of becoming old or about old people" (Doty, 1987, p. 213). Society's attitudes and beliefs about aging are culturally embedded and can have a profound effect on how people view themselves and others who are aging. Unfortunately, negative stereotypes about aging are still quite prevalent (Rowe & Kahn, 1987). Health care providers are not immune to these insidious stereotypes. This article reviews a number of ageism stereotypes in society generally and in the health care field. The aim is to demonstrate that ageism can negatively affect health care providers' professional training and service delivery and, ultimately, their clients' behavior and health outcomes.

For many years service providers used the World Health Organization (WHO, 1947) definition of health: "Health is a state of complete physical, mental, and social well-being, and not merely the absence of disease" (p. 16). This concept of health was a radical departure from the traditional model that saw health only as the absence of disease. WHO recognized that psychosocial well-being is an important component of health. However, health remained an abstract concept and, therefore, an ideal difficult to achieve. More recently, *Achieving Health for All* (Health and Welfare Canada, 1986) defined health in terms of "quality of life" and included in the definition the opportunity to make choices and to gain satisfaction from living despite functional limitations. This document suggested that health is a dynamic process of interaction between communities and individuals. Health involves freedom of choice: Communities (including health care providers) and individuals choose to take deliberate action to make the changes necessary for healthy aging.

Unfortunately, ageism can often affect the choices people are presented with and the decisions they make about those choices. If people believe that some of the "inevitable deterioration" of aging is preventable, they are likely to be more active in their own self-care. If health care providers believe that elderly people are valuable, equal members of society, then this belief should be reflected in professional training and service provision. Consequently, confronting ageism by enhancing positive beliefs about aging is a vital component of health promotion training and programming.

Effect of Ageism on Factors in Aging

Sociological Factors

Traditionally, aging has been viewed as a continual process of decline. Unfortunately, this stereotyping results in systematic discrimination that devalues senior citizens and frequently denies them equality (Butler, 1987).

In his review of the attitudes toward aging shown by humor, Palmore (1986) found that elderly people were often portrayed negatively. The humor tended to focus on physical and mental losses, as well as on decreases in sexual attractiveness and drive. Jokes about older women tended to be more negative than those about older men.

In North American culture, employability is often viewed as a primary measure of one's ability to contribute meaningfully to society and as a source of self-

identity and self-esteem (Moody, 1988). Botwinck (1984) reviewed the literature on the effects of ageism on employment. He found that although age was not an important factor in the evaluation of work competence, older age was given as one of the reasons for poor applicant quality if the person was not hired. When a younger applicant was not hired, lack of effort or inability was given as the reason.

Snyder and Barrett (1988) reviewed 272 federal court cases dealing with age discrimination and employment filed between 1970 and 1986. Sixty-five percent were decided in favor of the employer. The researchers found a number of problems with how these cases were decided. First, there was frequent use of generalities about the differences between older and younger workers' abilities, despite the fact that there was no documented evidence of consistent group differences in actual job performance. Often neither the employers nor the expert witnesses were asked for specific evidence concerning the plaintiff's actual physical capabilities and the specific job requirements. Second, the variability of decreased physical strength and fitness with age was frequently not addressed. Third, the possible effects of redesigning the workplace to accommodate older workers was often not considered.

These societal attitudes can affect not only how elderly people are perceived but also how they view themselves. Bodily (1991) surveyed inactive nurses to find out why they were not working. She was surprised to find that many respondents cited their age as the reason for not working without giving any other qualifiers. As Bodily stated,

What concerned me the most about the ways respondents were using "age" was that its meaning was being taken for granted; that is, as if the implications of phrases like "because of my age" or "I'm too old" were sufficiently obvious to require nothing more than a sympathetic nod on the part of the reader. While I was sympathetic, it was not because respondents were in fact too old, but because they were using "age" to disqualify themselves or otherwise limit their range of choices. (p. 248)

The quotation demonstrates the reciprocal nature of ageism. Negative stereotyping in society can lead to viewing elderly people in a depreciatory manner and as less valuable members of society. Elderly people who adopt these aging myths may see decline as inevitable and becoming more passive members of society as the only option available (Rodin & Langer, 1980). Unfortunately, when elderly people act according to these stereotypes, society's misperceptions about the aging process can be reinforced (Butler, 1987).

Physical Factors

Long-held beliefs in the health care field about the aging process are now being seriously questioned. Rowe and Kahn (1987) pointed out that much of what was considered to be inevitable deterioration is the result of individual behavior and environmental conditioning. They criticized researchers for perpetuating a narrow view of aging by concentrating on the central tendencies within a group and ignoring the substantial differences in functional aging (Troll, 1989).

Although changes in physiology are a part of aging, accumulated evidence indicates that many so-called usual disease processes can be modified and minimized (Rowe & Kahn, 1987). Diet and exercise have significant effects on carbohydrate metabolism, osteoporosis, cholesterol levels, diabetes, blood pressure, respiratory functioning, and hydration (Rowe & Kahn, 1987). Other studies have found that chronic pain can be greatly reduced through increased exercise and decreased medication use (Fordyce, 1976). Because musculoskeletal diseases account for 37 percent of all disabilities in the aged population (National Advisory Council on Aging, 1989b), increased mobility can have a significant effect on functional abilities and quality of life.

The lack of understanding about the aging process or the belief that continual decline is inevitable can lead to disease management as opposed to proactive intervention. Elderly people receive more medication prescriptions than younger people for equivalent symptoms (Rodin & Langer, 1980). Anxiolytic use more than doubles from 65 years of age on, and hypnotic medication use more than triples (Health and Welfare Canada, 1989). These statistics are quite disturbing given that 40 percent of all emergency department visits by elders are medication related.

Emotional Factors

It is well established that psychological well-being plays a significant role in the preservation of physical health and functional capacity (Zautra, Maxwell, & Reich, 1989). However, it has only recently been recognized that many of the variables that put elderly people at risk emotionally are responsive to intervention. In their review of the literature, Rowe and

Kahn (1987) showed that lack of or decrease in social support increases elderly people's mortality and morbidity rates and decreases adherence to health-promoting regimens. As an example, they cited studies showing that moving from familiar surroundings to a nursing home or institution increased mortality rates. Longitudinal studies in Sweden revealed that death rates increased by 48 percent for men and 26 percent for women within the first three months after losing a spouse (Svanborg, 1990). Other risk factors include the stress of managing on a fixed income, elder abuse, isolation, perceived health limitations, and the strain of being a caregiver (National Advisory Council on Aging, 1989a).

Unfortunately, psychological problems in older people can go untreated for a number of reasons. Emotional difficulties in elderly people can be difficult to diagnose because they are often masked by physical symptoms that can lead to further isolation and decreased activities. These important symptoms may be misdiagnosed and written off as part of the "normal aging process" (Katz, Curlick, & Nemetz, 1988). Compared to younger adults presenting with the same symptoms, elderly patients are referred less frequently for psychiatric assessments (Hillerbrand & Shaw, 1990). Elderly people themselves are often reluctant to seek assistance for emotional difficulties, even though there are many ways of relieving psychological distress and helping elderly individuals achieve a greater sense of well-being. Whether they attach a stigma to such help or lack knowledge about what type of help is available is unclear.

Cognitive Factors

There is strong evidence to suggest that a sense of well-being is in large part determined by a person's belief systems (Beck, 1991; Persons, 1989). Although a system involves a number of beliefs, two are seen as crucial: belief about control and belief about self-worth (that is, self-esteem). Although discussed separately, they are very much interrelated.

Sense of Control. The belief in the ability to exert control over an event influences how that event is appraised and subsequent coping activity (Lazarus & Folkman, 1984). A sense of control results from the belief that certain actions will lead to certain results and the conviction that one has the capacity to take the action necessary to produce those results (Bandura, 1977, 1982). This is an important concept when considering the aging process because sense of control can often be compromised in elderly people. If they see physical and mental deterioration as uncontrollable, the perceived lack of control is likely to reduce active coping behaviors (Rodin & Langer, 1980). A sense of helplessness in elderly people has been shown to decrease responsiveness, motivation, and self-esteem and eventually to increase illness, mortality rates, and memory problems (Parnham, 1987). Unfortunately, research has shown that increased contact with helping professionals can reinforce this sense of helplessness (Rodin, 1986).

Providing elderly people with the opportunity to increase perceived control over the environment leads to improved memory, alertness, activity, and physical health and decreased morbidity and mortality (Rodin,

1986). In one noteworthy study, alterations that increased residents' control of the environment in a nursing home demonstrated that even small changes can have a profound effect (Langer & Rodin, 1976). When the researchers returned 18 months after the intervention, they found that the experimental group (with increased control) had a 48 percent increase in subjective happiness; were increasingly active, alert, and social; and, perhaps most surprisingly, had a 50 percent lower mortality rate than the control group.

Successful aging cannot be equated with total independence and lack of reliance on others. Everyone maintains a balance between dependence and independence. The need for self-determination encompasses the right to choose not to exercise control. Therefore, service providers must be sensitive to the fact that it is the individual who chooses his or her level of dependence (Clark, 1988).

Self-Esteem. Self-esteem is a basic feeling of self-worth and a belief that one is fundamentally a person of value. In George's (1987) review of the literature on self-esteem and older adults, she suggested that the same factors that predict self-esteem in younger adults apply to elderly people: measures of personal achievement, success in interpersonal relationships, and meaningful leisure activities. However, correlates of self-esteem that were unique to older adults were health status and attitudes toward aging.

If aging is seen only in terms of the negative side of growing old and not as another stage of development, self-esteem can be seriously compromised. Rodin and Langer (1980) studied actions commonly seen as characteristic

of older people. The young and middle-aged participants saw elderly people as primarily involved in nonsocial behavior and passive activities and attributed to them unpleasant personal characteristics to a much greater extent than positive ones. They also found that all respondents, including the older ones, appeared to have a stereotype of elderly people that included the idea of senility. Ninety percent of the elderly respondents believed that there was a strong possibility they would become senile. However, medical estimates indicate that only 4 percent of people over 64 years of age suffer from a severe form of senility, and only another 10 percent suffer from a milder version (Katzman & Carasu, 1975).

Purpose and meaning in life influence self-esteem (George, 1987). For elderly people, this component is related to whether growing older is viewed as a time for continued contribution, goal setting, and purpose (Baltes, 1990). A perceived meaningless existence can lead to anxiety, depression, hopelessness, and physical decline, whereas meaning and purpose in life are associated with positive mental and physical health (Reker, Peacock, & Wong, 1987). Although meaning in life changes with each developmental phase, the need to be challenged and valued remains the same (Troll, 1989).

Effects of Ageism on Health Care Training and Service Delivery

Gatz and Pearson (1988) stated that although global negative attitudes of aging may not exist in the health care field, specific biases

may. Part of the responsibility for health care professionals' biases belongs to the educational institutions. Santos and VandenBos (1982) pointed out that few graduate programs in the social sciences offered training in gerontology. Whitbourne and Hulicka (1990) analyzed 139 psychology textbooks written over 40 years for evidence of ageism. They found that aging issues received little attention even in the later editions. When aging was addressed the texts tended to focus on problems rather than successes and described older adults as suffering from multiple deficits and handicaps that were attributed entirely to the aging process. The texts also only infrequently mentioned intellectual plasticity, the difference between normal aging and disease processes, and the ways in which individuals can compensate for losses associated with aging. The authors concluded that these texts exposed students to a narrow and permanently fixed view of the aging process.

Researchers argue that when others believe that an older person's range of physical and cognitive abilities is narrowing, there is a tendency to restrict individual freedom even further (Clark, 1989). These restrictions can lead to reinforcement of dependent rather than independent behavior by the helping professions (Baltes & Barton, 1979) and to symptom management rather than health promotion (Rodin & Langer, 1980). This behavior may best be conceptualized as "disabling support" versus "enabling support" (Rowe & Kahn, 1987).

One study exemplifies the impact of the two approaches.

When others believe that an older person's range of physical and cognitive abilities is narrowing, there is a tendency to restrict individual freedom even further.

Avorn and Langer (1982) divided residents in a nursing home into three groups and gave them a jigsaw puzzle to complete. One group was actively assisted by the staff to complete the puzzle (helped group), one was encouraged but received only minimal assistance (encouraged group), and one was left to complete the puzzle on its own (control group). All three groups were tested before and after puzzle assembly on ability to complete the task and on self-confidence ratings. The "helped" group's performance deteriorated posttest and they rated the task as more difficult, compared with the "encouraged" group, who improved their performance and felt more confident in their abilities. Even the control group, who received no help at all, increased their speed of performance slightly. It may be that the expectation of disability becomes disabling in and of itself. It could be argued that what has been termed "helpless behavior" in elderly people is an active attempt to cope with a system that reinforces adherence to stereotypes and dependent behavior.

Clarfield (1989) also pointed out that established practice defines physical diseases and psychological difficulties according to the way they typically present in 20- to 40-year-old individuals. Diagnosis and treatment of a more complex presentation in older people generally has received only minimal attention. Behavior that would warrant further investigation in a younger person may be less rigorously investigated in an elderly person. Elderly people are also more likely to receive less long-term therapy and to be institutionalized for the same symptoms that would be treated more aggressively in a younger population

(Rodin & Langer, 1980). A study of age bias in a general hospital (Hillerbrand & Shaw, 1990) found that compared to younger patients, geriatric patients were less likely to be referred for psychiatric consultation. The study also found that the suicidal ideation and past psychiatric history evaluations were not as complete for older patients. The authors found this oversight disturbing because the suicide rate for the elderly population is 50 percent higher than for younger populations.

Schaie (1988) criticized psychological research for having ageism undertones. He listed a number of methodological mistakes, including failing to operationalize the concept of the aging variable (that is, grouping everyone over 60 together as if they were a homogeneous group), not providing reasonable estimates of effect size in age comparisons, confounding findings with other concomitant age changes (for example, uncorrected peripheral sensory deficits), using test materials that are normed on young adults, and not considering the range of individual differences that result in overlapping distributions. He concluded that to avoid being accused of inadvertently supporting ageist biases, researchers in psychology need to address the above concerns and be as sensitive to these issues as they would to issues of race and gender.

Effects of Ageism on Health Care Policy

Subtle ageism may be partly to blame for the deficits in service delivery to the elderly population. In his review of the effects of ageism on public policy, Kimmel (1988) stated that 45 percent of U.S. community mental health centers reported having no spe-

cific programs for elderly people and that 41 percent did not have any clinical staff members trained to deliver geriatric services. Roybal (1988) called for an expansion of the federal response to mental health and aging. He pointed out that even though elderly people make up 12 percent of the U.S. population, only 6 percent of people served by mental health centers are older Americans.

The American Psychological Association and the American Psychological Society were cosponsors of a recent report entitled *Vitality for Life: Psychological Research for Productive Aging* (Adler, 1993). This report recognized that elderly people have been poorly represented in research and funding priorities. It lists four priorities in the area of aging: (1) learning how best to maximize elderly people's productivity at work, (2) developing mental health assessment and treatment strategies to enhance vitality, (3) learning how to change older people's health behavior, and (4) increasing research on how to optimize the functioning of those over 75. The report's sponsors will use the report to demonstrate to Congress the importance of providing more funding to agencies that support behavioral science research on aging.

Discussion

The recent acknowledgment that society needs to examine the whole concept of the aging process is long overdue. Studies demonstrating the effect of individual behavior and environmental conditioning on the aging process are exciting and challenging. Such research supports the contention that there is a strong interaction between individuals and their environment about health choices and responsibilities. There are a number of implications for professionals working with the elderly population. The first concern is individual professional responsibility. Because ageism can be quite subtle, service providers need to continually examine their own attitudes toward aging and elderly people. Health care professionals need to move away from using the term "age" as an explanatory variable and the assumption that after enough time certain "things" will happen to people. As Bodily (1991) pointed out, this assumption moves away from actual causes to the view that time is a sufficient cause and places the profession squarely in the biomedicalization model of aging. Instead, social workers and other health professionals need to focus on the causes of functional impairments, even the impairments that occur more frequently among older adults.

Professionals can also combat ageism through the types of programs offered and the way these programs are developed. Service providers need to actively involve elderly people in identifying what programs are needed and in designing, implementing, and managing the programs. Examples of such programs are Peer Counseling and Mentor Programs, where older people "buddy up" with high school students who are at high risk of dropping out. Programs could also be designed to target misconceptions about aging more directly in elderly people themselves. These programs would encourage them to examine how aging myths may be affecting their behavior and to experiment with acting differ-

ently. Such programs could have three main components: (1) direct challenge of aging myths, (2) skill-developing practice, and (3) a supportive environment for testing the new behavior. The advantage of this approach is that not only do participants learn new ways of responding, they also become more attuned to the manifestations of aging myths in society and the subtle effect they may be having on their own responses to aging and sense of well-being.

The second concern is professional training. Exposure to elderly people and to aging issues has been shown to reduce ageism (Gatz, Popkin, Pino, & VandenBos, 1984). Educational institutions in the health care and social sciences need to establish departments with subspecialties in gerontology, particularly at the graduate level (Storandt, 1983). These same educational institutions need to include aging issues in their continuing education programs, thus allowing working professionals to keep up to date on the gerontological literature and new trends in the field. Schaie (1988) criticized researchers and professionals working in gerontology for having a lack of awareness of relevant work in the existing aging literature.

The third area of concern is research. More research needs to be conducted on issues such as work and aging, individual differences in age-related change in behavior and performance, the magnitude of age changes and age differences, how to enhance health behaviors, and how to optimize the functioning of very old people. Research also needs to be aimed at identifying aging stereotypes and their effect on individuals and society, factors that contribute to

their development and maintenance, and ways they can most effectively be changed. Researchers need to be educated about the biases that may be influencing their own research. As Schaie (1988) pointed out, much of the current aging literature can be dismissed because of these biases.

Finally, professionals working with the elderly population have an obligation to make a concerted effort to confront ageism in society as a whole. Older people's failure to make health changes may often be the result of the barriers society creates to block successful change. The stereotypes of aging discussed in this article may prevent elderly people from initiating change or may defeat them before they start. Much can be learned from other groups, such as the women's movement, about how to raise awareness of stereotyping and unfair practices, including concerted lobbying efforts to change government policy at all levels. And service providers must actively target stereotypical beliefs in themselves, their professional organizations, and their communities to bring about lasting change.

References

Adler, T. (1993). Experts in aging outline research, funding focus. *APA Monitor, 4*(10), 18.

Avorn, J., & Langer, E. (1982). Induced disability in nursing home patients: A controlled trial. *Journal of the American Geriatrics Society, 20,* 297–300.

Baltes, M., & Barton, E. (1979). Behavioral analysis of aging: A review of the operant model and research. *International Journal of Behavioral Development, 2,* 297–320.

Baltes, P. B. (1990, October). *A psychological model of successful aging.* Paper presented at the 19th Annual Scientific and Educational Meeting of the Canadian Association on Gerontology, Victoria, British Columbia.

Bandura, A. (1977). Self-efficacy: Toward a unifying theory of behavioral change. *Psychological Review, 84*, 191–215.

Bandura, A. (1982). Self-efficacy mechanism in human agency. *American Psychologist, 37*, 122–147.

Beck, A. T. (1991). Cognitive therapy: A 30-year perspective. *American Psychologist, 46*, 268–375.

Bodily, C. L. (1991). "I have no opinions. I'm 73 years old!" Rethinking ageism. *Journal of Aging Studies, 5*, 245–264.

Botwinck, J. (1984). *Aging and behavior* (3rd ed.). New York: Springer.

Butler, R. N. (1987). Ageism. In G. L. Maddox & R. C. Atchley (Eds.), *The encyclopedia of aging* (pp. 22–23). New York: Springer.

Clarfield, A. M. (1989, November). *The geriatric imperative.* Paper presented at the 75th Annual General Meeting of the Pharmaceutical Manufacturers Association of Canada, Ottawa.

Clark, B. (1989, November). *The aging of North America: The shape of things to come.* Paper presented at the 75th Annual General Meeting of the Pharmaceutical Manufacturers Association of Canada, Ottawa.

Clark, P. G. (1988). Autonomy, personal empowerment, and quality of life in long term care. *Journal of Applied Gerontology, 2*, 279–297.

Doty, L. (1987). *Communication and assertion skills for older persons.* New York: Hemisphere.

Fordyce, W. E. (1976). *Behavioral methods for chronic pain and illness.* St. Louis: Mosby.

Gatz, M., & Pearson, C. G. (1988). Ageism revised and the provision of psychological services. *American Psychologist, 11*, 184–188.

Gatz, M., Popkin, S. J., Pino, C. D., & VandenBos, G. R. (1984). Psychological interventions with older adults. In J. E. Birren & K. W. Shaie (Eds.), *Handbook of the psychology of aging* (2nd ed., pp. 755–787). New York: Reinhold.

George, L. (1987). Self-esteem in later life. In G. L. Maddox & R. C. Atchley (Eds.), *The encyclopedia of aging* (p. 593). New York: Springer.

Health and Welfare Canada. (1986). *Achieving health for all: A framework for health promotion* (Catalog No. H39-102/1986E). Ottawa: Ministry of Supply and Services.

Health and Welfare Canada. (1989). *The active health report on seniors* (Catalog No. H-39-124/1988E). Ottawa: Minister of Supply and Services.

Hillerbrand, E. T., & Shaw, D. (1990). Age bias in a general hospital: Is there ageism in psychiatric consultation? *Clinical Gerontologist, 2*(2), 3–13.

Katz, I. R., Curlick, S., & Nemetz, P. (1988). Functional psychiatric disorders in the elderly. In L. W. Lazarus (Ed.), *Essentials of geriatric psychiatry* (pp. 113–137). New York: Springer.

Katzman, P., & Carasu, T. (1975). Differential diagnosis of dementia. In W. S. Fields (Ed.), *Neurological and sensory disorders in the elderly* (pp. 103–104). Miami: Symposium Specialist Medical Books.

Kimmel, D. C. (1988). Ageism, psychology, and public policy. *American Psychologist, 11*, 175–178.

Langer, E., & Rodin, J. (1976). The effects of choice and enhanced personal responsibility for the aged: A field experiment in an institutional setting. *Journal of Personality and Social Psychology, 34*, 191–198.

Lazarus, R. S., & Folkman, S. (1984). *Stress, appraisal and coping.* New York: Springer.

Moody, H. R. (1988). *The abundance of life: Human development policies for an aging society.* New York: Columbia University Press.

National Advisory Council on Aging. (1989a). *1989 and beyond: Challenges of an aging Canadian society* (Catalog No. H37-3/10-1989). Ottawa: Ministry of Supply and Services.

National Advisory Council on Aging. (1989b). *Understanding seniors' independence Report No. 1: The barriers and suggestions for action* (Catalog No. H37-3/11-1-1989E). Ottawa: Ministry of Supply and Services.

Palmore, E. B. (1986). Attitudes toward aging shown by humor: A review. In L. Nahemow, K. McCluskey-Fawcett, & P. McGhee (Eds.), *Humor and aging* (pp. 101–119). New York: Academic Press.

Parnham, I. (1987). Perceived control. In G. L. Maddox & R. C. Atchley (Eds.), *The encyclopedia of aging* (pp. 454–455). New York: Springer.

Persons, J. B. (1989). *Cognitive therapy in practice: A case formulation approach.* New York: W. W. Norton.

Reker, G. T., Peacock, E. J., & Wong, T. P. (1987). Meaning, purpose in life and well-being: A life span perspective. *Journal of Gerontology, 11*(1), 44–49.

Rodin, J. (1986). Aging and health: Effects of the sense of control. *Science, 233*, 1271–1276.

Rodin, J., & Langer, E. (1980). Aging labels: The decline of control and the fall of self-esteem. *Journal of Social Issues, 36*(12), 12–29.

Rowe, J. W., & Kahn, R. N. (1987). Human aging: Usual and successful aging. *Science, 237*, 143–149.

Roybal, E. R. (1988). Mental health and aging. *American Psychologist, 43*, 189–194.

Santos, J. F., & VandenBos, G. R. (1982). *Psychology and the older adult: Challenges for training in the 1980s.* Washington DC: American Psychological Association.

Schaie, K. W. (1988). Ageism in psychological research. *American Psychologist, 43*, 179–183.

Snyder, C. J., & Barrett, G. V. (1988). The Age Discrimination in Employment Act: A review of court decisions. *Experimental Aging Research, 14*(1), 3–47.

Storandt, M. (1983). Psychology's response to graying in America. *American Psychologist, 38*, 323–326.

Svanborg, A. (1990, October). *Aging, health and vitality: Results from the Gothberg longitudinal study.* Paper presented at the 19th Annual Scientific and Educational Meeting of the Canadian Association of Gerontology, Victoria, British Columbia.

Troll, L. (1989). *Continuations: Adult development and aging.* College Park: University of Maryland, International University Consortium.

Whitbourne, S. K., & Hulicka, I. M. (1990). Ageism in undergraduate psychology texts. *American Psychologist, 11*, 1127–1136.

World Health Organization. (1947). The constitution of the World Health Organization. *WHO Chronicles, 1,* 16.

Zautra, A. J., Maxwell, B. M., & Reich, J. W. (1989). Relationship among physical impairment, distress, and well-being in older adults. *Journal of Behavioral Medicine, 12*, 543–557.

 Article Review Form at end of book.

The author thanks Lory Block and Geoff Smith for their incisive comments and suggestions in the preparation of this manuscript and the members of the New Westminster Health Unit for their support, especially Pat Catton, Colleen Cameron, and Sandy Odin.

What are barriers to prevention and treatment of AIDS among minorities?

Concern about AIDS in Minority Communities

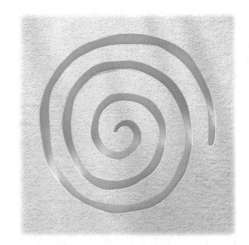

Alexandra Greeley

Alexandra Greeley is a writer in Reston, Va.

Although the spread of HIV seems to be relentless worldwide, and the virus that causes AIDS now affects men, women and children of every age and ethnic group, concern has been expressed that in this country, certain groups may not be receiving adequate health care due to cultural barriers.

Figures released from the national Centers for Disease Control and Prevention in Atlanta show that as of Dec. 31, 1994, there have been a total of 441,528 reported cases of AIDS in the United States since the epidemic began, and about 1 million people are infected with the virus. Although the number of new cases reported in 1994 (80,691) shows a decline from 1993 (106,618), when CDC expanded the AIDS surveillance case definition to include conditions—that is, opportunistic infections—that happen earlier in the disease, they are higher than in 1992 (47,572).

Now, rapid increases in HIV infection are showing up among minorities, specifically in the African American and the Hispanic communities. As CDC's *HIV/AIDS Surveillance Report* of December 1994 states, "Among reported cases, 1994 was the first year when blacks and Hispanics together accounted for the majority (53 percent) of all cases reported among men."

Infection rates are growing among the two other minority communities as well—the Asian American/Pacific Islander and the Native American (American Indian/Alaska Native) communities. According to CDC, of the total reported new cases (including men, women and children) of AIDS in 1994, 33,193 were among European Americans (not Hispanic); 31,487 among African Americans; 15,066 among Hispanics; 577 among Asian Americans/Pacific Islanders; and 227 among American Indian/ Alaska Natives.

Minority groups, or "communities of color," have been, for reporting purposes, classified into these four categories by the National Commission on AIDS. According to the 1992 study, "The Challenge of HIV/AIDS in Communities of Color" by the now disbanded commission, members of each community share some physical characteristics or ancestry. In addition, the study says, they also share the unfortunate position of being society's underdogs, facing, historically, "broad, sustained" racial discrimination. Other experts point out that those who live in poverty of any ethnic background, including European American, face the same kinds of problems accessing health care as do those classified as racial or ethnic minorities.

> **"Race and ethnicity are not risk factors, but they are markers for other factors that put people at increased risk, like lack of health insurance and limited access to care."**
> **—Paul Denning, M.D., CDC epidemiologist**

HIV's Spread Among Minorities

Even from the beginning of the epidemic, minorities were affected by the virus, says the commission's study. In fact, says Helen Fox, senior policy analyst, National Minority AIDS Council,

Source: From Alexandra Greeley, "Concern About AIDS in Minority Communities" in *FDA Consumer,* December 1995, U.S. Food and Drug Administration Office.

Washington, D.C., there has always been a higher incidence of HIV infection in communities of color than early statistics indicated, because people used to assume that AIDS was a gay white man's disease only and did not look for it elsewhere. "There was no understanding of the disease or of the relationship of injecting drugs and the transmission of the virus," she says.

"Race and ethnicity are not risk factors," says Paul Denning, M.D., epidemiologist in CDC's AIDS Surveillance Branch. "But they are markers for other factors that put people at increased risk, like lack of health insurance and limited access to care."

Indeed, say Brenda Lee and Lyvon Covington, public health specialists in the Food and Drug Administration's Office of AIDS and Special Health Issues, a number of common factors, many economic ones, affecting many minority groups contribute to the increase in AIDS: lack of medical insurance, which results in a lack of access to health care; a higher incidence of diseases or maladies in general; fear of medical care, particularly among illegal aliens; limited or no means of transportation to get to a health clinic; and for some, particularly in rural areas, too few doctors. And even when doctors are available, having Medicaid does not ensure adequate care says Denning. "You may have Medicaid," he says, "but many practitioners won't accept it."

Without routine medical care or testing, many people never suspect they are infected with the virus, says Fox. "There is such a long incubation period, and so many people feel pretty good," she says. "It is not until they come down with some kind of infection or [for women] yeast infection that doesn't go away that they

suspect something. Also people may be sick, but without access to health care, they won't do anything about it until they are very ill. Taking care of kids, housing and work—these basic needs are more important than worrying about HIV."

In addition, for many women, condom use can be a major domestic issue. Hispanic women, for example, often lack empowerment in sexual relationships, says Ledia Martinez, Hispanic HIV/AIDS coordinator, Office of HIV/AIDS Education, American National Red Cross. "Women may not be able to speak with their partners about condom use. . . . Such conversations are often interpreted as a sign that the female thinks the male is unfaithful. So even if you are unsure of your man, but he is putting food on the table, you risk losing him, pushing the condom-use issue. You put that aside because it is more important that the kids have a roof and that you are alive on a day-to-day basis." Besides, she notes, most Hispanics are Roman Catholics, and the position of the Catholic church, which opposes the use of condoms and other forms of contraception, is another barrier against condom use.

And, Denning points out, many minorities live in the inner city or urban areas, the foci of the epidemic. "Because the virus is very prevalent in the communities, the chances or odds that a person's sexual partner may be infected with HIV are increased," he says. "Also, one must consider the fact that injection drug use and other substance abuse, which are concentrated in disadvantaged, urban areas, have played a major role in the spread of HIV. Injection drug use serves as a direct mode of HIV transmission, while other substance abuse, like

crack cocaine use, may contribute to high-risk sexual behavior."

Some experts point to the "at-risk" factor as another reason why HIV has spread rampantly, a factor that knows no community boundaries. "I think the primary reason why people don't use protective measures—from abstinence to condoms—is that they don't see themselves at risk," says Owen McMaster, Ph.D., pharmacology toxicology reviewer, Center for Drug Evaluation and Research, FDA. "They think they know their sexual partner, or believe that this happens only to gay men who are not in a mutually monogamous relationship, or they think that there is no way that this beautiful, healthy-looking man or woman could have HIV."

Even understanding risk factors does not prevent risky behavior among some minorities, points out Rafael Chang, prevention education director, The Living Well Project, San Francisco. In a recent study of 260 gay Asian Pacific Islander men, he says, the researchers found that many people do understand the risk. "But they are not incorporating a sense of worthiness and self esteem," he says, since they feel they do not meet the American standard of beauty. As a result, he says, these men take great risks by not practicing safer sex if their partner does meet that standard of beauty.

Barriers to Treatment

For minorities, discrimination, poverty, and inadequate health care and education are barriers to meaningful prevention messages and to treatment. And often, so are traditional beliefs.

Homophobia and the belief that AIDS is a gay, white man's disease have helped both to spread

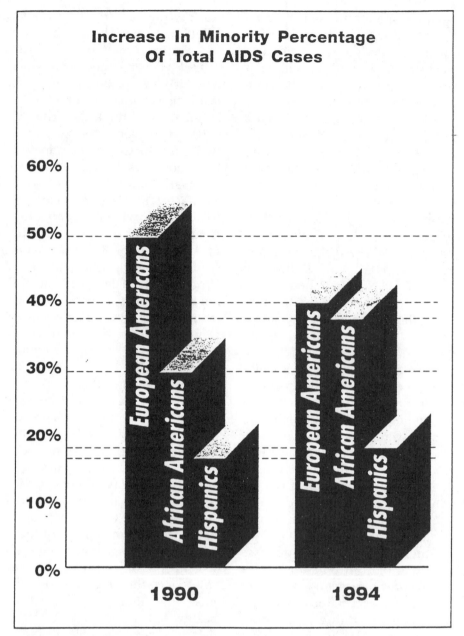

Increase In Minority Percentage Of Total AIDS Cases

1990

European Americans
African Americans
Hispanics

1994

European Americans
African Americans
Hispanics

In 1990, European Americans accounted for about 52 percent of AIDS cases while African Americans made up about 30 percent and Hispanics about 17 percent. By 1994, the proportion of African American and European American cases had become nearly equal: European Americans made up about 41 percent of AIDS cases and African Americans about 39 percent. The Hispanic proportion rose to about 19 percent. (Source: Centers for Disease Control and Prevention)

and to hide the disease. First, many minorities believe that the epidemic can't affect them or those in other communities of color, says Cherylene Showell, executive director of IMPACT (Intergroup Minority Project, AIDS Consortium and Trust) of D.C. in Washington, so they ignore its threat. Second, when HIV strikes and is associated with homosexuality, people deny its presence. This is true in some African American communities, she says, where families often hide and treat infected relatives as long as possible so outsiders cannot suspect the presence of homosexuality.

And it is true in many Asian American communities, adds Fox, where AIDS still often remains undiscussed and hidden and where many recent immigrants believe that homosexuality brings shame on the family. Among other immigrant populations, when men have sex with men, they do not consider themselves gay, she says—and if the men become infected, it's a real stigma.

"In most public health practices, once you know that there is something dangerous, you let the community know," says Showell. "And they can take whatever measures they need to protect themselves. But with HIV, people don't treat it like the flu, because it is tied to all these 'isms' [prejudices]." Instead, HIV becomes invisible with devastating results: no awareness of HIV, increased infection rates, limited medical treatment, and the spread of the epidemic. "It's really rather simple," she says. "I have seen this played out over and over again."

Other traditions provide roadblocks to medical care, too. In the Hispanic population, for example, the community's language isolation and culture may be part of the problem, according to Martinez. "Many Hispanics live in their own communities and remain connected to each other, but isolated from the mainstream," she says. "Even at school, there might be an HIV curriculum, but it is not taught in Spanish, so Hispanic children who speak only Spanish often never receive any HIV-prevention messages."

Add to that the Hispanic view of life, their fatalism, she says. "It is very common among

Hispanics to feel that people are born with their own cross to bear, and for some, having AIDS, or a son or sister with AIDS, is the cross."

Among African Americans, the epidemic has provided a greater sense of discrimination. "There is a denial [among African Americans] about the origins of the disease," says Darlene Washington, African American HIV/AIDS coordinator, Office of HIV/AIDS Education, the American Red Cross. "The disease was associated with Africa, and immediately, people said, 'I won't believe this. They are always blaming us for bad things. Why is Africa a deep, dark place of teeming germs?'"

But there is another level of denial, says Washington. The social, sexual and drug implications of HIV at first caused some African American faith communities to shy away from the issue, and as a result its members shied away, too. However, says McMaster, many African American congregations now do have HIV programs and are involved in HIV ministries.

In addition, Washington and others believe that for African Americans, the notorious 1970s Tuskeegee study, in which black men infected with syphilis were studied but not treated, stirred a fear of mainstream medicine. McMaster says this history seems to lead some African Americans to believe that AIDS was created by scientists to get rid of black people. "They think, 'If you made the disease to make me sick, why should I trust you to cure me?'" he says. This distrust keeps people from getting early treatment, from participating in clinical trials, and from using experimental drugs.

Finally, some minorities still prefer traditional medicines—such as herbs, massage, vitamins, and acupuncture—over Western medicines due to uncertainty about side effects of some drugs, says Chang.

Federal Response to the Epidemic

Numerous private, corporate, community, state, and federal agencies are trying to help stem the tide of HIV among minorities and assist and support outreach and education programs. Federal agencies, in particular can sustain broad prevention, research and education activities.

In its 1992 report, the National AIDS Commission recommended that federal health educators learn and take into account the cultural differences of minorities in order to target prevention messages successfully. CDC is applying this strategy in its new community collaboration and outreach efforts.

A special telephone line (1-800 TRIALS-A) provides information about how to get into clinical trials and how to get experimental drugs.

"We looked at the whole idea of communities and partnerships and community planning," says Dorothy Triplett, assistant director for Minority and Other Special Populations, Division of HIV/AIDS, CDC. "Community leaders and state and local officials sit at the same tables and are determining what the needs are," she says.

CDC is working with community gatekeepers to change risky behaviors and, she says, CDC also funds national minority organizations and community-based organizations. It has set up initiatives with the Minority Health Professions Foundation, all African American medical schools, and is working with the University of Puerto Rico.

At the National Institutes of Health in Bethesda, Md., which sponsors AIDS clinical trials, officials are extending their efforts to enroll minorities, which have historically been under-represented in trials and treatment studies. According to George W. Counts, M.D., an infectious disease specialist and director of the Office of Research on Minority and Women's Health in NIH's National Institute of Allergy and Infectious Disease (NIAID), it's important to make certain that trial results apply to the minority population, and to make certain that experimental therapies are equally available to minority groups.

To achieve these ends and to provide the best care to trial participants, he says, NIAID aims to ensure equal access to clinical trials and research programs and to dispel mistrust of those programs. Minority enrollments in AIDS clinical trials rose from 17 percent of enrolled subjects in 1988 to 44 percent in 1994.

FDA has developed and maintained numerous research and outreach efforts in the AIDS fight. Says FDA's Mary Beth Jacobs, director, division of life sciences, Center for Devices and Radiological Health, and the center's AIDS coordinator, FDA focused immediately on condoms and their testing and on fast-tracking the new Reality brand female condom as a barrier to virus transmission. A new test method was developed in FDA labs to evaluate barrier effectiveness for condoms and latex gloves. The new Reality brand female condom was fast-tracked for approval.

Elsewhere in the agency, the Center for Drug Evaluation and Research (CDER) actively facilitates the submission of investigational new drug applications, uses treatment INDs and other mechanisms to make drugs available as early as possible, and speeds the approval of AIDS drugs.

"We also send speakers to conferences to explain to researchers, particularly those in minority communities, how to access the FDA," he says. "While we have no minority-specific programs, FDA is making sure that minorities are getting the information about how to get into clinical trials and how to get experimental drugs." For example, a special telephone line (1-800 TRIALS-A) provides such information on an ongoing basis.

"We also encourage sponsors to include a diverse population in their clinical trials, but we have no specific regulatory requirement at this time," he says. "In fact, both CDER and the FDA's Office of AIDS and Special Health Issues give information to minority groups and minority physicians about which pharmaceutical companies are doing clinical trials so that minorities can enroll in the trials."

McMaster says that center officials are also studying the issue of pharmacogenetics—that is, the way in which a person's genetic makeup influences the efficacy of a drug and its side effects. The goal is to determine if certain genetic groups may benefit more, or have fewer side effects, when treated with certain classes of drugs. For example, such studies have shown that African Americans respond better to certain classes of antihypertensive drugs than to others. The hope is that similar information could be obtained for AIDS drugs. The agency is also meeting with representatives of other governments at the International Conference on Harmonization to establish a single set of regulations worldwide.

Without routine medical care or testing, many people never suspect they are infected with the virus.

FDA's David Feigal, M.D., division director for antiviral drug production in the center, says that FDA has responded in many ways, including approving 20 different treatments in, "the fastest review time of any group of products the agency has been responsible for."

As for the future? While many researchers and activists brace themselves for the uphill fight ahead, Feigal feels that everyone must be committed for the long haul. We can't wait for a vaccine, he says. Rather, victory will come in little steps, as happened in the national effort to cut the stroke rate among African Americans in the so-called "stroke belt" in the South. "Broad-based community programs took screening and health care into the black communities," he says. "So we need to do much of this with HIV. This won't make the problem go away over night, but we can chip away at it little by little."

 Article Review Form at end of book.

How have HIV/AIDS education and activism impacted health care?

Power to the Patient

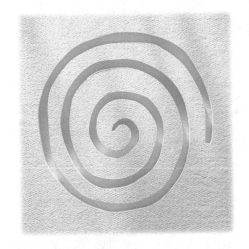

Mark Hagland

Mark Hagland is a contributing writer to Hospitals & Health Networks.

Hamilton Jordan vividly recalls the moment back in 1985, when, diagnosed with non-Hodgkin's lymphoma and lying in a hospital bed feeling sorry for himself, he received a visit from a doctor friend. His friend spoke bluntly. "You've got to take charge of your own health care. Nobody has more at stake in this than you do." With that, the former chief of staff in the Carter administration recalls, "I got up, got someone to help me into a wheelchair, went down to the medical library, and began to research my illness."

What sets Jordan apart from the average patient? The answer, increasingly, is less and less. Indeed, while the depths he reached in his search for answers remain the exception rather than the rule, Jordan personifies a new type of health care consumer: educated, interested, aware, and very active in charting the course of his or her own health care.

Jordan and millions of health care consumers like him want a new partnership, one in which pa-tients bring information of their own to the table, to discuss their treatment options in detail and make informed, consensual decisions. Many such judgments relate to personal values, lifestyle choices and calculations of health risk. The new trend will become particularly apparent in the context of diseases like prostate illness, which involve complicated judgments.

Case in point: Hamilton Jordan. A decade after his lymphoma had been in remission, he was given yet another shattering diagnosis—prostate cancer. Sensing something was wrong despite normal test results, Jordan prodded his doctors to do a prostate ultrasound and then a random needle biopsy. His persistence paid off with an early diagnosis—in fact, early enough to be potentially lifesaving.

It also sent him on another journey of learning, as he carefully researched his options. He eventually chose to have a radical prostatectomy. Today, several months after surgery, Jordan ap-pears to be cancer-free, and is satisfied with his control of physical functions.

If it sounds like Marcus Welby—the fatherly, white-haired doctor who ruled over our health care destinies—is dead, well, yes, he is. The old model of the doctor-patient relationship, in which doctors explained relatively little and patients did whatever they were told, is near dead, too. The onset of the Internet-laden information age, coupled with a growing awareness that "managed care" really implies the patient managing his or her own care, was its death knell.

So, instead, armed with an exploding array of information sources, from personal health books, magazines, and newspaper articles to the avalanche of information on the Internet, consumers are leaving behind the old do-what-the-doctor-ordered protocols. In many cases, it's the doctors who are listening— really listening— to the patients.

A cursory surf of the World Wide Web these days reveals that much of the information from

> **In a world where managed care is a misnomer, is it any wonder that consumers are taking charge of their own destiny? After all, it's not like they can rely on their doctors to do it for them.**

national and international journals, symposia and other forums on clinical advances and research, as well as a massive pile of more general health and medical information, is there for the downloading.

Baby boomers are fueling this fundamental change, as the best-educated and most independent-minded generation of health care consumers begins to face middle age. Add to this the growing awareness on the part of millions of health care consumers that treatment under managed health plans is not automatic, and that managing one's own health may often mean taking responsibility for understanding the economics, as well as the clinical aspects, of care.

In many cases, this is far from an academic distinction. Just ask Phillip Matthews, the executive director of the Manhattan-based People with AIDS Coalition of New York. Matthews, who was diagnosed as HIV positive in 1987, began educating himself in depth on HIV/AIDS when he became a staff member at the PWA Coalition. His education led him to switch doctors after his previous doctor refused to look into using an innovative Canadian HIV drug that Matthews had learned about through his own research.

But that only opened the door to a new dilemma. After switching to a physician whose board certification is in dermatology, but who is respected as one of the best HIV doctors in New York City, Matthews found himself up against his managed health plan. It strictly segregated the dermatologist and put multiple barriers in the way of Matthews seeing that doctor as his primary care physician, de-

spite the benefits of the arrangement. "In this context," says Matthews, "the managed care phenomenon is kind of scary, because it limits what I'm able to accomplish with my physician."

Multiply the experiences of Matthews and Jordan by several million, and it's easy to see what's coming next. It's almost as though the ground is shifting just when doctors and hospitals thought they were beginning to really understand what patients want out of health care.

The experience of Matthews, a man in his 30s facing a critical disease, illustrates a key point about the new health care consumer. If one historical development can be singled out as a harbinger of change, it's the arrival of HIV/AIDS as a widespread health epidemic in the mid-1980s. The AIDS crisis, for the first time, brought a complex and mysterious illness into the lives of large numbers of generally affluent, well-educated, urban men in their 20s, 30s and 40s. The combination of a dearth of information, intense interest in treatment and research, and a groundswell of political activism around the issue created the first model of a deeply participatory patient-provider relationship in 20th century health care.

Not surprisingly, HIV/AIDS education and activism offered inspiration to other advocacy movements, most notably the movement for funding, recognition and self-support for breast cancer.

Fran Visco, president of the Washington-based National Breast Cancer Coalition, herself a survivor of breast cancer, readily acknowledges the debt her movement owes to AIDS activism, in terms of bringing many health

care consumers to the realization that they need to be active in their own health care.

After all, she notes, in areas like HIV/AIDS and breast cancer, there are providers who don't have all the information they need, either. Early on in the history of bone marrow transplants, she points out, "there were a lot of doctors out there saying, 'Go out there and get a bone marrow transplant; that's the only thing that will save your life." But, says Visco, in truth, "we don't know that; it's just not evidence-based." Her solution? Intensive education. This is a good time, she says, for consumers to become more and more educated on their own, through advocacy and patient-driven organizations. "We're sort of taking up the slack there, and providing information that physicians can't or won't."

Consumers, though, aren't alone in fueling this new and powerful movement. After all, hospital executives and physicians have a big stake in patient awareness, too. "The best health care is care that's offered on a partnership basis," says Ned Calonge, M.D., director of preventive medicine at Kaiser Permanente–Colorado. In fact, he says, "I'm a big advocate for patient empowerment." But, he adds, "there's a very big issue— the filtering out of poor-quality information in this context. I worry about the information that consumers are accessing out there."

The media, Calonge says, don't understand the complexity of medical issues; they just report the latest research. A good example: mainstream coverage of cancer. The reporting on estrogen replacement for breast cancer suggested that during menopause the treatment might actually increase the chances of breast cancer. "What hasn't been widely noted is the possibility that estrogen replacement will reduce the chances of heart disease," Calonge says, "and the risk of a woman dying of heart disease is 10 times higher than of dying of breast cancer." In fact, many researchers think that women who live longer because of estrogen replacement therapy do so because of the reduction in heart disease risk.

William Osheroff, M.D., medical director at the Cypress-based PacifiCare of California, agrees, adding that another important factor is missing from the ready spread of consumer information: personal values. Every treatment "has its upsides and downsides," he says, and the quality-of-life calculations one needs to make, particularly in reference to diseases like prostate cancer, can be complex. "As doctors and patients, we need to become more comfortable talking about these kinds of issues," says Osheroff.

Many doctors, Osheroff says, are still very uncomfortable with the new dynamic of interaction among patients, physicians and hospitals. Some may never adjust. Each doctor-patient team, he adds, will have to determine which kind of communication they want to develop.

Mark Bricklin, editor of *Prevention* magazine, the nation's largest-circulation consumer health publication, says the proliferation of consumer health information offers doctors an opportunity for expanded dialogue with patients. Doctors and other health professionals can and should be interested in knowing what their patients are reading. Unfortunately, he says, "doctors tell us they have time constraints. They're not getting paid for this, and they often get very nervous, because they don't really want to answer patients' questions."

Still, a good number are beginning to do so, though electronically rather than face-to-face. There are dozens of hospital-based Web sites, sponsored by such prominent organizations as Harvard Hospital, Stanford University Medical Center, and the University of Illinois College of Medicine. The University of Iowa operates its full-fledged Virtual Hospital, a site that provides both health professional-oriented and patient-oriented interactive forums.

Such approaches can do a lot more than just assist in marketing efforts, says Janet Parodi, CEO of Long Beach (Calif.) Community Medical Center. "Health care today is about information and intervention," Parodi adds, "and nothing else." Her goal is to deliver high quality at low cost through "virtual" diagnostics, "virtual" intervention, "virtual" management, and "virtual" delivery. "That's why we're totally committed to exploiting the Internet, as well as other media venues, such as videoconferencing, for their potential links to patients and consumers."

Long Beach Community's Web site carries 200 pages, offering informational, educational and interactive opportunities for health care consumers; already 700 users a day are taking advantage of it.

The informed patient is the more successful patient, says Jeanne Donlevy, senior vice-president for patient care services at Good Samaritan Hospital, Lebanon, Pa. Good Samaritan's home care-based program has been successful. The program, designed for self-monitoring of patients discharged after treatment for congestive heart failure, used intensive education as part of an overall case management initiative.

It has resulted in a tremendous decline in readmissions for the disease among participating patients. When patients learned the science of their disease, Donlevy says, it encouraged them to take more personal responsibility for their own care, a vital aspect of the program's success. If Good Samaritan can be successful in such a venture, Donlevy adds, it shows a tremendous potential for improving patient and family participation.

In the end, it all comes back to this, says Hamilton Jordan. "Ten years from now, those health care professionals and businesses who are most successful will be the ones who have understood and found new ways to utilize patient knowledge, involvement and curiosity. And those who ignore this desire will suffer as businesses and as medical institutions."

After all, he asks, parroting the same question asked of him years ago: "Who's got more at stake than the patient?"

 Article Review Form at end of book.

WiseGuide Wrap-Up

- Access to healthcare is adversely influenced by poverty, discrimination, and inadequate healthcare coverage.

- Active participation in your own healthcare and in improving the healthcare system is necessary to improve access to healthcare for all.

R.E.A.L. Sites

The adjacent list provides a print preview of typical **coursewise** R.E.A.L. Sites. (There are over 100 such sites at the **courselinks**™ site.) The danger in printing URLs is that web sites can change overnight. As we went to press, these sites were functional using the URLs provided. If you come across one that isn't, please let us know via email at webmaster@coursewise.com. Use your Passport to access the most current list of R.E.A.L. sites at the **courselinks**™ site.

Site name: Office of Minority Health Resource Center

URL: http://www.omhrc.org/welcome.htm

Why is it R.E.A.L.? Provides easy and quick access to extensive databases on minority health documents, audiovisuals, organizations, programs, events, conferences, resource persons, and funding opportunities.

Key topics: governmental agency, minority health

Activity: Find out what program the Red Cross offers on African American and Hispanic HIV/AIDS education. Decide if you think the program would be successful in your community. Why or why not?

Site name: American Association for Retired Persons

URL: http://www.aarp.org:80/

Why is it R.E.A.L.? AARP is a highly reputable nonprofit organization dedicated to securing the rights of older adults. Wide variety of links serve the health advocacy and informational needs of older adults.

Key topics: aging, empowerment, activism & advocacy

Activity: Find out the benefits of membership and if you are eligible to become a member.

Site name: Human Rights Campaign

URL: http://www.hrcusa.orr/issues/index.html

Why is it R.E.A.L.? One of the nation's largest nonprofit organizations dedicated to lobbying and fundraising for lesbian and gay rights.

Key topics: human rights, community agency, activism & advocacy

Activity: Click on "Lesbian Health" to find out the issues then see how you can make a difference.

Site name: Department of Health and Human Services: Improving Services for Hispanics

URL: http://phs.os.dhhs.gov/about/heo/hispanic.html

Why is it R.E.A.L.? Consumer-oriented resource on Hispanic health issues, especially on cancer and diabetes, migrant and border health.

Key topics: governmental agency, minority health, consumer health, cancer

Activity: Find out why cancer and diabetes are special health concerns of Hispanics.

Site name: Healthy People 2000

URL: http://odphp.osophs.dhhs.gov/pubs/hp2000

Why is it R.E.A.L.? Government document regarding U.S. health goals and objectives for the year 2000, includes special population health risks for older adults, women, and minorities.

Key topics: governmental agency, health statistics, minority health

....

Site name: Women's Health Initiative

URL: http://www.womens-health.com

Why is it R.E.A.L.? Interactive and proactive effort to inform and empower women about their health issues. Includes various online health assessments on pregnancy, gynecologic symptoms, cardiovascular health, and bleeding.

Key topics: community agency, women's health

....

Site name: National Organization for Women

URL: http://www.now.org/

Why is it R.E.A.L.? Pioneer nonprofit organization dedicated to serving the needs of women.

Key topics: women's health, community agency, human rights, activism & advocacy

....

section

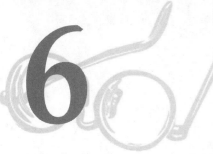

6

Key Points

- Duplication and gaps in the current healthcare system create excess that adds unnecessary costs and threatens access to care.

- Managed care plans provide varying degrees of benefits and limitations.

- Insurers have used genetic information to discriminate against people.

- Individual and combined effort from health consumers can make physicians and the healthcare system more accountable for providing equitable access to healthcare.

Making Your World a Healthier Place

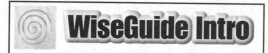

In order to make your world a healthier place, you must first identify the problems, then marshal resources and implement solutions. Health consumer groups have more information and power to promote positive changes to the healthcare system than ever before.

All the articles in Section 6 address the healthcare system. The first three articles outline specific problems with the current healthcare system in the United States. Lamm ("The Ethics of Excess") makes a case that duplication and gaps in healthcare, in the areas of medical technology, personnel, and institutional capacity, interfere with access and create ethical problems. The fifteen questions Davis ("Give Your HMO a Checkup") recommends health consumers ask before deciding on a managed care plan speak to many of the existing limitations of some plans. And concerns are raised about the health insurance industry's use of genetic information to discriminate in "Genetic Discrimination and Health Insurance: An Urgent Need for Reform." The last three articles ("Checking Up on Your Doctor," "Whatever Works," and "Partnerships: The Prescription for Healthier Communities") provide insight into possible solutions for health consumers, such as considering healthcare alternatives, investigating the qualifications of your physician, and forming community coalitions.

Questions

R34. Why is underutilization of medical resources an important concern for health consumers?

R35. Why is it important to know the right questions to ask when deciding on a managed care plan?

R36. How have insurers used genetic information to discriminate against people?

R37. How can patients investigate their doctors?

R38. What criteria could you use to judge the value of an alternative health product, service, or discipline?

R39. What is the purpose of coalitions?

Why is underutilization of medical resources an important concern for health consumers?

The Ethics of Excess

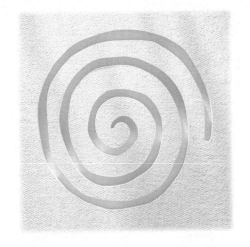

Richard D. Lamm, LLB CPA

Mr. Lamm was Governor of Colorado 1975 to 1987. He is currently Director of the Center for Public Policy & Contemporary Issues, University of Denver and Chairman for the Pew Health Professions Commission.

My wife had breast cancer in 1981 which was discovered by a mammogram. After her (successful) mastectomy, we made a practice of helping dedicate any mammography machine anywhere in Colorado. We were grateful and wanted to help expand this important service and, of course, every hospital loved to have either the Governor or the First Lady at their dedication.

In 1991, however, a study in the *Annals of Internal Medicine*[1] showed that although America had 10,000 mammography machines, we essentially utilized 2600 of them. The study postulated that if every woman had a mammogram every time the American Cancer Association suggested it was appropriate, we would utilize approximately 5000—still half as many as were

then in existence. The study further showed that because the underutilized machines had to be amortized, American women had to pay more than twice what the real cost was, and this was having the effect of driving American women away from mammograms. It also found sites that did not do a sufficient number of mammograms had more flawed readings of the results. Welcome to the new world of excess preventing access and quality. (There are now 16,000 mammography machines in the United States, six times as many as are fully utilized.)

Recognizing that you can never have perfect utilization, and such formulas are thus not perfect, the fact remains—in the case of mammography machines as elsewhere in the health care system—that excess is interfering with access.

I am increasingly disturbed by the number of well-intentioned people making what they think are health-producing decisions who are in fact adding duplicative, superfluous health care facilities to the system. The net effect of these actions has been to build

a great redundancy into our health care system at the same time great need exists in other parts of the system. Half-empty hospitals exist blocks from where children lack access to vaccinations. We have trained far too many medical specialists. Yet, a few streets away from every medical center, women go without prenatal care. Excess sits cheek-to-jowl with inadequacy.

I suggest the sheer magnitude of this problem has become an ethical one. We are all trustees of the U.S. health care system—whatever our roles. We must eventually take responsibility for the indirect as well as the direct consequences of our actions. A hospital administrator in Colorado, which has a statewide hospital occupancy of less than 50%,[2] cannot say that the 500,000 uninsured Coloradoans have nothing to do with his/her facility. That facility is consuming significant resources which are desperately needed elsewhere in the system.

Once a community, state, or nation builds up a medical infrastructure, it must pay for that

Source: From Richard D. Lamm, "The Ethics of Excess" in *Public Health Reports*, Volume 111, May/June 1996, U.S. Public Health Service, Department of Health and Human Services.

infrastructure. If it is too large, the citizens pay too much. The Government Accounting Office (GAO) has found:

Health spending per capital increases with the size of a state's health infrastructure, with hospital and physicians' services accounting for approximately two-thirds of the total personal health spending. States with greater health resources, including physicians as well as hospital and nursing home beds, have higher health care spending on the average.[3]

Supply seems to drive demand and create its own demand. Boston has twice as many hospitals per capita as New Haven, and it has twice as many hospital admissions with *no* difference in outcome.

A 50% increase in the capacity of the acute hospital sector decreases the threshold for admitting patients in a way that results in a 50% increase in hospital use.[4a]

The number of specialists often determines how many and what types of procedures are performed in the community. The biggest correlation to the number of tonsillectomies, prostatectomies, hysterectomies, and hernia repairs is not the underlying health of the population, but the number of specialists in the area. Rates for appendectomies, which is not an elective procedure, are nearly geographically uniform while elective procedures, where doctors have discretion, vary by disturbing amounts. The major determinant of how many procedures are done in a given area is the number of specialists in the area who can perform them.[1,5,6] One expert captured the dynamics perfectly:

. . . in order to gain competitive advantage, there are strong economic incentives for providers to develop new, state of the art facilities and services. This kind of development, in turn, encourages unnecessary or inappropriate utilization in order to generate sufficient revenue to cover the operating and capital costs of the new capacity.[7]

Much of what we do in health care serves the interests of the physician or a particular institution rather than the interests of the public. Well-meaning people continually turn away from facing the ethical implications of this dynamic.

Excess Physicians

There have been a number of studies[8] that have found that America is training too many physicians. These studies generally point out that training too many physicians can be as big a mistake as training too few. The medical profession has ignored report after report showing that it was training too many physicians. And it is clearly expensive. Ginzberg speculates:

If we would have increased physicians from 140 per 100,000 (1962) to 190 per 100,000 (1990) instead of the 250 per 100,000 which actually occurred, potential savings would amount to $173 billion out of the health spending of $660 billion.[9]

The Bureau of Health Professions estimates that the United States currently has 15,000 surplus physicians; and by the year 2000, they will have 50,000 surplus physicians.[10] There are other estimates which put this number considerably higher. Currently, we do know that America has 240 physicians per 100,000 people; and by the year 2000, our 126 medical schools will

raise that number to 260 per 100,000 people.[11,12]

On the other hand, Health Maintenance Organizations (HMOs)—one of the main models for managed competition—operate at 120 doctors per 100,000 subscribers.[13] Fee-for-service medicine commonly uses 450 to 500 doctors per 100,000 people,[14] but society is demanding more efficiency and is experimenting with 17 varieties of restructured delivery systems that will dramatically multiply the effectiveness of each physician.

Kissick at the University of Pennsylvania estimates that if we could serve all of America with the same efficiency that Kaiser Permanente serves its system, we would need less than half the number of existing physicians.[15] In the face of clear evidence, U.S. medical schools should dramatically reduce the number of physicians they train, while in fact they actually increased the number. "Cost containment may ultimately require constraints on the number of physicians allowed to enter the system," says John Hughes of Yale University School of Medicine.[12] Recognizing that one cannot serve rural America with the same efficiency as Kaiser serves its subscribers (Kaiser's demography is somewhat different also), Kissick suggests this comparison clearly shows that America will experience tremendous dislocation among physicians as Adam Smith restructures the marketplace and more and more physicians go to work in groups or for salaries in large systems.[16] Those physicians unwilling or unable to make an arrangement with a health care system will be forced to go to a

We are all trustees of the U.S. health care system—whatever our roles.

rural or inner city area, retire, or leave the practice of medicine. Many specialists will seek retraining in the growth sector of primary care.

There is other evidence of this surplus. The Medical Economics Continuing Survey finds that 45% of doctors reported they were not practicing at their full capacity.[16] All the empirical evidence we have confirms that America has too many physicians and that this problem will grow worse before it gets better.

Specialists. We have not only trained too many doctors, we have trained the wrong types.[18–20] Simply stated, other developed industrial countries for many years have practiced medicine with roughly 50% of physicians in primary care and 50% in specialties and subspecialties.[18–20] In the United States, however, we train and employ about 32% primary care physicians (such as general practitioners, family physicians, general internists, general pediatricians, and some obstetrician/gynecologists and emergency medicine physicians), and about 68% specialists and subspecialists.[18–20] Other developed countries, however, do as well or better than the United States at providing care at much lower cost (whether cost is measured as the amount per capita per year, or as a percentage of the GNP). Yet, the situation in the United States is rapidly getting worse. The percentage of physicians graduating from U.S. medical schools who are declaring generalist fields has drastically declined during the last decade, from 36% of the graduating class of 1982 to only 14% in 1992.[18–20]

Comparing the 50:50 specialist-to-generalist ratio desired and the existing 68:32 ratio, one finds a shortfall of approximately 100,000 generalist physicians and an over-supply of 100,000 specialists and subspecialist physicians.[21–23] Compounding this excess, existing models of managed care show that if the Federal Government, individual states, or the private marketplace creates health alliances or accountable health partnerships for everyone, we will need a work force that more closely approximates a 35% specialist and 65% generalist physician distribution, according to Sokolov. Using such models and some basic arithmetic, one can demonstrate a shortfall of 200,000 generalist physicians between current physician supply and what may be needed in the near future. The Pew Health Professions Commission did not accept the number, but it did the trend. Few people argue that we do not have too many specialists.

Wennberg has made a similar analysis:

If the hiring practices of prepaid group practice HMOs had been in force throughout the United States in 1988, more than half of all specialists would not be unemployed.[4b]

He further adds:

. . . if radiology residency programs were completely eliminated, it would still take about twenty years before the numbers per capita in the national economy approached the numbers now hired by prepaid group practice HMOs. Under the same policy, it would take more than twenty-five years for the supply of neurosurgeons and about seventeen years for the supply of urologists to approximate the numbers employed by these HMOs.[4c]

An example of the excess in specialties is found in a recent study by Leape where he looked at the number of surgeons the United States as compared to

> **All the empirical evidence we have confirms that America has too many physicians and that this problem will grow worse.**

what is likely to be needed under the new health care delivery systems. He pointed out that the AMA projected the total supply of surgeons will increase 14% between 1986 and 2010, with most of the growth occurring in surgical specialties. Using productivity standards that are widely agreed upon, he finds that half of the surgeons in the United States are presently significantly underutilized. He points out that staff model HMOs use surgeons two or even three times more efficiently than fee-for-service medicine.[24] At the same time, they perform significantly fewer operations. Fewer surgeons will, in the future, perform fewer operations and yet produce more health.

Medical Schools. In the face of clear evidence, U.S. medical schools should dramatically reduce the number of physicians they train. If America comes anywhere near achieving the efficiency of an HMO in its entire health care system, there will be no need for medical schools to turn out approximately 16,000 physicians a year. An unneeded medical school is an expensive luxury which cannot be tolerated in an efficient system.

The remaining medical schools should recognize that they have an ethical obligation to dramatically increase the number of primary care physicians they graduate, and to reduce the number of specialists. Supply and demand have never heretofore been a concern to medical schools. As a tragic result, a generation of young professionals are being prepared, at great public and personal expense, for careers where employment will be limited and perhaps not even available. Left unchanged, in fact, the 25 billion public dollars we devote to training health professionals will give our society professionals we simply do not need.

The future system will require medical schools to take much more into consideration the community needs for health manpower, and require them to match their output to what the market needs.

Recognizing that there are many rural and inner city areas which are not adequately served by doctors, one nevertheless has to predict that there will be a considerable surplus of doctors after health care reform takes effect. This conclusion is reached after looking at a number of comparisons with other health care organizational models.

Excess Institutional Capacity

It is axiomatic that a nation must pay for its medical infrastructure. Once a hospital is built, or a doctor trained, or a piece of medical technology put in place, it almost inevitably has to be funded. America has too much health care infrastructure that is draining too many dollars from other important needs. This costs America dearly.

Hospital Beds

Most industrialized nations put strict limits on hospitals, hospital beds, and medical technology. European countries seem to recognize that once hospital beds are in place and once doctors and specialists have graduated, they will be used. There is a Parkinson's Law to hospital beds and medical technology: *The work expands to fill facilities available.* Even though the United States actually has a smaller number of

hospital beds per capita than most nations, we deliver by far the most intensive treatment while in that bed. We may have fewer beds per capita than other countries, but our beds are often dramatically underoccupied, and a large number of patients in a hospital do not really need to be there. The United States averages 3.8 hospital beds per 1,000 people.[2a] Yet, some experts estimate that because of outpatient surgery, drug therapy, and other medical advances, we only need 1.8 beds per 1,000 people.[13] We have massive underutilized capacity in most metropolitan areas. The United States seems to have a "7–11" theory of hospitals where we want a hospital on every corner filled with every marvelous machine and open 24 hours a day. This is a terribly expensive luxury—one we can no longer afford.

Excess capacity creates its own demand. Health economists have an axiom called Roemer's Law which states: "A built bed is a filled bed."[25] Not totally true, of course, but a built bed is a magnet that does create demand. As Evans has noted:

. . .overall bed capacity emerges from study after study as the single most important factor influencing hospital inpatient utilization, and the level of bed capacity at which use would appear to stop responding to increases is double or triple current capacity or need estimates.[26]

At any given time, approximately one-third of America's 924,040 staffed hospital beds are empty.[27] This is staffed beds—licensed beds are actually a much higher figure. Large HMOs in the United States operate with only 1.5 beds per 1,000 members.[13] Put another way, HMOs operate with less than half the hospital beds per capita as now exist, and yet keep their subscribers every bit as healthy as fee-for-service medicine.

America may have over 1000 unnecessary surplus hospitals which think they are contributing to the nation's health, but actually consume resources desperately needed elsewhere in the system.

"There is clearly excess capacity in the system," says Richard Wade, spokesman for the American Hospital Association. He predicts 20% to 25% hospital capacity will be cut, along with many of the 3.5 million people employed in hospitals. In 1992, 39 of the country's 5,000 hospitals closed with many more shrinking their staff.[28]

Of course, many uninsured will be brought into the U.S. health care system; but since many of them are already inefficiently served in emergency rooms, this is unlikely to save the large scale closure of hospitals.

Centers of Excellence

America has 850 hospitals doing open heart surgery,[29] less than half do the minimum number (250) to meet federal standards. A hundred of these hospitals do less than one heart surgery a week. Under an efficient health care system, many of these institutions will close. There is no way, for instance, that the Denver metropolitan area needs 14 open heart surgeries,[30] or that Colorado needs four hospitals doing heart transplants. HMOs either own their hospitals or contract with one highly efficient hospital. If America follows the experience of European countries, it will close some of its redundant hospitals, and create centers of excellence which consolidate specific operations in specialized centers.

Intensive Care Beds

It is estimated that $62 billion of the $809 billion of health care in 1992 was for the expense of intensive care units.[31,32] The United

States has approximately three times more intensive care beds as do other developed countries. For instance, our intensive care unit (ICU) utilization is 2.5 times that of Canada.[31,33] Whereas 8% of the total Canadian inpatient costs were allocated to ICU units, the United States had 20% of its inpatient care costs allocated to ICU units. Intensive care units employ about 19% of the nurses who worked in general specialty bed units.[31]

The reason that the United States has so many more intensive care beds is that we have different standards about who we put in an intensive care bed. By the standards of other nations, we put many people into an intensive care bed for whom there is no happy outcome. And, conversely, we often put people in an intensive care bed who are not sick enough to really need such a level of care. Eight percent of patients in intensive care units consume 92% of the inpatient hospital resources; and of those 8% high cost patients, 70% died in the hospital.[31-33] It would seem clear from the statistics that other developed countries with very similar standards and culture with regard to death and dying are much more thoughtful about the categories of people who have access to an intensive care bed.[30-33] In America, we expend massive resources often only to give someone an expensive death.

The Myth of Medical Technology

Americans love technology of any type. Much of this is justified and has led to our being a world leader in the manufacture and use of technology. It is deeply ingrained into our culture. But there is a widespread belief that *medical technology saves money*. Alas, it does not. Here's what one study found on medical technology:

. . . most technological innovations in the health service industry have added to, rather than reduced costs. This *added* cost reflects a qualitative difference in what the client receives. For example, today's treatment for a particular ailment will almost certainly include a set of therapeutic procedures that is markedly different from what would have been received 25 years ago. . . . In short, the question is not whether recent technological developments have added to health costs. They have. The real question is whether the benefits exceed the costs, and in at least some instances, they may not.[31-33]

Some critics question whether hospitals actually add technology to save health care costs. Evans observes:

Technological innovations that really reduce costs, simultaneously and by definition, reduce sales and income as well. That is not the end most health providers seek when adding a new technology.[34]

Newhouse, an economist at Harvard, estimates that half of the increase in the national bill for medical care now goes to pay for new technology.[35] Whatever the motivation, medical technology does not come cheap and seldom saves money. Our miracles are often very expensive.

The United States has far more medical technology than it can effectively utilize. With 4.7% of the world's population, we have one-half of the world's CT scanners, and about two-thirds of the world's magnetic resonance imagers (MRIs). In 1987, the United States had 7.4 times as many radiation therapy units and 8 times as many MRIs per million people as did Canada, and had 4.4 times as many open heart surgery units and 2.8 times as many lithotripter units as did Germany.[36]

The state of Colorado has 22 stationary MRIs in hospitals—three on the same block in Denver.[37] Although Canada has the same number of MRIs as Colorado, Canada has nine times our population. Colorado has a myriad of unmet social needs. Yet, it is wasting resources on duplicative, redundant medical technology that often exists in a hospital which is itself not needed for the health of the state.

Conclusion

I would suggest that the sheer size of the health care system has become an ethical issue. It is filled with highly trained (and highly paid) people who believe they are adding to the nation's health. Often they are not. They are utilizing resources desperately needed elsewhere in the system. The opportunity costs of those resources could go a long way toward correcting the inadequacies in the system. Excess is interfering with access and ethical people should work to correct both.

References

1. Is the supply of mammography machines outstripping need and demand? Ann Intern Med 1990;113:547
2. Facts about Colorado hospitals. Denver: Colorado Hospital Assn 1991:1–2.
3. State health care spending factors. Publication No. B-2446979. Washington DC: Government Accounting Office, 1992;Feb. 13.
4. Wennberg J et al. Health Affairs 1993 12(2):(a) 94; (b) 95; (c) 97.
5. Schroeder SA. Health care reform: a special report. Med Econ New York: 1993, p. 32.
6. Phelps C, Health economics. New York: Harper-Collins, 1993.

7. Coddington D et al. The crisis in health care. Jossey-Bass 1990:6.

8. Pew Health Professions Commission staff report. 1993.

9. Ginzberg E. JAMA 1992 Feb. 2.

10. Improving access to health care through physician workforce reforms: dimensions for the 21st century. New York: Council on Graduate Medical Education, October 1992.

11. Rising health care costs: causes, implications, and strategies. Congressional Budget Office Washington, DC: April 1991, p. xii.

12. Hughes JS. Wall Street J, 1991 May 8, Sect B:1.

13. World development report. The World Bank 1993, chap. 6, p. 6.

14. Reinhardt UE. Health manpower forecasting: the case of physician supply. In E Ginzberg, editor. Health services research: key to health policy. Cambridge: Harvard University Press, 1991.

15. Schroeder SA. Physician supply in the U.S. medical market place. Health Affairs, spring 1992, p. 235.

16. Kissick WL. Medicine's dilemmas. New Haven: Yale University Press 1994.

17. Owens A. How low can productivity go? Med Econ 1987:64 (25) 172–203.

18. Petersdorf RD. The doctor is in. Washington, DC: Association of American Medical Colleges, 1993.

19. Levinsky NG. Recruiting for primary care. N Engl J Med 1993:328:656–60.

20. Politzer R, Harris DL, Gaston MH, and Mullan F. Primary care physician supply and the underserved. JAMA 1991: 266:104–109.

21. Council on Graduate Medical Education. Improving access to health care through physician workforce reform: directions for the 21st century. Rockville (MD): Health Resources and Services Administration, Public Health Service October 1992.

22. Lundberg GD and Lamm RD. Solving our primary care crisis by retraining specialists to gain specific primary care competencies. JAMA 1993:270(3):380–381.

23. Lundberg GD. Caring for the uninsured and underinsured. JAMA 1991:266:2079–2080.

24. Leape LL. The future of surgery. In RJ Blendon and TS, Hyams eds. Reforming the system: containing health care costs in an era of universal coverage. 1992: p. 213

25. Roemer M. Bed supply and hospital utilization: a natural experiment. J Am Hosp Assn 1961:35:36–42.

26. Evans RG. Strained mercy. Butterworthy 1984.

27. Inglehart J. The American health care system. N Engl J Med 1993: July 29 372.

28. Wade R. Wall Street J 1993: July 13, Sect A:2

29. Medicare tries to save with one fee billing. Wall Street J 1992: Sect. A-1.

30. Excess capacity. Report. Rocky Mountain Health Institute 1991: Dec. 7.

31. Schapera DV, et al. Intensive care: survival and expense of treating critically ill cancer patients. JAMA 1993:269:783–786.

32. Jacobs, Roseworthy. Crit Care Med 1990: November vol. 13:11.

33. Siro CA et al. An initial comparison of intensive care in Japan and the U.S. Crit Care Med 1992:20:1207.

34. Evans RE. Illusions of necessity: evading responsibility for choices in health care. J Health Polit Policy Law fall 1985:10:453.

35. Newhouse J. New York Times 1993:March 21, Sect F:5.

36. Cordes S. The economics of health services. Cooperative Extension Service, Pennsylvania State University.

37. Aaron HJ. Serious and unstable condition: financing America's health care. Brookings Institute 1991:p.86.

38. Division of Shortage Designation. Rockville, MD: Bureau of Health Care Delivery and Assistance, Public Health Service, 1992.

Article Review Form at end of book.

Tearsheet requests to Richard Lamm, Director, Center for Public Policy & Contemporary Issues, University of Denver, 2301 S Gaylord, Denver CO 80208; tel. 303-871-3400; fax 303-871-3066; e-mail <rlamm@aol.com>.

Why is it important to know the right questions to ask when deciding on a managed care plan?

Give Your HMO a Checkup

Ask these 15 questions to make sure you get maximum benefits from your health-insurance plan

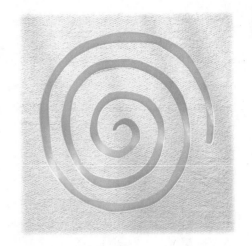

Flora Davis

Flora Davis, based in Princeton, N.J., wrote about short-term psychotherapies in the February issue.

Irene McDade of Medford, N.J., needed a life-saving operation last fall to remove a tumor on her spinal cord. Neurosurgeon Fred Epstein of the New York University Medical Center was expert in the surgery, but McDade's health maintenance organization insisted on sending the 30-year-old woman to a Philadelphia surgeon who had never performed the procedure. Because he and his hospital were part of the HMO's network, they would cost the health plan less. Epstein volunteered to perform the $12,000 operation for free if the HIP Health Plan would pay the hospital bills. It refused, caving in only after local newspapers headlined McDade's dilemma. The surgery went well, but three months later McDade's condition began to worsen. To recover, according to Epstein, she needed months of physical therapy, but the HMO was willing to cover only 60 days. At press time, the issue was still unresolved. "It's a disgrace," says Epstein.

Lately, troubling reports like this one seem to be cropping up everywhere. "What we have today is not managed care but managed *cost*," says Dr. Kimberly Yeager, chief of the Office of Women's Health, a California state agency. While employees recognize the need to cut health-care costs, anecdotal experiences—ranging from caps on mental-health visits to prolonged waits to see specialists—are fueling consumer protest over the quality of care given by HMOs.

Nevertheless, managed care is booming. Just four years ago, more than half of employer-insured Americans were covered by traditional, fee-for-service (FFS) plans, according to Foster Higgins, a New York employee-benefits consultancy. By 1995, however, only 29% fell into that category; 41% were enrolled in HMOs and 29% in preferred provider organizations (PPOs).

PPO and HMO plans regulate your choice of doctors, tests and treatments. Join a PPO and you'll be given a list of approved doctors and hospitals that have agreed to treat members at a discount; you can stay with a non-member doctor in many cases, but you'll have to pay more. An HMO

How Eight Big Plans Compare

HMO and region studied	NCQA-accredited?	Hospital stay after normal childbirth; after C-section	Drugs by formulary?	Gag rules?	How doctors are paid	Percentage of children immunized
AETNA Northern California	Has 3-year accreditation	Decided by physician	Yes	No	Some fee-for-sevice, mostly capitation with bonuses for meeting targets in providing preventive care. Capitated fee must cover tests, procedures and referrals.	70.8%
CIGNA HEALTHCARE Phoenix	3 years	Decided by physician	Yes	No	Salary, discounted fee-for-service. capitation. Bonuses for "quality care and cost-effective practices." Capitation covers routine care but not referrals.	91%
FHP California	3 years	Decided by physician	Yes	No, although contract asks physicians not to criticize the plan	Discounted fee-for-service, capitation. In some contracts: capitation must cover referrals, tests and procedures.	66.3%
HEALTH NET California	1 year	1.5 days; 2 days	Yes	No	Mostly capitated fees to medical groups, which may in turn capitate their physicians, though some pay salaries. Groups must pay for all medical procedures, specialists and tests, except for AIDS and transplant cases. Annual competition rewards best preventive care.	79.3%
HUMANA Kansas City	1 year	Decided by physician	Yes	No	Salary, capitation and discounted fee-for-service. Bonuses based on quality, member satisfaction and cost-effectiveness.	N/A
KAISER PERMANENTE Northern California	Pending	Decided by physcian	Yes	No	Salary.	85.8%*
PRUDENTIAL Houston	3 years	Decided by by physcian	Yes	No	Salary. Bonuses linked to productivity, cliet satisfaction and other factors.	73%*
US HEALTHCARE Pennsylvania	3 years	2 days; 4 days	No	No	Capitation. Amount based on quality of care and, to a lesser extent, cost reduction. Covers only physician's own services.	87.6%*

If your HMO isn't covered here, you many be able to learn more about it by calling the National Committee for Quality Assurance at 202-955-3515. The NCQA, an independent accrediting organization, has now examined approximately half the HMOs in the U.S. Those that meet all its standards get full, three-

is still more regulated. In the most common variety, a medical practice gets a prepaid, flat fee for providing all your medical care, from shots to surgery, either in a central facility or through a network of similarly affiliated doctors. If you go outside the plan, you must pay in full yourself.

But managed care definitely has benefits. The cost of premiums and routine doctor's visits is usually much lower, prescription drugs may be free and there's often a welcome emphasis on disease prevention and healthy living. While FFS medicine is fragmented, many HMOs are integrated—their doctors work together to treat patients—and tightly managed plans screen physicians before signing them up, monitor them and sometimes drop unpopular ones.

Furthermore, the massive databases accumulated by big HMOs can be used to learn which treatments really work. Eventually, studies of medical outcomes will also reveal which health plans are particularly good at managing asthma, for example, or treating breast cancer.

For now, though, surveys show that sicker people are more dissatisfied with managed plans.

Percentage of women aged 52 to 64 receiving mammograms	Percentage of women receiving Pap smears	Percentage of pregnant women receiving prenatal care in first trimester	Cap on annual mental-health outpatient visits	Covers "nonemergency" ER visits?	Co-pay higher for emergency care?
47.3%	54%	N/A	Determined by employer	Case-by-case	Determined by employer, waived if hospitalized
80%	82%*	86%*	45	No penalty for "reasonable judgement"	Co-pay is $25 to $50 (determined by employer), waived if hospitalized
60%	62.2%	61.6%	Determined by employer	If "member perceived situation as potentially life -threatening"	Co-pay is typically $35 to $40 higher
77.9%	81.3%	72.5%	Determined by employer	Case-by-case	Co-pay up to $25, waived if hospitalized
N/A	N/A	N/A	Determined by employer	No penalty for using "reasonable judgement"	Determined by employer, waived if hospitalized
73.5%*	76%*	90%*	20	Case-by-case	Determined by employer
71%*	71.3%*	75.6%*	20	If "a reasonable layperson would have considered it an emergency	Co-pay is $25 to $75 (determined by employer) waived if hospitalized
72%*	75.8%*	84.4%*	20 (a seriously ill member can swap up to 10 inpatient hospital days for increased outpatient visits)	Only for "sudden severe symptoms requiring immediate care"	Determined by employer

year accreditation; those with room for improvement get one-year or partial approval; about 12% flunk. *Percentage derived from a new, stricter scoring system devised by the NCQA. Not all plans have yet adopted this system.

"Managed care can be terrific if you don't get [really] sick," says John Canham-Clyne, research director at Congress Watch, a division of the national advocacy group Public Citizen. "But once you begin to need access to a lot of services, the problems crop up."

When choosing health insurance, consumers and companies need to consider more than the cost. Foster Higgins estimates that 48% of large firms offer employees at their biggest work sites a choice of plans. Here are 15 questions you should ask before making a decision.

1. What incentives does the plan offer physicians for cutting costs? Insurers use incentives to keep costs down. The primary one is capitation: Providers are paid so much for each enrollee. The fee is the same whether the individual never gets sick or is chronically ill. Theoretically, that means the provider has an incentive to keep its members well so that illnesses don't get out of hand and require expensive treatment. In practice, however, capitation can also be an incentive to withhold costly treatment.

In older HMOs—such as Kaiser Permanente, which has 6.8 million members in 16 states—

doctors are on salary. Despite capitation, they don't run any financial risk themselves if they prescribe costly care for patients. Newer HMOs, by contrast, tend to pay physicians flat, capitated fees, so a doctor with a number of very sick patients could lose money caring for them. "You don't want the doctors who make decisions about your health to have their income directly affected by what they decide," says Peter Lee of the HMO Consumer Protection Project at the Center for Health Care Rights in Los Angeles.

Some insurers shift even more of the financial risk of capitation onto primary-care physicians. They pay the doctors flat fees for treating plan members, and the physicians are also required to pick up the tab if they order tests or send a patient to a specialist. This can produce a dangerous conflict of interest, says Mark Hiepler, a California attorney and patient advocate. In a celebrated case, Hiepler represented the Agoura, Calif., family of Joyce Ching, who died of colon cancer at 35 after her physicians failed to refer her to a specialist. The Chings sued the doctors, arguing in part that their financial arrangement with Met Life had encouraged them to put their income ahead of her health. The physicians received a capitated fee of about $28 a month for her care; if they had referred her to a specialist, done outside testing or hospitalized her, they would have had to pay the first $5,000 of those costs. Last November, a jury awarded the Ching family nearly $3 million. (Because of limits set by the state, the family eventually received $700,000.)

Some health experts contend, however, that not all managed-care incentives are as bad as they sound. Health economist Robert H. Miller of the University of California at San Francisco says that it generally makes little difference to a physician's income if a few patients need expensive treatments, since the doctor has many others who need little care and whose fees are paid anyway. Many physicians also belong to large medical groups that collectively assume the risks of capitation, so the financial hazard to any one member of the group is small. In addition, HMOs often present physicians with a bundle of incentives, including some designed to promote good medical care, such as a bonus if patients say they're satisfied. "There are many ways to put checks and balances into the system," Miller says. But Lee notes that in some plans, doctors can lose a lot by not controlling costs and gain only a little by providing good care.

2. What is the procedure if I need to have tests, see a specialist or be hospitalized? In a further effort to control costs, many health plans require patients to get approval from their primary-care doctor before seeing a specialist or having procedures done. In some plans, the doctor must check with a central office before giving a referral; others allow physicians to make such decisions freely, but may drop those who fail to keep costs down.

Many HMOs and PPOs and most FFS plans insist that doctors get approval before admitting patients to the hospital. The person giving the approval (often a nurse) goes by plan guidelines (you might ask to see these) and never actually sees the patient.

Some plans sign up very few specialists—one way to limit expensive care

3. What benefits does the plan offer? In particular, ask for details about coverage for childbirth, emergency care and psychotherapy— they're problem areas. In a controversial policy trend, many new mothers are forced to leave the hospital just 24 hours after childbirth because their insurance doesn't cover a longer stay. According to Carol Lockhart, an Arizona health-policy specialist, early discharge isn't necessarily a bad thing, provided there's good follow-up care, such as home visits by an experienced nurse. But some plans won't pay for this, and in some areas home care isn't available. Last year, a New Jersey couple left the hospital with their baby after 24 hours. The infant was fidgety and wouldn't eat, and because of a mix-up, the visiting nurse who was supposed to check on mother and child didn't come. The baby died of a massive infection when she was two days old. After this tragedy, New Jersey passed a law requiring insurers to pay for two days in the hospital after a vaginal delivery, four after a cesarean. Maryland, Massachusetts, New Mexico, New York and North Carolina have passed similar laws, and others are considering legislation.

Emergency-room care can be another problem—not getting the care itself (by law, the ER must screen and stabilize you) but getting your health plan to pay for it. That's true even of some fee-for-service plans. Jill Simon, 52, a Miami nurse, was rushed to the emergency room last year with tachycardia: Her heart was beating wildly, 180 to 200 times a minute, because of a congenital defect. For more than six months, her HMO refused to pay the $600 ER bill because she hadn't contacted her primary-care doctor first; the insurer also argued that her tachycardia wasn't an emergency. Simon knows her condition was life-threatening—she works in an ER—and finally convinced the plan to pay up. Arkansas, Maryland and Virginia have now passed laws requiring insurers to pay ER bills if a "reasonable layperson" would consider the situation a medical emergency.

Mental-health benefits are also being limited in new ways. If you're depressed, for example, your insurer may say you're not depressed enough for treatment to be medically necessary. Or your plan may agree to pay for medication but not for psychotherapy, and it may require your physician to prescribe less expensive antidepressants rather than newer drugs with fewer side effects. HMOs commonly cover 20 visits to a therapist; FFS plans often set a cap of $1,000. Some mental-health experts say these arbitrary limits do not provide sufficient care for everyone.

4. If I get sick away from home, will the plan pay for my medical care? Almost every insurer covers emergency treatment; in nonemergency cases, arrangements vary.

5. Will I see the same primary-care doctor every time? With some centralized HMOs, you always go to the same clinic, but you may see different doctors. If you do have an assigned physician, find out whether you can switch if you're not happy, and how.

6. How long will I generally have to wait to get an appointment with my primary-care doctor? Long waits are sometimes a problem. A 1994 study in the *Journal of*

the American Medical Association found that 37% of HMO enrollees were unhappy with long waits, compared with 18% in FFS plans. Ask if you can talk to the doctor by phone and reach him or her nights and weekends.

7. How long is the usual wait to see a specialist? Delays can be extensive since some plans sign up very few specialists—one way to limit expensive care. The Center for Health Care Rights wants state governments to set maximums of one day for urgent problems and two weeks for all other appointments except routine screenings.

8. Will I have to pay for prescription drugs if they're not in the formulary? Ninety-five percent of managed-care plans now ask their doctors to prescribe drugs using a formulary, a list of medications the plan can obtain at discounts. Sometimes the formulary is presented simply as a guideline, but often it's restrictive: If your physician prescribes a drug not on the list, you must pay the whole cost unless the plan agrees to the switch. If that's true of a plan you're considering, ask whether medications you regularly use are on its list.

Formularies are intended to steer doctors into using less expensive medications that work as well. Supposedly, the money saved enables the insurer to pay for prescriptions. But critics complain that in some plans, when medications in the formulary don't work, it takes weeks for a doctor to get permission to prescribe a drug not on the list.

Susan Horn, senior scientist at the Institute for Clinical Outcomes Research in Salt Lake City, analyzed the formularies of six HMOs. Some excluded three-quarters of the drugs available to treat certain conditions. Horn concluded that, ironically, "the more

you limit drugs, the more you spend" in some cases, because if the patient doesn't get the right medication immediately, more office visits and more prescriptions may follow.

Some formularies require doctors to prescribe generic drugs rather than more costly brand-name versions, yet generics don't always work as well. Horn's father-in-law has Parkinson's disease. When his health began to deteriorate recently, the family assumed it was the course of the disease—until someone mentioned to Horn that his new health plan had switched his medication to a generic. At her suggestion, he began taking the brand-name drug again and quickly improved.

Some health plans refuse to answer questions about their incentive system or formulary. Arizona recently passed a law that requires HMOs to tell prospective enrollees about both.

9. What is the grievance procedure, and how long does it take? Virtually all insurers have a grievance system so that patients can appeal the plan's decisions. However, these systems often work very slowly. In 22 states, you can take a complaint to a state agency. You can also sue, unless your plan required you to agree to binding arbitration when you signed up—rare on the East Coast but common out west. According to Mark Hiepler, arbitrators are usually big-business lawyers, less sympathetic to patients than a jury would be.

10. How many complaints against the plan, filed with the state, were upheld last year? What were they? If plan officers aren't willing to answer this question, contact the state agency that regulates health insurance.

11. Does the plan have a gag clause in its contracts with physicians? Aynah Askanas, legal counsel for the California Medical Association, reviews managed-care contracts for doctors. She says that perhaps one in five has a clause forbidding the physician to say anything negative about the plan. These HMOs argue that gag clauses are meant to encourage doctors to discuss their concerns with the plan, not with their patients, but New York neurologist Carolyn Martin asserts that doctors are silenced; if they disagree with an HMO's decision, they can't talk about it honestly with a patient. Because of negative media coverage, Askanas says, outright gag clauses are becoming less common.

12. Has the plan been accredited by the NCQA (the National Committee for Quality Assurance)? The NCQA, an independent, nonprofit investigative body, has now examined about half of all HMOs as part of its accreditation process. It considers 50 criteria, and one in eight plans fails. The findings are available free of charge; to order, call 202-955-3515 or check the group's Web site at www.ncqa.org.

13. How many of the plan's physicians are board-certified? If 85% or more of a plan's primary-care physicians are board-certified, that's considered pretty good; with specialists, you'd hope for more.

14. What percentage of doctors leave the plan every year? Four percent is about average for HMOs and PPOs. If the proportion is much higher than that, ask why.

15. May I see the results of a patient-satisfaction survey? If you don't like the answers to these questions, do you have any leverage? Yes, if you work through your employer. The competition for corporate business is increasingly fierce, and employers have begun to focus on high-quality health care. Last year, 30 big corporations, including AT&T, GTE and PepsiCo, formed the Foundation for Accountability to study how well HMOs perform. For our diagnosis of how eight of the largest regional plans stack up, consult the chart on pages 166-167.

 Article Review Form at end of book.

How has genetic information been used by insurers to discriminate against people?

Genetic Discrimination and Health Insurance: An urgent need for reform

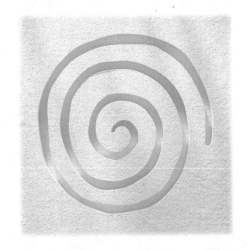

Kathy L. Hudson, Karen H. Rothenburg, Lori B. Andrews, Mary Jo Ellis Kahn, Francis S. Collins

The accelerated pace of gene discovery and molecular medicine portend a future in which information about a plethora of disease genes can be readily obtained. As at risk populations are identified, research can be done to determine effective prevention and treatment strategies that will lower the personal, social, and perhaps the financial costs of disease in the future. We all carry genes that predispose to common illnesses. In many circumstances knowing this information can be beneficial, as it allows individualized strategies to be designed to reduce the risk of illness. But, as knowledge about the genetic basis of common disorders grows, so does the poten-

tial for discrimination in health insurance coverage for an ever increasing number of Americans.

The use of genetic information to exclude high-risk people from health care by denying coverage or charging prohibitive rates will limit or nullify the anticipated benefits of genetic research. In addition to the real and potentially devastating consequences of being denied health insurance, the fear of discrimination has other undesirable effects. People may be unwilling to participate in research and to share information about their genetic status with their health care providers or family members because of concern about misuse of this information. As genetic research progresses, and preventive and treatment strategies are developed, it will be increasingly important that discrimination and the fear of

discrimination not be a roadblock to reaping the benefits. To address these issues, the National Institutes of Health-Department of Energy (NIH-DOE) Working Group on Ethical, Legal, and Social Implications (ELSI) of the Human Genome Project and the National Action Plan on Breast Cancer have jointly developed a series of recommendations for state and federal policymakers which are presented below.

In the past, genetic information has been used by insurers to discriminate against people. In the early 1970s, some insurance companies denied coverage and charged higher rates to African Americans who were carriers of the gene for sickle cell anemia (1). Contemporary studies have documented cases of genetic discrimination against people who are healthy themselves but who have a gene that predisposes them or their children to a later illness such as Huntington's disease (2). In a recent survey of people with a known genetic condition in the family, 22% indicated that they had been refused health insurance coverage because of their genetic status, whether they were sick or not (3).

As a case example, Paul (not his real name) is a healthy, active 4-year-old, but he has been twice denied health insurance. Paul's mother died in her sleep of sudden cardiac arrest when Paul was only 5 months old. Paul's maternal uncle also died of sudden cardiac arrest when he was in his twenties. After these sudden and unexpected deaths, Paul's family began a hunt to discover the cause. Their search finally led to a research geneticist who was able to determine that several family members, including Paul and his mother, carried an alteration in a gene on chromosome 7. This gene is one of several genes that causes the long QT syndrome, so-called because of the distinctive diagnostic pattern on an electrocardiogram.

Several years ago, Paul's father, Bob, lost his job and with it the group policy that provided health insurance coverage for Paul and him. Paul's father has repeatedly applied for a family health insurance policy with a major insurance company. The company agreed to cover Bob but refused to issue a family policy that would cover Paul because he has inherited the altered gene for the long QT syndrome from his mother.

The story of Jackie and Emma further illustrates the social, ethical, and legal dilemmas presented by the revelation of genetic information. Sisters Jackie and Emma, along with many other members of their family, have been tested as part of a research protocol for alterations in the gene, BRCA1, that confers hereditary susceptibility to breast and ovarian cancer. Both were offered an opportunity to learn the results of their genetic tests and both accepted. They each learned they carry an altered form of the gene, putting them at increased risk for breast and ovarian cancer.

After finding out the results of her genetic test, Emma had a mammogram that showed a very small lesion in her breast. A subsequent biopsy revealed carcinoma, and Emma decided to proceed with a bilateral mastectomy because of the substantial risk of cancer arising in the opposite breast. Her lymph nodes were negative for cancer, so her prognosis for cure is very good.

Emma's sister Jackie also tested positive for the same alteration in the BRCA1 gene, though no cancer was detected. Although the benefit of prophylactic mastectomy in reducing the risk for breast cancer is not yet known, she decided to have a bilateral prophylactic mastectomy. Emma and Jackie feel strongly that they have benefited from knowing this genetic information but are fearful that it will be used against them and their family by insurers and employers. They both keep their genetic status secret and are so fearful of losing their health insurance that they used assumed names when sharing their story at a recent workshop on genetic discrimination (4).

Emma and Jackie's story is not unique. An estimated 1 in 500 women carry a mutation in the BRCA1 gene that may confer as much as an 85% chance of breast cancer and a 50% chance of ovarian cancer (5). Although substantial uncertainty exists about the relative value of the available options (surgery compared with intensive surveillance) for a woman with a BRCA1 mutation, it is likely that ultimately this information will be medically useful.

Health Insurance in the United States

Because of high costs, insurance is essentially required to have access to health care in the United States. Over 40 mil-lion people in the United States are uninsured (6). Group insurance, individual insurance, self-insurance, and publicly financed insurance (for example, Medicare and Medicaid) are the principal forms of health insurance in the United States for the 240 million Americans with coverage. Most people get their health insurance through their employer.

Many employers provide health insurance coverage through self-funded plans in which the employer, either directly or through a third party, provides health insurance coverage. For individuals and small groups, insurance providers use medical history as well as individual risk factors, such as smoking, to determine whether to provide coverage and under what terms. This is known as underwriting. Insurers argue that underwriting is essential in a voluntary market to prevent "adverse selection," in which individuals elect not to purchase insurance until they are already ill or anticipate a future need for health care. Insurers fear that individuals will remain uninsured until, for example, they receive a genetic test indicating a predisposition to some disease such as breast or colon cancer.

In the absence of the ability to detect hereditary susceptibility to disease, the costs of medical treatment have been absorbed under the current health insurance system of shared risk and shared costs. Today, our understanding of the relation between a misspelling in a gene and future health is still incomplete, thus limiting the ability of insurers to incorporate genetic risks into actuarial calculations on a large scale. As genetic research enhances the ability to predict individuals' future risk of diseases, many Americans may become uninsurable on the basis of genetic information.

State and Federal Initiatives

A recent survey has shown that a number of states have enacted laws to protect individuals from being denied health insurance on the basis of genetic information (Fig. 1) (7). (Figure 1 omitted) The first laws addressing genetic discrimination were quite limited in scope and focused exclusively on discrimination against people with a single genetic trait such as sickle cell trait (8). Since the Human Genome Project was launched in 1990, eight states have enacted some form of protection against genetic discrimination in health insurance. The recently enacted state laws are not limited to a specific genetic trait but apply potentially to an unlimited number of genetic conditions. These state laws prohibit insurers from denying coverage on the basis of genetic test results, and prohibit the use of this information to establish premiums, charge differential rates, or limit benefits. A few of these states, including Oregon and California, integrate protection against discrimination

in insurance practices with privacy protections that prohibit insurers from requesting genetic information and from disclosing genetic information without authorization.

Two factors limit the protection against discrimination afforded by current state laws. First, the federal Employee Retirement Income Security Act exempts self-funded plans from state insurance laws. Nationwide, over one-third of the nonelderly insured population obtains health insurance coverage through a self-funded plan. Second, nearly all of the state laws focus narrowly on genetic tests, rather than more broadly on genetic information generated by family history, physical examination, or the medical record (7). Limiting the scope of protection to results of genetic tests means that insurers are only prohibited from using the results of a chemical test of DNA, or in some cases, the protein product of a gene. But insurers can use other phenotypic indicators, patterns of inheritance of genetic characteristic, or even requests for genetic testing as the basis of discrimination. Meaningful protection against genetic discrimination requires that insurers be prohibited from using all information about genes, gene products, or inherited characteristics to deny or limit health insurance coverage.

No federal laws are currently in place to prohibit genetic discrimination in health insurance (9). The Clinton Administration's proposal to reform the health care system and provide health insurance for all Americans did prohibit limited access or coverage on the basis of "existing medical conditions or genetic predisposition to medical conditions" (10). Congressional efforts to reform the health care system in 1995

have been much more modest and are targeted at guaranteeing access, portability, and renewability of coverage and at leveling the playing field in the insurance market so that the same rules apply to insured and self-funded plans. Recent federal health insurance reform proposals attempt to guarantee the availability of health care by prohibiting insurers from denying coverage on the basis of health status, medical condition, claims experience, or medical history of a participant. Most of the proposals permit exclusions for pre-existing conditions, but these are time limited.

It is not clear if the current health insurance reform proposals would prohibit insurers from denying coverage on the basis of genetic information. Genetic information is distinct from other types of medical information because it provides information about an individual's predisposition to future disease. In addition, genetic information can provide clues to the future health risks for an individual's family members. If enacted, current health reform proposals would prohibit denying insurance to those currently suffering from disease or with a past history of disease. But these proposals may not protect people like Paul, who are healthy but have a genetic predisposition to disease, from being refused insurance coverage. Current proposals also may fail to protect couples who, although healthy themselves, carry the gene for a recessive disorder such as cystic fibrosis that might affect their children or future children.

Recommendations

Planners of the Human Genome Project recognized from the beginning that maximizing the medical benefits of genome research would require a social environment in which health care consumers were protected from discrimination and stigmatization based on their genetic make-up. Genome programs at both the DOE and the National Center for Human Genome Research, a component of NIH, have each set aside a portion of their research budget to anticipate, analyze, and address the ELSI of new advances in human genetics. The original planners also created the NIH-DOE ELSI Working Group, which has a broad and diverse membership including genome scientists; medical geneticists; experts in law, ethics, and philosophy; and consumers, to explore and propose options for the development of sound professional and public policies related to human genome research and its applications. The ELSI Working Group has long been involved in discussions about the fair use of genetic information. In a 1993 report, "Genetic Information and Health Insurance" (11), the ELSI Working Group recommended a return to the risk-spreading goal of insurance. The Working Group suggested that individuals be given access to health care insurance irrespective of information, including genetic information about their past, current, or future health status. Because denial of insurance coverage for a costly disease such as breast cancer may prove to be a death sentence for many women, the National Action Plan on Breast Cancer (NAPBC), a public-private partnership designed to eradicate breast cancer as a threat to the lives of American women, has identified genetic discrimination in health insurance as a high priority (12).

Building on their shared concerns, the NAPBC (13) and the ELSI Working Group (14) recently cosponsored a workshop on genetic discrimination and health insurance (4). Scientists, representatives from the insurance industry, and members of the ELSI Working Group and the NAPBC participated in the 1-day session. On the basis of the information presented at the workshop, the ELSI Working Group and the NAPBC developed the following recommendations and definitions for state and federal policymakers to protect against genetic discrimination.

1) Insurance providers should be prohibited from using genetic information, or an individual's request for genetic services, to deny or limit any coverage or establish eligibility, continuation, enrollment, or contribution requirements.

2) Insurance providers should be prohibited from establishing differential rates or premium payments based on genetic information or an individual's request for genetic services.

3) Insurance providers should be prohibited from requesting or requiring collection or disclosure of genetic information.

4) Insurance providers and other holders of genetic information should be prohibited from releasing genetic information without prior written authorization of the individual. Written authorization should be required for each disclosure and include to whom the disclosure would be made.

The definitions are as follows. Genetic information is information about genes, gene products, or inherited characteristics that may derive from the individual or a family member. Insurance provider means an insurance company, employer, or any other entity providing a plan of health insurance or health benefits including group and individual health plans whether fully insured or self-funded.

These recommendations have been endorsed by the National Advisory Council for Human Genome Research (NACHGR) (15). The NACHGR stresses the positive value of genetic information for improving the medical care of individual patients and the need to ensure the freedom of patients and their health care providers to use genetic information for patient care. The NACHGR views the elimination of the use genetic information to discriminate against individuals in their access to health insurance as a critical step toward these goals.

The ability to obtain sensitive genetic information about individuals, families, and even populations raises profound and troubling questions about who will have access to this information and how will it be used. The recommendations presented here for state and federal policy-makers are intended to help ensure that our current social, economic, and health care policies keep pace with both the opportunities and challenges that the new genetics present for understanding the causes of disease and developing new treatment and preventive strategies.

References and Notes

1. L. Andrews, Medical Genetics: A Legal Frontier (American Bar Foundation, Chicago, IL, 1987).
2. P. R. Billings et al., Am. J. Hum. Genet. 50, 476 (1992).

3. E. V. Lapham (Georgetown University) and J. O. Weiss, The Alliance of Genetic Support Groups, Human Genome Model Project, preliminary results of a survey of persons with a genetic disorder in the family.

4. "Genetic discrimination and health insurance: A case study on breast cancer," Bethesda, MD, 11 July 1995, workshop sponsored by the National Action Plan on Breast Cancer (NAPBC) and the NIHDOE Working Group on the Ethical, Legal, and Social Implications of Human Genome Research.

5. D. F. Easton et al., Am. J. Hum. Genet. 52, 678 (1993); D. Ford et al., Lancet 343, 692 (1994).

6. Employee Benefit Research Institute Special Report SR-28, issue brief number 158, February 1995.

7. K. H. Rothenberg, J. Law Med. Ethics, in press.

8. North Carolina, NC ST: 58-65-70 (1975), Florida, FL ST: 626.9707 (1978), Alabama, AL ST: 27-5-13 (1982). In 1987, Maryland passed a law, Art. 48A, 223(b)(4), prohibiting health insurers from discrimination in rates based on genetic traits unless there was "actuarial justification."

9. In March 1995, the U. S. Equal Employment Opportunity Commission (EEOC) released official guidance on the definition of the term "disability." The EEOC's guidance clarifies that protection under the Americans with Disabilities Act (ADA) extends to individuals who are discriminated against in employment decisions solely on the basis of genetic information about an individual. For example, an employer who makes an adverse employment decision on the basis of an individual's genetic predisposition to disease, whether because of concerns about insurance costs, productivity, or attendance, is in violation of the ADA because that employer is regarding the individual as disabled. Issuance of the EEOC's guidance is precedent setting; it is the first broad federal protection against the unfair use of genetic information.

10. Health Security Act, Section 7516, S. 1757/HR 3600.

11. "Genetic information and health insurance: Report of the task force on genetic information and insurance" (NIH-DOE Working Group on the Ethical, Legal, and Social Implication of Human Genome Research, 10 May 1993).

12. The NAPBC has as its mission to reduce the morbidity and mortality from breast cancer and to prevent the disease. Specific goals include the following: (i) to promote a national effort to establish and address priority issues related to breast cancer etiology, early detection, treatment, and prevention; (ii) to promote and foster communication, collaboration, and cooperation among diverse public and private partners; and (iii) to develop strategies, actions, and policies to improve breast cancer awareness, services, and research.

13. NAPBC steering committee: Susan J. Blumenthal (co-chair), Zora Kramer Brown, Doris Browne, Anna K. Chacko, Francis S. Collins, Nancy W. Connell, Kay Dickersin, Arlyne Draper, Nancy Evans, Harmon Eyre, Leslie Ford, Janyce N. Hedetniemi, Mary Jo Ellis Kahn, Amy S. Langer, Susan M. Love, Alan Rabson, Jane Reese-Coulbourne, Irene M. Rich, Barbara K. Rimer, Susan Sieber, Edward Sondik, and Frances M. Visco (co-chair). NAPBC hereditary susceptibility working group: Kathleen A. Calzone, Francis S. Collins (co-chair), Sherman Elias, Linda Finney, Judy E. Garber, Ruthann M. Giusti, Jay R. Harris, Joseph K. Hurd Jr., Mary Jo Ellis Kahn (co-chair), Mary-Claire King, Caryn Lerman, Mary Jane Massie, Paul G. McDonough, Patricia D. Murphy, Phillip D. Noguchi, Barbara K. Rimer, Karen H. Rothenberg, Karen K. Steinberg, and Jill Stopfer.

14. ELSI working group: Betsy Anderson, Lori Andrews (chair), James Bowman (dissenting), David Cox, Troy Duster, (vice chair), Rebecca Eisenberg, Beth Fine, Neil Holtzman, Philip Kitcher, Joseph McInerney, Jeffrey Murray, Dorothy Nelkin, Rayna Rapp, Marsha Saxton, and Nancy Wexler.

15. NCHGR council members: Anita Allen, Lennette J. Benjamin; David Botstein, R. Daniel Camerini-Otero (dissents with recommendation 3), Ellen W. Clayton, Troy Duster, Leroy E. Hood, David E. Housman, Richard M. Myers, Rodney Rothstein, Diane C. Smith, Lloyd M. Smith, M. Anne Spence, Shirley M. Tilgham, and David Valle.

K. L. Hudson is assistant director of Policy Coordination, National Center for Human Genome Research, National Institutes of Health (NIH). K. H. Rothenberg is Marjorie Cook Professor of Law and director of the Law and Health Care Program, University of Maryland School of Law, and member of the National Action Plan on Breast Cancer (NAPBC). L. B. Andrews is chair of the NIH Department of Energy Working Group on Ethical, Legal, and Social Implications and professor at Chicago-Kent College of Law. M. J. Ellis Kahn represents the Virginia Breast Cancer Foundation and the National Breast Cancer Coalition and is co-chair of the Hereditary Susceptibility Working Group, NAPBC. F. S. Collins is director of the National Center for Human Genome Research, NIH, and co-chair of the Hereditary Susceptibility Working Group, NAPBC.

 Article Review Form at end of book.

How can patients investigate their doctors?

Checking Up on Your Doctor

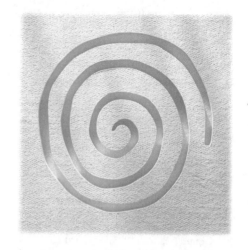

Stephanie Wood

Stephanie Wood is a Blauvelt, NY, writer who checked up on her family practitioner after reporting this story.

Two small rooms in a drab state office building in downtown Boston are an unlikely setting for a revolution in health care. Yet the phones haven't stopped ringing here since last November, when Massachusetts became the first state in the country to provide citizens with easy access to the disciplinary and malpractice payment records of its 27,000 actively licensed physicians.

Four days into the new program, the volume of calls was so heavy that organizers had to add extra phone lines. Today staffers average 600 to 700 calls per day. On the other end of the line are citizens taking advantage of a unique opportunity to investigate their doctors' backgrounds and safety records. Some are managed-care newcomers hoping to choose a physician with a clean bill of health; others are checking up on a doctor they're suspicious of. Malpractice lawyers call. So do doctors seeking information about their peers. Like consumers, they want access to data on hospital discipline, malpractice payments, legal settlements and criminal convictions—information that until very recently was out of reach.

The Secrets Doctors Keep

M.D.'s on drugs. Botched surgeries. Rapes under anesthesia. Medical horror stories have become as commonplace as the weather report on the evening news. But even more frightening is the fact that more than two-thirds of the nation's 13,000-plus questionable doctors—those disciplined by state and federal agencies—still practice freely, according to the Public Citizen's Health Research Group (PCHRG), a Washington nonprofit organization that fights for health consumers. This is particularly threatening to women, who see physicians more than men do and who change doctors more often. The Massachusetts program is a glimmer of hope for the nation's 400,000 annual victims of medical negligence. "For too long, consumers have been denied information about the professionals they trust most," says PCHRG director Sidney Wolfe, M.D.

Indeed, the medical community has made it nearly impossible to investigate a doctor's record. In most states the only way is to call the licensing board. (Some states refer to it as the Board of Registration, others the Department of Professional Regulation. If in doubt, contact the secretary of state's office in your state capitol.) The board will reveal whether or not a doctor has a license to practice. In some states, you may also learn the outcome of any litigation brought against the doctor. But rarely will you be informed of pending lawsuits or disciplinary action taken by a state or hospital medical board.

Nor will you learn the names of doctors like the one who treated Leslie Tiller, 46, of Atlanta. Tiller saw an endocrinologist after becoming convinced that her weight gain, high blood pressure and other syptoms were caused by Cushing's disease, the result of a pituitary gland tumor. But when she asked the doctor to test for Cushing's, he dismissed her request. Instead he tested her for a

> Are you putting your health in good hands? Medicine's latest breakthrough turns out to be the new, supersleuth ways you can investigate your physician's vital statistics

thyroid problem and prescribed medication.

Three years and thousands of dollars later, Tiller had ballooned to 350 pounds, developed facial hair, stopped menstruating and had a beet-red face and a body temperature so high she didn't need a coat in the winter. Terrified, she consulted a different endocrinologist, who found her condition to be a classic case of Cushing's disease.

After surviving a high-risk surgery, Tiller successfully sued the endocrinologist who had failed to diagnose her in spite of more than 20 examinations and repeated requests for tests for Cushing's. She later heard that he suffered from attention deficit disorder, which no doubt hampered his ability to make sense of her symptoms. But other patients will never be privy to this. "As part of the legal settlement, I had to agree never to give out his name," says Tiller. "He's still practicing, and it really bothers me that other people can go to him and not know."

Why all the secrecy? "Doctors don't trust the public to understand that being sued is not necessarily a sign of incompetence," explains Michael Donio, spokesman for the People's Medical Society, a consumer advocacy group in Allentown, PA. "But we all know that people often sue when the results of a treatment aren't what they hoped for."

In addition, specialists who deal with particularly sensitive conditions seem to invite lawsuits. "Obstetrician/gynecologists and neurosurgeons pretty much expect to get sued," notes Timothy McCall, M.D., a Cambridge, MA, internist and author of *Examining Your Doctor: A Patient's Guide to Avoiding Harmful Medical Care.* "Other doctors are

vulnerable because they take on high-risk cases."

More than two-thirds of physicians disciplined by state or federal agencies still practice freely

Putting such physicians under a malpractice microscope would indeed seem unfair. But while experts like Dr. McCall feel that malpractice lawsuits don't always correlate closely with incompetence, a *pattern* of being sued is something a patient should have the right to know about.

The issue of whether the public needs to know about malpractice suits is at the heart of the debate over government-controlled National Practitioner Data Bank. Established in the '80s, it contains legal and disciplinary information about every physician in the United States, but only the medical community has access to it. The American Medical Association has lobbied to keep the data bank closed to consumers. "It would be inflammatory to provide liability information to the public without context," says Dan Maier, spokesman for the AMA.

Dr. Wolfe favors letting the public decide. It was in protest to the secrecy surrounding the National Practitioner Data Bank that PCHRG began publishing *Questionable Doctors* in 1990. The

most recent directory contains the names of 13,012 physicians disciplined by the state or federal government (see "AH Address Book," page 102*).

The Disciplinary Dilemma

While malpractice isn't always a reliable basis for drawing conclusions, even many physicians agree

Four Signs of Malpractice

Most victims of negligent medical care never take legal action. Consider these red flags when deciding whether you have a justifiable complaint:

• Your hospital stay or recuperation lasts much longer than you were told it would.

• Your physician has to bring in another doctor during a procedure (an indication that a repair may need to be made).

• You suffer a totally unexpected adverse result from a treatment or procedure.

• Your physician won't give you a reasonable explanation for adverse consequences or is reluctant to talk about them.

If your thinking about suing, you can find an attorney through your local bar association. Most will screen your case for free. Even if you decide not to pursue a case, report the doctor to your state medical board.

What "Board-Certified" Really Means

Go into any physician's office and you'll see an impressive array of certificates hanging on the wall. But which credentials signal quality? According to the American Board of Medical Specialties, the official certifying organization located in Chicago, 70% to 75% of the nation's doctors are board-certified in one or more of 24 approved specialties. There are, however, another 125 unofficial organizations that provide certification. Some require rigorous training, but others don't even demand a medical degree. On top of that, many doctors claim credentials

without really having them. Others say they're "board-eligible," meaning they completed the course work but never took the exam. The only way you can know for sure is to check with the ABMS at 800-776-2378.

Certification is voluntary, and many competent physicians practice without it. Still, most hospitals and many managed-care networks require it. And since any M.D. can call herself a specialist, it is often the only way to prove that a physician has the expertise she claims.

*Not included in this publication.

that disciplinary action is. "If a doctor's peers on a medical board discipline him, that's significant," says Nicholas Soldo, M.D., of Phoenix, past chairman of the Arizona State Medical Board. When a doctor's license is suspended or revoked, the Federation of State Medical Boards is informed; licensing records are supposed to be checked before the physician can practice in another state.

The trouble is, unlicensed doctors still slip through the cracks. When Laura Link, 30, of Jacksonville, FL, had a back injury, she decided to try a new clinic. All went well until one day when she stopped by and the physician who had treated her wasn't in. Another doctor on staff offered to perform an exam. Moments later, she was horrified to feel his hands grope her breasts. As she knocked them away, a nurse walked in and the physician fled the room.

Hours later, Link and her husband confronted the clinic owner, who countered that she had misinterpreted the incident. Only then did she call the Florida Department of Professional Regulation. She was shocked to learn that neither of the doctors she had dealt with was currently licensed; the one who had molested her was supposed to be retired, and the other had been suspended because of pending complaints.

Link's case was unusual in that the doctor had already been suspended. Of the 25,069 disciplinary actions taken against physicians named in *Questionable Doctors*, only 26.5% led to the removal, even temporarily, of a doctor's license. Perhaps one reason so many dangerous doctors escape detection is that their conduct is reviewed by other doctors.

Says Jim Perdue, a medical malpractice attorney in Houston, "Medicine has a good old boys' network like every other business."

New Avenues to Access

So let's say you want to check up on a physician's record. Where should you begin? One of the best places is the AMA's Internet service called Physician Select, which includes the names and credentials of more than 650,000 doctors (see "AH Address Book," below*). The site doesn't provide legal or disciplinary information, but the organization has eliminated the names of those with licensing problems, those convicted of felonies, and anyone who has been kicked out of the AMA. "All the doctors in Physician Select are professionals we would feel comfortable with, and consumers can too," says Maier. The AMA's *American Medical Directory*, which contains basically the same information—albeit less current—is available in most libraries.

You should also consider taking advantage of the Medi-Net (see "AH Address Book"): This service provides background on a doctor's age, education, licensing and board certification and detailed explanations of disciplinary action. Medi-Net's database has over 20,000 names of disciplined physicians and is updated daily.

If you don't obtain a Medi-Net report, you can call the American Board of Medical Specialties certification line in Atlanta to determine if the doctor is board-certified in her specialty (see "What 'Board-Certified' Really Means," page 64*, for details). Certification is optional, but "the odds are better that a board-certified physician will be competent," notes Dr. McCall.

*Not included in this publication.

You may want to dig deeper if you want to feel especially secure—or you have reason to suspect that something is amiss. Visit the courthouse in the county where the physician practices or resides. Ask for the plaintiff-defendant tables and scan them for the physician's name. Dr. Soldo notes, "In most states, medical boards can't discuss a case unless it's first posted in a public agenda." You can get the agenda by calling the state medical board office, then either attend the hearing in person or request a copy of the minutes.

Good-Sense Guidelines

Of course a clean record is no guarantee that you'll be happy with a physician. Plenty of other factors come into play: Doctors should be willing to listen to your viewpoint and treat you with respect. They should use drugs sparingly and offer the least expensive option whenever possible. The amount of time a doctor spends with you is also important. "An office visit shouldn't feel like an Indy 500 pit stop," notes Dr. McCall.

Many managed care organizations promote the idea that their physicians are carefully selected, but you can't simply cede power to an insurance company or even a licensing board. "Doctors guilty of negligence or sexual misconduct may ultimately lose their licenses," says Dr. McCall. "But when it comes to outdated procedures and lousy communication, the consumer is the final check. By doing your homework, you can weed out bad doctors and keep the good ones on their toes."

 Article Review Form at end of book.

What criteria could you use to judge the value of an alternative health product, service, or discipline?

Whatever Works

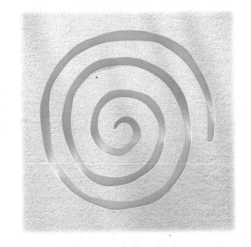

Emily Friedman

Is a healthcare writer, lecturer, and policy analyst based in Chicago. She is adjunct assistant professor at Boston University School of Public Health. Her anthology, The Right Thing: Ten Years of Ethics Columns from the Healthcare Forum Journal, *was published by Jossey-Bass in April.*

I guess you could say that I was there at the new beginning.

I wasn't there at the real beginning; that was thousands of years ago, in places I have never been. And in some of those places, that beginning became an unbroken path of healing—from Asia to Hawaii, from the Navajo lands to the inner city. That path was the way of alternative healthcare. Of course, those healers did not consider themselves alternative to anything; for these cultures, their ways of healing were the mainstream.

But the predominant healthcare culture in the United States became what we called "Western" (actually, European) medicine, which was rooted in institutional, largely secular or Christian, acute, procedure- and technology- and pharmaceutical-based care. Other approaches fell by the wayside.

Native American and African-American healing were condemned as quackery. The heyday of public health nursing was at the turn of the century; the vision of care for the chronically and incurably ill as a natural part of health services faded before this century was born. Prevention, which has always had a hard time of it, didn't have a chance.

There were those who lived in the mainstream culture but who believed in wheat germ and *tai chi* and spiritual approaches to personal health, but they were generally considered weirdos.

And Then Came the Sixties

As regular readers of this column know, I was a Berkeley hippie. And in the course of that, I became infatuated with the health foods, the non-peanut nut butters, yoga, meditation, and everything else that became acceptable once many of us had rejected the Prime Directive: Do as Your Parents Did.

It helped, of course, that this occurred in California, the home of avocado sorbet, where in many places, it was herbs and not antibiotics that have long been seen as the magic bullet against disease—and where ex-hippie (or perpetual hippie) parents in some northern counties don't believe in immunizing their children against infectious disease because immunization is a tool of the Establishment.

It also helped that I was in my late teens, and as a result was observing and experiencing all kinds of things. I could just as easily have observed and experienced them in Toledo, had I been there. Nonetheless, I observed, I experienced, and I learned. And as a result, there are things that I take as gospel that do not fit entirely into traditional medical mode. I learned how to combat certain diseases and conditions in ways that have nothing to do with traditional medicine or pharmacology:

Grapefruit—particularly its juice—strengthens the immune system. A friend of mine who had a liver transplant a couple of years ago told me she had to give away her Christmas present from me: a case of grapefruit. "Bolstering my immune system is not what we're trying to accomplish here," she explained. Her physician concurred.

From Emily Friedman, "Whatever Works" in *Healthcare Forum Journal*, November/December 1996, 39(6), pp. 10-13. Reprinted by permission of Healthcare Forum.

Cranberry juice is great for clearing up women's urinary tract infections. A freshly picked aloe leaf is a good poultice for a burn. My friends who drink herbal tea claim that some forms of it are the best sleeping potions ever created. I think even regular tea helps to ameliorate a host of ailments. Many of us have been aided during rough times by the simple peace of meditation. And quite a few of us believe that consistent exercise—even mild exercise—is as effective an antidepressant as there is.

And, although I haven't used the stuff in almost 30 years, there is certainly a committed community of people who believe that cannabis—marijuana—is a terrific treatment for a number of conditions ranging from glaucoma to the side effects of traditional therapies for AIDS and cancer. Indeed, this past summer in San Francisco, there were public protests when California state law enforcement authorities raided a cannabis buying club whose leaders claimed (perhaps truthfully, perhaps not) that they only supplied the drug to people in medical need. There is an initiative on the November ballot in that state that would legalize the use of marijuana for medical purposes, however those may be defined.

Personally (not that you asked), I oppose the legalization of marijuana, at least in a smokeable form; I think it's very potent, the quality and purity of every batch varies, and smoking it is bad for your lungs. Maybe I would change my mind if a consistently reliable form of it were developed; but even then, I would only support its use for strictly medical purposes—and we all know widespread abuse would occur. That issue aside, my belief in certain nonpharmaceutical ap-

proaches to care are not an article of faith or dogma for me; in my personal experience, they have worked. So, I might add, have aspirin and antibiotics.

A Visceral Distrust

So I was there when what is now called "alternative healing" had its renaissance in the Sixties. And I am amused—and impressed—by the fact that what motivated us then is a powerful motivation for the alternative healing movement today; an almost visceral dislike and distrust of the Establishment. If it comes from Authority, it must be bad; if it is part of the rebellion, it must be good. Such were, and are, the labels.

I was offered accidental proof of this while I was writing this column. I was putting some thoughts together on my faithful laptop computer while riding on an airplane. The woman seated next to me was, unbeknownst to me, watching me write. She interrupted me and explained that she was eavesdropping (eaves-watching?), and that she was an alternative healer involved in therapeutic touch and related disciplines. She told me of several successes, including one involving her son, and then began to tell me about conspiracies against alternative approaches. The one that troubled me the most was the story she told of a man in California who, in the Fifties, developed an herbal cure for cancer that was cheap and easy to produce. She insisted that the American Medical Association and pharmaceutical interests had quashed its development.

Now, many people have had problems, even severe conflicts, with organized medicine, but it is beyond my comprehension that physicians, faced with the possi-

bility of a cure for cancer, would deep-six it. Furthermore, why would the pharmaceutical manufacturers see to it that the "cure" disappeared? Why not seize control of it and patent it instead?

Her deep belief that this had actually happened reminded me of a "B.C." cartoon I saw once. A caveman runs up to another caveman and says, "I've found it! A cure for cancer! It's a plentiful weed!" The other caveman says, "Not so fast; how do we turn it into a drug we can patent?"

I do not believe in the quashed cancer cure; it sounds to me like one of the standard body of urban folk tales that also includes the perpetual light bulb and the indestructible panty hose whose development was prohibited by evil light bulb and panty hose manufacturers.

Nonetheless, I, like many other people, am tired of everything being medicalized, usually for profit: No treatment or therapy or answer for a condition could possibly be cheap or free or easy, because there is money to be made, so if it can't be patented, copyrighted, controlled, and charged for, it couldn't possibly work. And if people can't afford the price of the solutions we patent and copyright and control, well, heck with them if they can't take a joke—even if the joke is that they will die.

No More "Me Doctor, You Patient"

There are other motivations for the pursuit of alternative approaches besides anti-Establishment thinking and the search for profits. One is patient empowerment, a natural reaction to the uncomfortable healthcare tradition of "Me doctor, you patient." A person has a disease or condition and, after a cursory explanation of the situation, is given a slip of paper and told to purchase a drug—sometimes a very expensive drug. It isn't exactly the most positive consumer experience the patient is ever going to have.

And then someone comes along who says, "Here's something you can concoct yourself, or that grows wild, or is available at your local health food store, and you don't need a prescription of Doctor Pooh-Bah giving you permission to use it." It's very seductive.

This is not new, either. In his brilliant rumination on the 100th anniversary of the discovery of X-rays (*Journal of the American Medical Association*, September 20,1995), Dr. Ronald Evens tells of the hopes the dicovery inspired: that radiologic images would be so self-explanatory that doctors would no longer be needed. The film, he writes, "would show the 'obvious' to even the untrained eye, and the sufferer could then obtain the medication or rehabilitative treatments needed. To a population regularly poked, prodded, and dosed with alcohol- and narcotic-based medications, the notion of eliminating the diagnostic physician from the scene was not without its appeal."

> **In the Twenties, a patent medicine marketed as a ginger in concentrate was in fact, an industrial lubricant. It paralyzed 50,000 Americans.**

A Cut of the Pie

Another reason for courting public (and payer) acceptance of alternative treatments, approaches, and practitioners is more sinister: a desire to get a cut of the huge healthcare pie. Many healthcare professions make a whole lot of money, much of it through the relatively painless (for the patient) process of third-party payment. A great many people who work at the margins of healthcare would like a slice of that, just as nurse practitioners, physical therapists, and many other nonphysician professionals fought to get recognition from payers. (It seems a pity that it is recognition from payers, rather than from patients or other practitioners or outcomes research, that seems to be the gold standard, but that's healthcare in America.)

Certainly, some of the new disciplines are not only popular, but also seem to have produced good outcomes in a significant number of patients. Indeed, more and more insurers and HMOs are beginning to cover certain practices and practitioners.

That's old hat for the Indian Health Service and other healthcare entities that serve patients who belong to other cultures. It is an everyday occurrence for a shaman to perform healing rituals in some hospitals serving Native Americans, just as more and more hospitals and other sites of care are learning to allow families to provide favorite foods, prayers, and other ways of supporting a loved one who is ill. If surgeons are allowed to engage in Christian prayer before performing an operation, why shouldn't other faiths be allowed their place at the bedside?

However, there is a difference between practitioners of a venerable and demonstrably effective therapy such as, say, acupuncture, and quick-buck artists who prey on the frightened when their approaches are untested or even discredited. I was quite horrified, earlier this year, to read that Los Angeles Dodger player Brett Butler, who has been diagnosed with a rare form of cancer, is visiting Tijuana, Mexico, twice a week to undergo coffee enemas and to ingest Laetrile "to bolster his immune system."

Both of these "therapies" have been thoroughly examined and found worthless—and the coffee enemas may do the patient harm. Those who peddle them are not only outside the bonds of traditional medicine; they are also outside the bonds of the Hippocratic oath, which exhorts practitioners to do no harm.

Culture Influences Outcome

Approaches such as acupuncture raise a profound complication, however; the cultural specificity of many therapies. We all know that the *context* of healthcare is cultural: In some groups, patients are left alone; in others, the entire family wants to be in on the experience. In some cultures, the patients wants to know everything; in others, he or she is kept in the dark. Some cultures support organ donation; others consider it defilement of the dead. And different religions view dying and death quite differently indeed.

Culture, then, undoubtedly influences the outcome and given alternative therapy—as well as its perceived effectiveness. For example, many Southeast Asian immigrants practice coin rubbing, a therapy that involves running the edge of a coin along the ribs or other bones of a sick person. It raises welts, but is painless and harmless.

Nonetheless, in this country, emergency department staff are required to report any potential child abuse, and many coin rubbings have been reported as such. In one case, a father, accused of abusing his child by using coin rubbing, committed suicide.

By the same token, much as I hold in deep respect the living tradition of Hawaiian religion and its attendant traditional healers, I doubt that they would be as effective with me as with someone who was born and raised in that culture.

The point is that a therapy that is mainstream in one culture may be seen as kooky in another culture, and we should be very careful before we either embrace or condemn a healing practice that is not from our particular way of life.

Hope: A Great Therapy

There is one other motivation for seeking alternative treatment, and that is the oldest reason of all: when mainstream approaches offer no hope. Probably the largest natural experiment in this regard, other than cancer patients going to Mexico, has been the experience of persons with AIDS.

Confronted by a society that was lackadaisical about the epidemic, and then played fast and loose with research funds, I was particularly thrilled by the study that received AIDS money because it was scrutinizing PCP—except that it turned out to be focusing on the drug PCP, not the pneumonia, many AIDS patients turned to folk medicines and patent cures, ranging from herbs to illegal drugs to home-brew concoctions to pharmaceuticals used in other countries but not approved here.

Hope is as great a therapy as there is, and if the mainstream system can offer none—or, worse, doesn't particularly care to look for one—patients will naturally look elsewhere.

No One Is Above the Law

All these are powerful forces. And, whatever the reason, I certainly understand the enthusiasm for alternative healthcare services and products—the belief that there is a universe, or at least a wide selection, of means of addressing diseases and hurts that fall outside the mainstream pathways of healthcare.

However, some of what is going on is troubling, and the most worrisome aspect of the alternative healing movement to me is the desire on the part of its adherents that its products, services, and practitioners be above the law. That they should not be regulated. That the substances sold for ingestion or injection or whatever should not be subject to scrutiny or testing. A long parade of movie stars and celebrities goes to Washington, demanding that alternative care not be held accountable for its activities—or its outcomes.

In a pig's eye. To those who say the Food and Drug Administration has no jurisdiction here, I say, what is it you are offering as cures, if not foods and drugs? To those who say approval takes too long and valuable products would be taken off the market, I say the FDA—learning from and pressured by the AIDS community—has put a great many products on the fast track. To those who say the pharmaceutical manufacturers will seek to dominate the market by patenting the drugs, I say, how do you patent cranberry juice?

> **If surgeons are allowed to engage in Christian prayer before performing an operation, why should not other faiths be allowed their place at the bedside?**

To those who say that regulation, testing for purity, standards for ingredients, and requirements for truth in advertising are not necessary, I have two words for you: thalidomide, l-tryptophan.

In our zest to find non-Establishment answers, in our desire to do an end run around arrogant, unresponsive providers, in our anger against the drug manufacturers, let us not cut our throats to spite our faces.

A Few Handy Rules

So I would like to propose a few handy rules for judging the value of an alternative product, service, or discipline.

1. **Differentiate among approaches.** Those that do harm must be banned, no matter whether someone believes in them or profits from them or not.

Those that do no harm should be treated cautiously. A psychiatrist whom I heard speak recently said that if his depressed geriatric patients thought they were helped by melatonin, he had no objections to their using it. However, there is a danger— a very great one—when patients seek alternative therapies *in place of* demonstrably effective mainstream therapies, simply because the standard treatments are more expensive, painful, or scary.

Alternative therapies that help, or even cure, should be

welcomed and made readily available, hopefully at affordable prices.

2. **Insist on oversight.** The FDA isn't perfect, but it has protected Americans from a great many unproved, and sometimes horrific, substances that were tantamount to poison. When a substance is trumpeted as an alternative cure, but the manufacturer is accountable to no one as to what's in it, everyone is at risk. A recent report found that many substances being marketed as melatonin contained none of it.

In the Twenties, a patent medicine marketed as a ginger concentrate was, in fact, an industrial lubricant that happened to be a central nervous system toxin. It paralyzed more than 50,000 Americans permanently.

3. **Subject alternative approaches to the disciplines of data reporting and outcomes research.** We need to know what works and what doesn't, not just for reasons of cost and resource conservation, but because there is no point in offering treatments that don't work. There should not be two tiers of therapies: those that are subject to outcomes-based quality assessment, and those that are not.

4. **Forget ancient bigotries, standard teachings, and turf wars, and develop multiple-modality approaches to healing.** The situation is no longer one of "scientific" doctors squaring off against hippies chomping on peyote buttons. Rather, it's practitioners—medical or not—who have learned the value of humor, faith, meditation, herbs, exercise, and other approaches squaring off against pain, disease, and suffering.

Patients should not be the victims of turf wars, personal bigotry, ignorance, or political squabbles. Healthcare folk—all healthcare folk—should be united in seeking what is best for the people who seek their services. Thus, the principle that should unite hippie, alternative healer, and mainstream physician alike is simple enough; whatever works.

Article Review Form at end of book.

What is the purpose of coalitions?

Partnerships: The Prescription for Healthier Communities

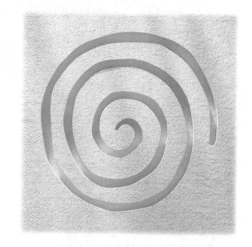

Melissa A. Rapp and Rona Wotschak

Melissa A. Rapp is a senior account executive with Paul Werth Associates, a Columbus, Ohio, public relations firm.

Rona Wotschak is an account executive with Paul Werth Associates.

As government funding shrinks and competition for nonprofit contributions intensifies, working together in community partnerships is the best—perhaps the only—way to eliminate preventable illness in our communities.

Whether the goal is to increase infant immunization rates, reduce the number of smokers, or increase the number of women receiving mammograms, forming coalitions to tackle the problem is a workable solution.

A coalition is a union of people or organizations working to influence outcomes on a specific problem. Sometimes coalition members are from a single industry; other times they're from the same geographic area. They seldom share the same views on all matters. In fact, members may not

agree on much at all, but they are all committed to a common goal.

For example, a coalition on unintended pregnancy may include both abortion-rights groups and Catholic social-services representatives. Needless to say, both organizations have very different ethical and philosophical views on such topics as abortion, sterilization, and birth control. But they can agree that a large number of adult and adolescent pregnancies are unintended. And they may be able to agree, in part, on how to address the issue in terms of health and sexuality education, the role and responsibility of the male, and other significant aspects. All parties know there is no simple solution to the problem and that it must be addressed on many fronts. By pooling resources and avoiding duplication of efforts, they hope to make a greater impact.

Forming a coalition offers several advantages, including: financial support; greater human resources with varied levels of expertise and creativity; intangibles such as prestige, clout, and access to important contacts and

constituencies; physical resources; credibility; and strength in numbers.

Although the advantages generally outweigh the disadvantages, working as a part of a coalition has drawbacks, most notably the shared control of leadership and the need to compromise and reach consensus. Getting the approvals of the many parties involved often slows the decision-making process.

Although the impetus behind forming a community coalition may vary, the following steps are key to building a successful coalition:

- Determine if you need a coalition. Do you need additional help to accomplish your goal? Are there other organizations in the community that share your views on the importance of this goal? Are there other organizations addressing a part of this need?

- Recruit the right people or groups for your coalition. Identify groups that share your commitment. Think outside the

Reprinted with permission from *Journal of Health Care Marketing*, by Melissa A. Rapp and Rona Wotschak, "Partnerships: The Prescription For Healthier Communities" published by American Marketing Association, 1996, 16(4) 43-44.

box. They don't have to be just hospitals, government agencies, or social service organizations. Consider businesses whose products are aimed at your target audience, insurance and managed care providers, companies known as profamily employers, service clubs, trade associations, and organizations owned or managed by someone with a special interest in health care. Should anyone approach you, don't turn them away. Successful coalitions can always find a role for a willing volunteer.

- Let coalition members get to know each other before tackling the big issue. A coalition needs to work together as a team, so members need to develop a trust level. Introductory or ice-breaking exercises during the first session can be helpful. Brief bios can be sent to coalition members in advance of the meeting to reinforce their introductions. Begin the first meeting by developing a shared vision of what the community will be like when your goal is reached. If you have a fairly large coalition, you may want to divide into a steering committee and task groups or various subcommittees.

- Make your first project or task a fairly simple one. The first step should be one the group can complete relatively quickly to gain a sense of accomplishment and confidence.

- Make sure the coalition's lead organization is able to fulfill its commitment. (The lead organization is usually the one providing the bulk of the coordination and administrative support.) Be realistic. Just keeping the coalition together takes time.

- Monitor progress and evaluate the coalition's efforts. How well did the coalition process work? Did your strategies achieve the objectives? If not, make adjustments as needed.

Project L.O.V.E.

To demonstrate how coalitions can work together to resolve health care issues, consider the example of a coalition formed in 1992 to increase infant immunization rates in Columbus, Ohio.

Widespread belief that childhood immunizations were no longer needed since diseases such as measles and mumps were no longer a threat had produced a crisis in Columbus. Nearly 60% of the city's two-year-olds were not fully immunized. Recognizing that the old methods of encouraging immunizations were failing, the city's 11 hospitals launched a community partnership called Project L.O.V.E. (Love Our kids— Vaccinate Early!)

Establishing the goal of a 90% immunization rate for two-year-olds by 2000 was the easy part. Various obstacles threatened the partnership from the beginning. The hospitals had never worked cooperatively on such a major project, even in the days when competition was not as intense. This project also required the participation of city and county health departments, whose agendas often conflicted with those of the hospitals. Additionally, support and participation from private physicians was needed if the coalition was to achieve its goal.

In conducting the initial research to determine why so many Columbus two-year-olds were not fully immunized, it became apparent that all the partners had a role to play and that additional partners would be needed to reverse the trend.

A Gallup poll of parental attitudes, Centers for Disease Control reports, and numerous medical journals confirmed that parents did not realize unprotected children were in danger. Parents failed to complete immunization schedules because they did not like to see their children given shots. Public health workers cited limited clinic hours and inconvenient locations as barriers to an improved immunization rate. Most surprisingly, physician interviews showed many were not proactively immunizing their patients and were not aware of recommended immunization schedules and practices.

This research demonstrated that parent education programs alone would not solve the problem. Physician education, increased access to immunizations, heightened public awareness, and improved linkage of children to primary care would also be necessary.

A strategic planning process was used to identify partners, involve them in the project, and keep them involved despite their conflicting views. The partners' planning committee included a public-relations firm, hospital representatives, physicians, and public health officials. Together they have written two complete strategic plans (1993-95 and 1995-97).

With a core goal to increase the infant immunization rate to 90% by the year 2000, the partners identified three initial objectives: (1) to increase awareness of the importance of immunization and educate parents and physicians about the immunization schedule, (2) to improve access to immunizations, and (3) to expand the partnership to increase resources.

As planning progressed, they identified additional objectives: (1) to devise a system to track immunizations, (2) to improve children's access to primary care, (3) to improve working relationships between the 11 hospitals, (4) to position the hospitals as committed to the well-being of the community, and (5) to create a model project that could be replicated elsewhere.

The project targeted expectant parents, parents of infants, and physicians and their staffs. Secondary targets included childcare providers, project partners, and potential partners. Together, the partners launched an immunization effort that included parent education, physician education, special events, media relations, and regular partner communication.

In a two-year period, the Project L.O.V.E. partnership raised immunizations of children under age two by 117%. It secured additional business and community partners, whose cash and in-kind contributions more than doubled the project's budget. Project L.O.V.E. also acquired a large grant from a local physicians' foundation to continue community education and outreach efforts, as well as a grant to aid in the development of the Immunization Information System, among other achievements.

The Project L.O.V.E. coalition is a model of how a well-planned and creatively executed coalition can help solve a challenging public health problem.

 Article Review Form at end of book.

WiseGuide Wrap-Up

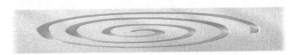

- Problems with the current healthcare system include duplication and gaps, inequitable access to care, lack of accountability by physicians, and misuse of patient genetic records.

- Solutions to problems in the healthcare system require vigilance and combined efforts from health consumers.

R.E.A.L. Sites

The adjacent list provides a print preview of typical **coursewise** R.E.A.L. Sites. (There are over 100 such sites at the **courselinks**™ Site.) The danger in printing URLs is that web sites can change overnight. As we went to press, these sites were functional using the URLs provided. If you come across one that isn't, please let us know via email at webmaster@coursewise.com. Use your Passport to access the most current list of R.E.A.L. sites at the **courselinks**™ Site.

Site name: Office of Alternative Medicine - NIH
URL: http://altmed.od.nih.gov
Why is it R.E.A.L.? Searchable government site from the Office of Alternative Medicine, National Institutes of Health with information on alternative health issues and links to resources, program areas, news and events, research grants. Includes information on bioelectromagnetics, diet changes, herbal medicine, manual health methods, mind/body interventions and pharmacological treatments.
Key topics: alternative medicine, governmental agency
Activity: Find out when and where the next conference on alternative health will be held. Would you attend if you had the time and money?

Site name: HMO Page
URL: http://www.hmopage.org
Why is it R.E.A.L.? Sponsored by Physicians Who Care to inform the public about managed care issues and health fraud.
Key topics: managed care, HMO, activism, health insurance
Activity: Find out how HMOs work and review "National Legislation." Then email Congress with your factually supported opinions on the matter.

Site name: AMA Health Insight
URL: http://www.ama-assn.org/insight/
Why is it R.E.A.L.? Highly credible and comprehensive source of information on specific conditions, general health, child health, adolescent health, women's health and human anatomy. Interactive features allow you to view the human musculature and skeleton as well as check up on your doctor.
Key topics: professional organization, medicine
Activity: Click on "AMA Physician Select" to find your doctor by name. See if she or he is licenced to practice in the U.S.

Site name: American Public Health Association Legislative Affairs and Advocacy
URL: http://www.apha.org/legislative/index.html
Why is it R.E.A.L.? The APHA is one of the largest and oldest professional organizations for public health workers. The site provides an opportunity to become a member, subscribe to professional journals, identify important public health issues, and actively participate in promoting public health advocacy.
Key topics: professional organization, advocacy, public health

Site name: Blue Cross and Blue Shield

URL: http://www.bluecares.com/

Why is it R.E.A.L.? Information about the health insurance and health care industry is provided here, along with a virtual tour of the human body.

Key topics: health insurance & managed care

Activity: Enter your zip code to find out about health insurance coverage where you live. Then go to "What's New" and "From Capitol Hill to the State House" to find answers to frequently asked questions about what health care reform will mean for you.

....

Site name: Community Tool Box

URL: http://ctb.lsi.ukans.edu/

Why is it R.E.A.L.? Serves the mission to promote "community health and development by connecting people, ideas, and resources." Provides strategies for delivery of health education programs including grantwriting, building coalitions, and preparation of materials, as well as success stories and inspirational quotes for community organizers.

Key topics: activism and advocacy, empowerment

Activitys: Take a guided tour of the website, then decide what core skills for doing community work and forming coalitions that you could improve by visiting this website.

....

Site name: Medscape

URL: http://www.medscape.com/

Why is it R.E.A.L.? Highly acclaimed web site providing interactive Internet publication on issues related to medicine and healthcare. Comprehensive, free access to Medline literature search.

Key topics: medicine, healthcare, general health and wellness

....

Site name: Association for Worksite Health Promotion On-line

URL: http://www.awhp.com/

Why is it R.E.A.L.? Homepage of professional organization for worksite health promoters. Opportunities for becoming a member, information about conferences.

Key topics: professional organization, worksite health

....

Site name: Environmental Protection Agency: Students and Teachers

URL: http://www.epa.gov/epahome/students.htm

Why is it R.E.A.L.? Governmental web sites designed specifically for students and teachers, to discover more about environmental health and how to protect the environment.

Key topics: environmental health, governmental agency

Activity: Go to "Surf Your Watershed" to investigate enviromental issues about the watershed in your own community. See what specific ways you can help to protect your watershed.

....

Index

Notes:

Entries in boldface type are authors of Readings.

emotional problems among, 143
helpless behavior among, 145
nutrition for, 18, 143
as targets of health fraud, 109–10
See also Aging
Electric currents, clinical trials of, 108
Ellis Kahn, Mary Jo, 171
Embarrassment risk, and health behavior, 51, 52
Emergency care, insurance coverage issues, 168
Emotional problems, in elderly people, 143
Employability, and stereotypes of elderly, 142
Employee Retirement Income Security Act, exempting self-funded plans from state insurance laws, 173
Environmental Protection Agency: Students and Teachers, R.E.A.L. site, 188
Equal Employment Opportunity Commission
definition of disability, 175
definition of sexual harassment, 62
Equanimity, and meditation, 128
Erectile difficulties, causes of, 73
Estrogen replacement therapy
and cancer risk, 125
conflicting views of, 155
Ethnicity
and circumcision rates, 87, 89, 91
and HIV/AIDS infection, 148–52
European Americans, HIV/AIDS among, 148, 150
Evans, R. G., on surplus hospital beds, 162
Exercise
importance for elderly people, 143
to reduce cancer risk, 124
role in new weight management paradigm, 7, 8
self-presentational motives for, 57
Exercise machines, effectiveness of, 29–31

F

Facts about Sexual Harassment, R.E.A.L. site, 70
Fat
and cancer risk, 16–17
CSPI campaigns over, 21–25
health effects of reductions to, 19
nutritional requirements for, 23–24
as percentage of calories in American diet, 20
and stroke risk, 17
Federal government, response to HIV/AIDS, 151–52
Federal health initiatives, and genetic discrimination in insurance, 173
Female condom, 76, 151
Fiber, and cancer risk, 16–17
Firearms, as cause of death, 123
FitLife, R.E.A.L. site, 32
Flat-earth paradigm, 3
Folic acid
and birth defects, 16, 18, 19
and coronary heart disease, 16, 19–20

Food and Drug Administration (FDA)
approval process of, 107
guide to choosing medical treatments, 107–11
response to HIV/AIDS, 151–52
Food Finder, R.E.A.L. site, 32
Formularies, for prescription drug coverage, 169
Francis, Bev, and strength in women, 27–28
Frazão, Elizabeth, 16
Freda, Margaret Comerford, 78
Friedman, Emily, 179
Fruits and vegetables, and cancer risk, 122, 124

G

Gag clauses, in managed care plans, 169
Gay and lesbian physicians, discrimination against, 99
Gay men, influence of self-perception on condom use among, 52
Gays and lesbians
and AIDS, 149–50
domestic violence among, 98
health insurance for, 98
inferior health care for, 98–99
mental health of, 96–97
misconceptions about, 97
suggestions for improving health care for, 101
violence against, 98
Gender, and body strength, 27
Gender bias
in insurance coverage, 139–40
in medical research, 137–38
Genetic discrimination, in health insurance coverage, 171–74
Genetic information, ethical use guidelines, 174
Genital mutilation, of women, 135, 136
Gerontology, training in, 146
Gonorrhea, effect of circumcision on contraction of, 91
Good Samaritan Hospital, patient education program, 155
Grant, Lynda D, 141
Grapefruit, medicinal effects of, 179
Greeley, Alexandra, 148
Grievance procedures, in insurance plans, 169
Guide to Locating Health Statistics, R.E.A.L. site, 70

H

Hagland, Mark, 153
Harmony, and meditation, 128
Harshbarger, Scott, in lawsuit against tobacco industry, 66–67
Hate crimes, against gays and lesbians, 98
Health
defining for people with chronic disabilities, 105–6
effect of conventional and alternative therapies on, 107–11
effect of self-presentation on, 50–59

of elderly people, improving, 141–46
sexual, protecting, 72–73
WHO definition, 141
of women, 135–36, 137–38
Health A to Z, R.E.A.L. site, 32
Health behavior, role of self-presentation, 50–59
Healthcare
ageism in, 141–46
barriers for minorities, 149–51
costs of, 160
lower quality for gays and lesbians, 98–99
quality of information about, 154–55
redundancies in system, 159–63
role of patient in, 45–46, 153–55
Healthcare practitioners, ageism among, 144–45
Healthfinder, R.E.A.L. site, 69
Health fraud, examples of, 108–11
Health insurance
coverage for women vs. men, 139
for gays and lesbians, 98
genetic discrimination in coverage, 171–74
Health maintenance organizations
assessing, 165–70
long waits for appointments with, 169
physician-patient interactions in, 40
provider/client ratios, 160
use of specialists, 161
Health problems, forming coalitions to address, 184–86
Health risks, and self-presentation, 50–59
Healthy People 2000, R.E.A.L. site, 156
Heart attacks, incidence of, 16
Heart disease
incidence in women, 120–21
screening for, 113
Heart rate, as monitor of exercise intensity, 30–31
Hepatitis, effect of circumcision on contraction of, 91
Hepatitis B virus, vaccination against, 124
Herpes, effect of circumcision on contraction of, 91
Hiepler, Mark, and Ching conflict of interest case, 167–68
Hip fractures, incidence of, 18
Hispanics, HIV/AIDS among, 148, 150, 151
HIV/AIDS
concealing infections, 150
effect of circumcision on contraction of, 91
federal government actions on, 151–52
fraudulent therapies for, 110–11
incidence of, 148
among minorities, 148–52
prevention program funding, 100
and promoting safer sex, 80–83
research funding for, 99–100
rise of alternative therapies for, 182
risk factors for, 149
role in changing patient-doctor relationships, 154
self-presentation and risk of contracting, 51–52
social support and resistance to, 97

effect of circumcision on, 88, 90, 93
influence of self-presentation on, 51–52
initiating, 72
oral sex, 88, 93
pressure for, as harassment, 63
problems with, 72–73
safer sex study, 80–83
Sexual desire, inhibited, 72
Sexual dysfunction
effect of circumcision on incidence of,
87–88, 90, 92
in National Health and Social Life
Survey data, 85
among older men, 88
Sexual harassment
defined, 62–63
on campus, 62–64
Sexual health
and mistreatment of women, 135, 136
protecting, 72–73
Sexually transmitted disease
and safer sex study, 80–83
effect of circumcision on incidence of,
87, 89, 91
influence of self-presentation on risk of
contracting, 51–52
mistreatment with over-the-counter
products, 94
and number of partners, 87, 91
underreporting of, 89–90
Sexual orientation
in anti-discrimination policies, 100
awareness of, 97
conversion therapy contraindicated, 101
See also Homosexuality
Sexual partners, number of
and circumcision status, 91
and HIV/AIDS risk, 82
and STD risk, 87, 91
Sexual satisfaction, effect of circumcision
debated, 85
Shape Up America, R.E.A.L. site, 32
Shapiro, Martin F., 80
Shivery, M., sexual harassment study by, 64
SIECUS (Sexuality Information and
Education Council), R.E.A.L. site, 103
Skalko, Thomas K., 105
Skin cancer
incidence of, 52
influence of self-presentation on
occurrence, 52–53
screening for, 114
Sleath, Betsy, 38
Smokeless tobacco, reasons for using, 55
Smoking
effects on sexual functioning, 73
as heart disease risk factor, 16
self-presentational motives for, 55–56
Smoking cessation, to reduce cancer risk,
124
Snake venom, as fraudulent arthritis
therapy, 110
Snyder, C. J., study of age discrimination
cases, 142

Snyder, Karyn, 94
Sodium, dietary, and hypertension, 18
Specialists
effect on services performed, 160
surplus of, 161
waits for appointments with, 169
Stairstepper, exercise effectiveness of, 29, 30
Starch, in baby food, 25
State laws, prohibiting genetic
discrimination in insurance, 173
Stationary bike, exercise effectiveness
of, 29, 30
Steen, R. Grant, 122
Stehlin, Isadora B., 107
Steinem, Gloria, 26
Steroid use, self-presentational motives for,
57
Stethoscope examination, purpose of, 113
Stool sample, purpose of, 112
Strength training, for women, 26–28
Stress
and cancer risk, 122–23
among gays and lesbians, 97–98
Stress test, purpose of, 113
Stroke, 16, 17
Substance abuse, among homosexuals, 98
Success stories, and health for people with
chronic disabilities, 105–6
Sugar, in baby food, 25
Suicide, among elderly, 145
Sunbathing, and skin cancer, 52–53
Support groups, for information on
alternative therapies, 111
Supreme Court, definition of sexual
harassment, 63
Surgeons, surplus of, 161
Surgery, cosmetic, and self-presentation, 58
Syphilis, effect of circumcision on
contraction of, 91

T

Tanning, and self-presentation, 52–53
Tchividjian, Lydia R., 50
Tea, benefits of, 180
Technology, costs of, 163
Teenagers, as targets of health fraud,
109–10
Terms of Endearment, 129
Tests, obtaining under managed care, 168
Thinness, cultural paradigms about, 4, 5
Third World, prescription drug availability,
134
Tiller, Leslie, malpractice victim, 176–77
Title IX, and sexual harassment policies, 63
Tobacco, new restrictions on, 65–67
Tobacco companies, settlement with states,
65–67
Tobacco use
as cause of death, 123
self-presentational motives for, 55–56
Tolerance, and meditation, 128
Toxic agents, as cause of death, 123
Treadmill, exercise effectiveness of, 29, 30

Triaminic, acetaminophen in, 37
Triphasic birth control pills, and sex drive,
75
Tubal ligation, 76–77
Tuskeegee study, 151
Type I diabetes, 17
Type II diabetes, 17

U

Underwriting, 172
Uninsured, number in United States, 172
United States Pharmacopeia, on hazardous
effects of OTC medications, 36–37
University of Iowa
sexual harassment policy excerpt, 63
Virtual Hospital, 155
University of Massachusetts at Amherst,
sexual harassment study, 64
Unplanned pregnancy, reducing, 78–79
Uric acid test, 114
Urinalysis, 114

V

Vaginal deodorants, misuse of, 94, 95
Vaginal disorders, improper self-
medication for, 94–95
Vaginismus, incidence of, 72
Venous leak syndrome, 73
Violence, against gays and lesbians, 98
Virginity testing, of women, 135, 136
Viruses, as cause of death, 123, 124
Visco, Fran, on importance of patient
education, 154
*Vitality for Life: Psychological Research for
Productive Aging,* 145

W

Weakness, as female gender image, 27
The Web as a Research Tool: Evaluation
Techniques, R.E.A.L. site, 69
Weight
and body-image dissatisfaction, 11–14
relation to psychological problems, 6–7
Weight loss
as basis of weight management
paradigm, 3–5
failure of, 3–4
Weight management
approaches to, 3–8
current paradigm, 3–5
defining success of, 8
new paradigm for, 5–8
regaining lost weight, 3–4
Wenger, Neil S., 80
Wennberg, J., on specialist surplus, 161
Whitbourne, S. K., on psychology texts'
portrayals of aging, 144
White women, body-image dissatisfaction
among, 12–14
The Whole Nine Months, R.E.A.L. site, 103

Putting it in Perspective
-Review Form-

Your name:_____   Date: _____

Reading title: _____

Summarize: provide a one sentence summary of this reading: _____

_____

_____

_____

Follow the Thinking: how does the author back the main premise of the reading? Are the facts/opinions appropriately supported by research or available data? Is the author's thinking logical?

_____

_____

_____

_____

_____

_____

Develop a Context: answer one or both questions: how does this reading contrast or compliment your professor's lecture treatment of the subject matter? How does this reading compare to your textbook's coverage?

_____

_____

_____

_____

_____

_____

_____

Question Authority: explain why you agree/disagree with the author's main premise?

_____

_____

_____

_____

_____

_____

_____

COPY ME! Copy this form as needed. This form is also available at http://www.courselinks.com Click on: "Putting it in Perspective"